Essentials of
DENTAL
RADIOGRAPHY

for Dental Assistants and Hygienists

Fifth Edition

Essentials of
DENTAL
RADIOGRAPHY

for Dental Assistants and Hygienists

Fifth Edition

Wolf R. de Lyre, BA, DDS
*Professor Emeritus of Dental Assisting
and Dental Hygiene
Cerritos College
Norwalk, California*

Orlen N. Johnson, BS, DDS, MS
*Associate Professor of Dental Radiology
University of Nebraska College of Dentistry
Lincoln, Nebraska*

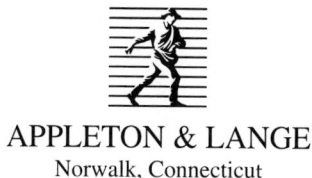

APPLETON & LANGE
Norwalk, Connecticut

95 96 97 98 99 / 10 9 8 7 6 5 4 3 2 1

Prentice Hall International (UK) Limited, *London*
Prentice Hall of Australia Pty. Limited, *Sydney*
Prentice Hall Canada, Inc., *Toronto*
Prentice Hall Hispanoamericana, S.A., *Mexico*
Prentice Hall of India Private Limited, *New Delhi*
Prentice Hall of Japan, Inc., *Tokyo*
Simon & Schuster Asia Pte. Ltd., *Singapore*
Editora Prentice Hall do Brasil Ltda., *Rio de Janeiro*
Prentice Hall, *Englewood Cliffs, New Jersey*

De Lyre, Wolf R., 1912–
    Essentials of dental radiography for dental assistants and
hygienists / Wolf R. de Lyre, Orlen N. Johnson. — 5th ed.
        p.   cm.
    Includes bibliographical references and index.
    ISBN 0-8385-2025-1
    1. Teeth—Radiography.   2. Dental auxiliary personnel.
I. Johnson, Orlen N.   II. Title.
    [DNLM: 1. Radiography, Dental.   WN 230 D367e 1994]
    RK309.D44   1994
617.6'307572—dc20
DNLM/DLC
for Library of Congress   94-15693
                                                  CIP

Acquisitions Editor: Cheryl L. Mehalik
Production Editor: Karen W. Davis
Designer: Penny Kindzierski

PRINTED IN THE UNITED STATES OF AMERICA

ISBN   0-8385-2025-1

90000

9 780838 520253

Contents

Preface

Technique and equipment changes, as well as greater concern with quality control, infection control, sterilization, and protection from possible exposure to hepatitis, AIDS, and other infectious diseases, make another revision of this book essential. We have also updated this text to include the latest trends in research and clinical methods.

Interest in dental radiography continues at an all-time high. Each year witnesses the passage of more legislation to control the use of x-radiation in medicine and dentistry. More and more states are permitting dental auxiliaries to perform x-ray duties but are also requiring them to take examinations to prove their competence. As most radiographs are exposed by dental auxiliaries, the auxiliary assumes a responsibility to safeguard the patient by using only the minimum radiation required to accomplish the task, by following correct development procedures, and by avoiding technique errors that make it necessary to reexpose the patient. Operators additionally have the responsibility to follow all radiation safety rules to protect the patient, themselves, and anyone near the x-ray source.

The benefits that the patient derives from x-ray procedures are numerous. These include the early detection of dental caries, changes in the bony structures that support the teeth, and abnormal soft and hard tissue changes. Radiation, however, may also cause damage within the body cells. That is why it is essential that every user of x-radiation understands the theoretical aspects of how x-rays are produced and used, as well as the clinical procedures necessary to make diagnostically acceptable radiographs. There must be an awareness that each exposure to x-rays is accompanied by a small degree of risk to the cell structures but that the potential benefits to the patient far outweigh the risks. Our two goals are (1) to create a sense of responsibility for the use of x-radiation in each operator of x-ray equipment, and (2) to present and describe practical techniques for consistently producing radiographs of high quality.

This book attempts a balanced, flexible approach that presents a clearly written treatment of one of the most important techniques used in dental diagnosis. This basic text provides an excellent balance of both the essential fundamental theories and the day-to-day clinical procedures practiced in the modern dental office. The inclusion of learning objectives and review questions in each chapter makes it easier for both teachers and students to use. The chapters contain the kind of coverage that will find application in self-improvement programs or on-the-job training, or as a convenient reference and basic text.

Topical stress is focused on four interrelated areas:

- the benefit the patient derives from preventive radiation, patient education, and radiation safety procedures;
- the clinical techniques to produce high-quality radiographs;
- the recognition of anatomic structures, common pathologic lesions, and preliminary radiographic interpretation; and
- the information needed by the student to prepare for licensing, registration, certification, and radiation safety examinations.

This book is an in-depth introduction to dental radiography—the art or science of producing and using x-rays to make pictures that the dental practitioner requires to make a diagnosis and complete the patient's treatment plan. Whereas the book is written primarily for college students of dental assisting and dental hygiene, the important topics with which it deals concern everyone who works in the vicinity of equipment that produces x-radiation. It is appropriate for one- and two-semester lecture–laboratory classes in introductory and advanced dental radiographic techniques. Although the dentist now seldom exposes or processes radiographs and is usually limited to interpreting them, the dental student benefits by studying the same procedures as the dental auxiliary. Without such training the dentist would be unable to provide the required supervision and maintain the necessary quality control.

The book is also adaptable for courses of various lengths offered by commercial dental assisting training schools and may serve as a handy review for dentists, dental hygienists, dental assistants, and dental radiography technicians who must prepare for radiation safety or licensing examinations. It is also useful to the on-the-job trainee who is unable to enroll in a formal training program and must rely on self-study. This book will be a valuable addition to the library of any dental practitioner or dental auxiliary.

The basic organization followed in the fourth edition has been retained. The 22 logically organized chapters cover theories, basic principles, and the entire spectrum of common radiographic procedures.

The initial chapters introduce the use of radiation in dentistry, the characteristics of radiation, the technical aspects of radiation production, and the components and functions of the dental x-ray machines. A study of these chapters provides the student with the background necessary to understand the following chapters that concern the effects of radiation, radiation safety, and infection control. Next described are the types of x-ray films and how they are processed, identified, and mounted. Then the chapter on quality control is presented. The next section includes the radiographic appearance of anatomic landmarks, pathologic lesions, restorative materials, and errors caused by faulty techniques. This is followed by chapters describing intraoral techniques using periapical, bitewing, and occlusal films. Special techniques for children and edentulous patients are described. Two chapters are devoted to extraoral radiographic techniques. The first of these is limited to techniques that can be employed using conventional x-ray machines, whereas the second chapter is devoted entirely to panoramic radiographic techniques. The final chapter, on patient education, includes methods for establishing radiation education programs for patients.

Teachers who have used former editions of this text in their classes will recognize immediately that a thorough revision has taken place. Each change, whether brief or complex, has been made to eliminate data that are no longer pertinent, to improve the presentation, or to add information that is required to qualify the student in the latest acceptable radiographic techniques.

Major specific improvements in this edition include the following:

- Forty-four new radiographs, diagrams, charts, or photographs have been added or improved to replace outdated illustrations and to clarify new techniques.
- Twenty-nine existing radiographs were redone in Chapters 10 and 11 to improve their quality.
- Two completely new chapters (Chapter 7, Infection Control, and Chapter 10, Quality Control) were written to fully explain these important subjects.
- Chapter 6 (Radiation Protection) was updated with four new illustrations and an explanation of the latest units of radiation and the new Protection Guides from the National Council on Radiation Protection and Measurements (NCRP).
- A new section was added in Chapter 9 (Dental X-ray Film Processing) explaining the disposal of radiographic wastes. Also, five pictures and illustrations were updated.
- Chapter 11 (Identification of Anatomical Landmarks for Mounting Radiographs) was revised by adding eight new drawings and improving the quality of the radiographs.
- Six new illustrations were added to Chapter 20 (Extraoral Radiography) to clarify extraoral techniques.
- Chapter 21 (Panoramic Radiography) was revised and updated to present the latest theories and techniques.
- Changes were made to the Glossary. Obsolete terms were removed and new terms were added. Many terms have been redefined to clarify their meaning.
- Objectives and review questions have been revised, added, or deleted where deemed necessary. The chapter bibliographies have been updated.

Flexibility should be the keynote for using this book. Some may wish to study the chapters in a different sequence or omit the ones that do not conform with the course outline. Some teachers prefer to begin with the chapters on radiation safety; others begin with the clinical phases and cover the theory last. The decision on where to start may hinge on the number of hours available for radiography, whether there is a separate lecture and laboratory class, and the type of students enrolled.

No claim is made to presenting original knowledge or techniques in this text. In many instances the material presented has been known for many years and is common knowledge in dental radiography; in some instances new subject matter has been derived from a condensation of lecture presentations and syllabuses made available at the workshops and symposiums conducted at the annual meetings of the American Dental Association and the American Academy of Oral and Maxillofacial Radiology.

Many authors have permitted the use of materials and illustrations from their writings. These are all gratefully acknowledged. Though it is virtually impossible to thank all who have so generously helped with this edition, we are grateful to Dr. Allan G. Farman, University of Louisville School of Dentistry; Dr. William C. Scarfe, University of Louisville School of Dentistry; Dr. Curtis Kuster, University of Nebraska Medical Center (UNMC); and Dr. Donald T. Waggener, UNMC, retired, for their reviews and suggestions. We want to express particular appreciation to Dr. Debra Gander, UNMC, for her assistance with the chapter on Infection Control and Christine E. Essay, RDH, Southeast Community College, Lincoln, Nebraska, for her extensive review of the manuscript and expert advice. In addition, we thank Mr. Kim Theesen, UNMC, artist, for new artwork and Margaret A. Cain, UNMC, photographer, for photographic illustrations.

Credit is also due to Eastman Kodak Company, Gendex Corporation, Polaroid Corporation, Rinn Corporation, and Siemens Medical Systems, as well as other manufacturers, for technical assistance and permission to use their illustrations and diagrams.

Credit is also due to the editorial and proofreading staff of Appleton & Lange.

We give special thanks to Joelene I. Johnson for spending many hours on the computer, skillfully typing much of the manuscript, correcting grammar and misspelled words, and suggesting constructive changes.

And finally, we wish to express our appreciation to our wives, Elva and Joelene, for their patience, encouragement, and support.

Wolf R. de Lyre, BA, DDS
San Antonio, Texas

Orlen N. Johnson, BS, DDS, MS
Lincoln, Nebraska

Essentials of
DENTAL
RADIOGRAPHY

for Dental Assistants and Hygienists

Fifth Edition

CHAPTER 1

Radiography in Dental Practice

By the end of this chapter the student should be able to

1. Trace the progress of radiography from its discovery to the present.
2. Name the pioneers of radiography and identify their contributions.
3. Identify techniques that have helped to make x-ray a safe and reliable diagnostic tool.

INTRODUCTION

As the twenty-first century approaches, many exciting things are happening in the dental profession. Modern dentistry is progressing so rapidly that changes in equipment and methods of practice are constantly taking place. One of these methods is radiography, the art and science of making x-ray pictures, called **radiographs.**

For over half a century, the dental profession has recognized that radiographs are valuable tools for diagnosing questionable clinical findings. Because correct diagnosis forms the basis for adequate dental treatment, the dentist requires radiographs of satisfactory quality. Although many new diagnostic aids have been developed during the past decades, x-ray continues to be the basis for most diagnostic procedures and has become an essential procedure in the practice of dentistry.

As public demand for dental services increases, dentists are expanding the duties of their trained auxiliaries to include the exposure, processing, and mounting of x-ray films. The diagnosis of the radiographs is never done by the auxiliaries; that is the sole responsibility of the dentist. Although the laws vary from state to state, the authority

1

to expose radiographs is either given or implied, provided the procedures are carried out under the dentist's supervision.

Good radiographs seldom happen by chance—they are the result of comprehensive education and practice of skills. All auxiliaries working with radiographic equipment should be thoroughly trained and versed in the theory of x-ray production. They should know how x-rays are used for getting the best diagnostic results, the operation of the x-ray unit, the various techniques commonly used to expose and process the films, as well as patient management, quality control, infection control, and radiation safety procedures. Radiographs produced by good modern techniques allow the dentist to diagnose accurately. At the same time, they protect the patient and the dental auxiliary from receiving unnecessary exposure to radiation. Both of these considerations are important.

DISCOVERY OF THE X-RAY

The discovery of x-rays, unlike man's first steps on the moon, was not watched by millions of people. Only one person witnessed the event in a darkened room, but the words of Neil Armstrong about his Apollo mission that it was "one small step forward for man and a giant leap for mankind" can apply to this discovery as well. Professor Wilhelm Conrad Roentgen's (pronounced rent' gun) experiment in Bavaria (Germany) on a Friday afternoon, November 8, 1895, produced a tremendous advance in science.

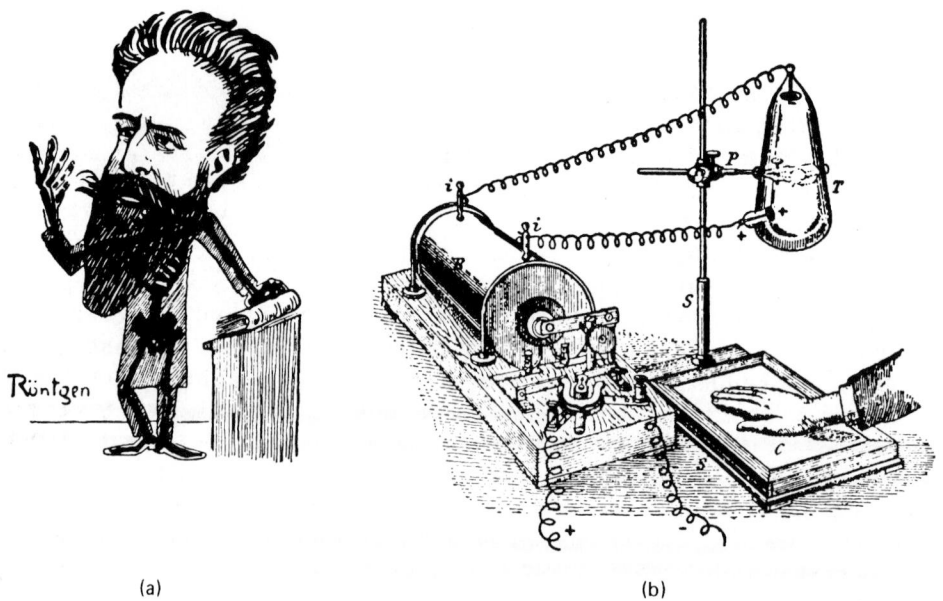

(a)   (b)

Figure 1–1. Early sketches. **(a)** Caricature of Professor Roentgen. **(b)** Roentgen's initial equipment. *(Courtesy of Heinz Moos Verlag, Munich, and Siemens Corporation, Dental Division, Germany.)*

During an experiment with a low-pressure discharge tube covered with black paper, Professor Roentgen's curiosity was aroused when he observed that a fluorescent screen near the tube began to glow when the tube was activated by passing an electric current through it. Examining this strange phenomenon further, he noticed that shadows could be cast on the screen by interposing objects between it and the tube. Further experimentation showed that such shadow images could be permanently recorded on photographic film (Fig. 1–1).

In the beginning Roentgen was uncertain of the nature of this invisible ray that he had accidentally discovered. When he later reported his findings at a scientific meeting he spoke of it as an "x-ray" because the symbol x represented the unknown. After his findings were reported and published, fellow scientists honored him by calling the invisible ray the **roentgen ray** and the image produced on photosensitive film a **roentgenograph.** Whether the image is called an x-ray picture, a roentgenograph, or a radiograph makes no difference—the terms are interchangeable. The patient is best acquainted with the word x-ray; scientists and professionals generally prefer radiograph. Because there is a basic similarity between a photographic negative and an x-ray film, and the x-ray closely resembles the radio wave, the prefix *radio* and the suffix *graphy* have been combined into **radiograph.** The latter term is used in professional offices because it is more descriptive than x-ray and easier to pronounce than roentgenograph.

EARLY PROGRESS AND DEVELOPMENT

Little of the progress achieved by medical and dental science would have been possible without **radiography,** which can be defined as the science of generating and directing x-radiation to sensitized film for the purpose of making a shadow picture. A few weeks after Professor Roentgen announced his discovery, Dr. Otto Walkhoff, a German physicist, exposed a prototype of a dental radiograph. This was accomplished by covering a small, glass photographic plate with black paper to protect it from light and then wrapping it in a sheath of thin rubber to prevent moisture damage during the 25 minutes that he held the film in his mouth. A similar exposure can now be made in 1/10 second. The resulting radiograph was experimental and was of little diagnostic value because it was impossible to prevent film movement, but it did prove that the x-ray would have a role in dentistry. The length of the exposure made the experiment a dangerous one for Dr. Walkhoff, but the dangers of overexposure were not known at that time.

We will probably never know who made the first dental radiograph in the United States. It was either Dr. William Herbert Rollins, a dentist and physician of Boston, Dr. William James Morton, a physician of New York, or Dr. C. Edmund Kells, a dentist of New Orleans.

Dr. Rollins was one of the first to alert the profession to the need for radiation hygiene and protection and is considered by many to be the father of the science of radiation protection. Unfortunately, his advice was not taken seriously by many of his fellow practitioners for a long time. Several years passed before the potential benefits and hazards of Professor Roentgen's discovery were fully appreciated.

Because x-rays are invisible, the pioneers in the field of radiography were not aware that exposure to them produced accumulations of radiation effects in the body and, therefore, could be dangerous to both patient and radiographer. When radiography was in its infancy, it was common practice for the dentist to help the patient hold the film in place while making the exposure; thus the dentist was needlessly exposed to unnecessary radiation. Frequent repetition of this practice endangered the dentist's health and occasionally led to permanent injury or death. Fortunately, although the hazards of prolonged exposure to radiation are not completely understood, we have learned how to reduce them drastically by proper use of fast film and safer x-ray machines. Placing a protective lead apron over the patient's lap decreases the risks, and the practice of having the radiographer stand six feet from the patient's head or behind lead shielding affords protection from scattered radiation.

Today, when almost half the radiation-producing equipment used in the United States is in dental offices, it is worth noting that initially few hospitals and only the most progressive physicians and dentists possessed x-ray equipment. One of the earliest users, and a strong advocate of dental radiography in this country, was Dr. C. Edmund Kells, of New Orleans. He made numerous presentations to organized dental groups and was instrumental in convincing many dentists that they should use dental radiography as a diagnostic tool. Unfortunately, he lost his life—as did some other pioneers in radiography—from excess radiation. At that time it was still customary to send the patient to a hospital or physician's office on those rare occasions when dental radiographs were prescribed.

This limited use of dental radiography can be attributed both to the fact that the early equipment was primitive and sometimes dangerous and to its widespread use as a means of entertainment by charlatans at fairgrounds. People often associated it with quackery. Resistance to change, ignorance, apathy, and fear delayed the widespread acceptance of radiography for years.

EQUIPMENT IMPROVEMENTS AND NEW TECHNIQUES

The quality of all x-ray units has improved steadily throughout the years. The newer units are more powerful than the old ones and produce better radiographs. Among recent developments are panoramic units, which are capable of exposing a radiograph of the entire dentition on a single film. Improved film emulsions and processing chemicals have also enabled the radiographer to secure better radiographs and, at the same time, to shorten the exposure time. And the automatic film processor, which completely processes radiographs in four minutes or less.

Many innovations in dental radiography have led to improved techniques. Two of the major problems that plagued the dental radiographer were (1) obtaining radiographs in which the teeth and related structures were shown in true anatomic relationship and size with minimal distortion, and (2) prevention of the radiation beam from spreading to areas the dentist did not want to study. Both of these problems have been partly solved.

The first breakthrough took place in 1920 when Franklin McCormack improved the right angle or paralleling technique, which greatly reduced dimensional distortion. Many others, notably Dr. G. M. Fitzgerald and Dr. William J. Updegrave, refined this technique and made it more practical. Dr. Updegrave designed a series of film-positioning devices and wrote several booklets describing methods of simplifying the exposure of dental radiographs. Within the last 20 years major progress has been made in restricting the size of the x-ray beam. One such development is the replacing of the pointed cone through which x-rays pass from the tube head toward the patient with open cylinders. When the pointed cones were first used, it was not realized that many of the x-rays were deflected through contact with the material of the cones, thus producing scatter radiation. Because cones were used for so many years, many still refer to the open cylinders or rectangular tubes as **cones**. A newer term that is more descriptive of its function of directing the x-rays, rather than of its shape, is **position indicating device (PID)**.

A further improvement has been the introduction of rectangular lead-lined PIDs, limiting the size of the x-ray beam that strikes the patient to the actual size of the dental film. Such a PID is shown in Figure 1–2. Naturally, such devices are only effective if

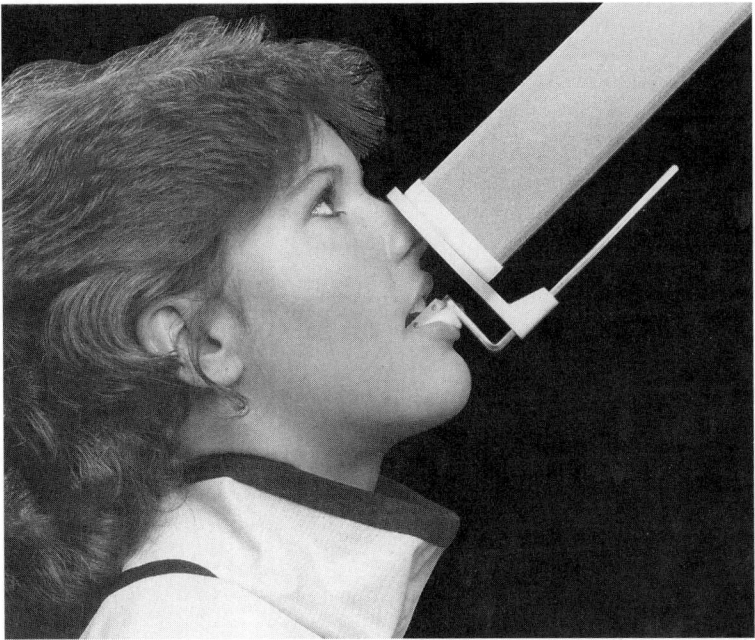

Figure 1–2. Improved rectangular instrumentation for reduced tissue exposure. The radiographer first places the x-ray film on a holder and positions it in the oral cavity, and then brings the position indicating device (PID) into alignment with the aiming device. The lead-lined PID limits the size of the x-ray beam to an area just large enough to expose the film. Note that the patient is draped with a leaded apron and thyroid collar. (Courtesy of Rinn Corporation, Elgin, IL.)

properly used and if all film exposure times and other factors that control radiation intensity are held to minimum required levels.

MODERN USE OF DENTAL RADIOGRAPHY

Few offices today are without x-ray units; many even have a unit in each operatory. In fact, most dentists have supplemented their conventional-type x-ray unit with a panoramic-type x-ray machine (Fig. 1–3B) that can produce a radiograph of the entire dentition and surrounding structures on a single film. The use of radiography enables the dentist to practice better dentistry. This obviously benefits the patient but also protects the dentist in the event of a dispute with the patient. Radiographs are visible evidence of prior conditions or the nature of work performed and furnish legal evidence of the patient's dental condition or need for treatment.

Most dental insurance companies or governmental agencies request to see the radiographs before authorizing dental treatment or paying for it. To avoid the release of the original radiographs, many dentists use film duplicating techniques or obtain duplicate films by using packets containing two films. Occasionally a patient will request possession of the radiographs taken. Although the policy on this may vary from den-

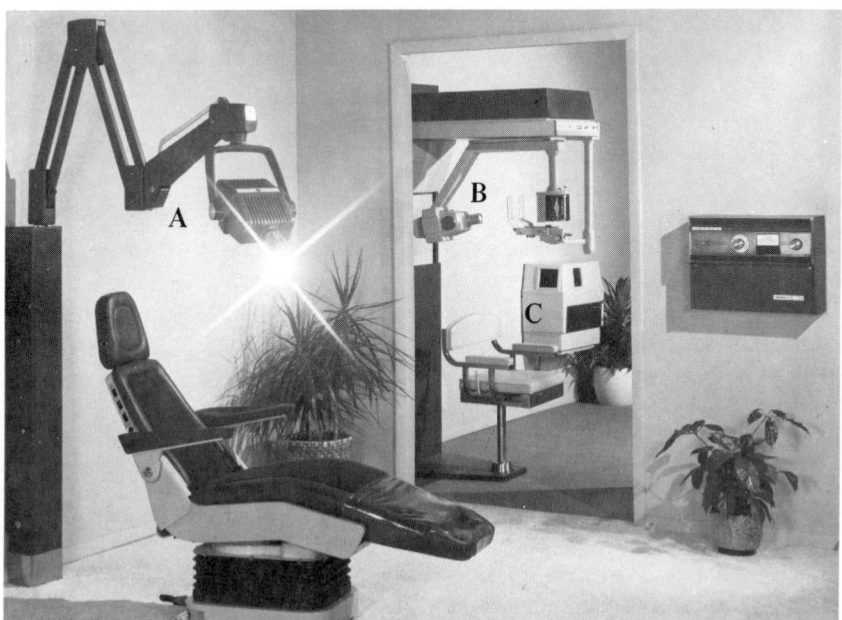

Figure 1–3. X-ray room in modern dental office showing dental chair with **A.** conventional x-ray unit in foreground and **B.** panoramic-type x-ray unit and **C.** automatic processor suitable for daylight use in background. *(Courtesy of General Electric Company, Medical Systems Division.)*

tist to dentist, it is best not to release the radiographs to the patient. Instead, such radiographs should be mailed to the dentist designated by the patient.

The dental auxiliary must be made aware of the importance of protecting, preserving, retaining, and properly filing all original radiographs and must be familiar with the office policy for their release to a third party.

The courts have ruled that radiographs are the property of the dentist; the patient pays only for the diagnosis. However, patients may have access to their films. They may request a copy of their radiographs if they decide to change dentists or request a consultation with a dental specialist. The original films, however, belong to the dentist. A related legal question is the frequency and number of radiographs that may be exposed. There is no set rule on this; the health and needs of the patient are the determining factors.

A few words of caution! Occasionally, for a variety of reasons, patients express opposition to the dentist's proposal that "x-rays be taken." Typically these patients believe that such radiographs are unnecessary and just add to the cost or that they have been exposed too many times in the past year or two and are fearful that additional x-ray exposure will be hazardous to their health. When this happens, the dentist or radiographer must carefully explain in clear terms why the suggested radiographs are needed to complete the diagnosis, prognosis, or treatment plan and therefore are of benefit to the patient.

Frequently a patient may say, "I will assume the responsibility for not taking x-ray pictures if something later goes wrong because of this." At this juncture the dentist must inform the patient in a diplomatic manner that legally, even if the patient agrees, it may be considered malpractice to render services that are below the standards of care in the community. Thus, if radiographs are necessary in the dentist's opinion, failure to take them may result in becoming vulnerable in a subsequent malpractice suit.

It is difficult to imagine how any modern dental practice could be carried on without radiography (Fig. 1–3). At the same time no diagnosis can be based only on radiographic evidence. A visual and digital examination must always be made as well. But aside from helping the dental general practitioner make a diagnosis, radiographs help the prosthodontists and orthodontists to measure the head and to determine space relationships of the face. One type is called a **cephalometric radiograph** (from the Greek words *kephale*, meaning "head," and *metricus*, meaning "measurement"). The oral surgeon depends on radiographs to locate fractures, impactions, foreign objects, and benign and malignant tumors. Every dental specialist makes use of radiographs at some time.

Radiography, aided by the introduction of transistors and computers, is benefited by the incorporation of minicomputer technology that permits significant radiation reduction in modern x-ray units. Hospitals employ radioisotope scanners (not presently suitable for dental use) that give a highly detailed picture of internal organs. A radioactive isotope is injected into the body. A special camera picks up the radioactivity as it scans across the body. A computer then reconstructs a highly detailed, almost three-dimensional picture of the organ or body section involved.

The use of tomography in medicine and dentistry is increasing. **Tomography** is a method of radiography by which a single selected plane is radiographed, with the outlines of structures in other planes eliminated (this principle is used in most panoramic-type x-ray machines).

Magnetic resonance imaging (MRI) is another new technique for obtaining cross-sectional pictures of the human body without exposing the patient to x-rays. The patient is placed within a large MRI machine that generates a static magnetic field. The nuclei of certain atoms within the body react to the magnetic field, and a picture is obtained.

A revolution equal in magnitude to the introduction of the air-turbine handpiece is under way in dentistry. The introduction of a computed approach with instant images (both radiographic and photographic) has the potential to greatly improve the quality of dental care. This most recent and exciting advance in dental radiography is called **digital imaging.**

Currently, there are four digital intraoral radiographic systems available in the US market, namely, RadioVisioGraphy (Trophy Radiology, Atlanta, Georgia), Sens-A-Ray (Regam Medical Systems AB, Sundsvall, Sweden), VIXA/Visualix (Gendex, Milwaukee, Wisconsin) (Fig. 1–4), and Computed Dental Radiography (Schick Technologies, Inc., Long Island City, New York). Undoubtedly more will come on the market in the near future.

All currently available digital imaging systems use the modern computer. The computer serves to acquire, store, process, retrieve, and display the digital image. A

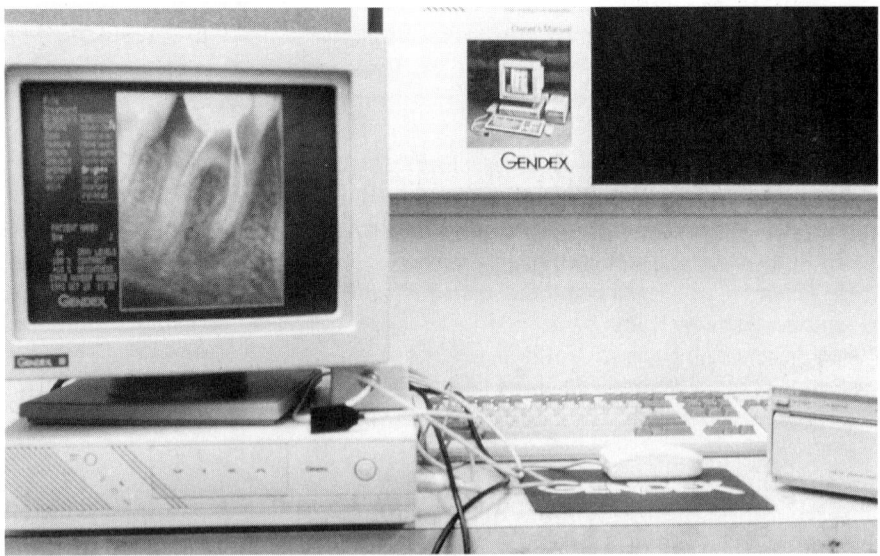

Figure 1–4. VIXA/Visualix digital intraoral radiographic system. Instead of a film packet, *a detector (sensor)* is placed in the patient's mouth and exposed to x-rays. The picture is immediately available on the video monitor. The image can be adjusted for brightness and contrast levels. *(Courtesy Dr. Allan G. Farman and Dr. William C. Scarfe, School of Dentistry, University of Louisville, Louisville, Ky).*

detector converts the transmitted light of a conventional radiograph or the remnant x-ray beam into an electronic signal. This signal is then converted to a digital form that is stored in and displayed by the computer. Digital x-ray systems are so new that standards have not been set. It seems certain that future generations of digital sensors will be greatly improved over those presently available.

The discovery of x-radiation has already revolutionized the practice of dentistry, and future technological advances undoubtedly will increase the use of radiography in the years ahead and make it safer.

CHAPTER SUMMARY

Roentgen's discovery of the x-ray revolutionized the methods of practicing medicine and dentistry by making it possible to visualize internal body structures. Although the usefulness of x-ray as a diagnostic tool was recognized almost immediately, the methods of control to avoid tissue damage were delayed. The use of radiographs in medical and dental diagnostic procedures is now essential. Most patient exposures are now made by trained technicians, dental assistants, or dental hygienists, but the responsibility for making the diagnosis rests with the dentist. It is of vital importance that the person making the x-ray exposure understands how x-rays are produced, controlled, and used to achieve the best diagnostic results. Improved equipment, advanced techniques, and better-trained personnel make it possible to obtain clearer radiographs with high diagnostic value and minimal risk of unnecessary radiation to patient or operator.

KEY WORDS

Cephalometric radiograph	Radiograph
Cone	Radiography
Digital imaging	Roentgen ray
Magnetic resonance imaging (MRI)	Roentgenograph
Panoramic radiography	Tomography
Position indicating device (PID)	X-ray

REVIEW QUESTIONS

1. Who discovered the x-ray? _W.C. Roentgens_ When? _Nov 8 1895_.

2. Define PID. _Position   Indicating   Device_.

3. The courts have ruled that radiographs are the property of the _Dentist_.

4. Who has the responsibility to diagnose the radiograph? (a) the dental assistant, (b) the dental technician, (c) the dental hygienist, (d) the dentist.

5. Who discovered the x-ray? (a) C. Edmund Kells, (b) Franklin McCormack, (c) Wilhelm Conrad Roentgen, (d) William Rollins.

6. Who is believed to have exposed the prototype of the first dental x-ray film? (a) William Rollins, (b) Otto Walkhoff, (c) Wilhelm Conrad Roentgen, (d) C. Edmund Kells.

7. Who is considered by many to be the father of the science of radiation protection? (a) William Rollins, (b) William Morton, (c) C. Edmund Kells, (d) Franklin McCormack.

8. What proportion of all x-ray equipment in the United States is believed to be owned by dentists? (a) 15 percent, (b) 35 percent, (c) 50 percent, (d) 85 percent.

9. What is the most important use of radiography in dental practice? (a) for therapy, (b) for diagnosis, (c) for patient education, (d) for control of pain.

10. In which method of radiography is a single plane selected to be radiographed? (a) digital imaging, (b) tomography, (c) radioisotope scanners, (d) magnetic resonance imaging.

BIBLIOGRAPHY

Goaz PW, White SC: *Oral Radiology Principles and Interpretation*, 3rd ed. St. Louis, MO: CV Mosby, 1994

Eastman Kodak: *Radiation Safety in Dental Radiography*. Rochester, NY, 1993

CHAPTER 2

Characteristics of Radiation

OBJECTIVES

By the end of this chapter the student should be able to

1. Differentiate the various atomic and molecular structures important to radiography.
2. Explain background radiation.
3. Identify the electromagnetic spectrum.
4. Identify the common characteristics of radiation.
5. Compare x-ray wavelength to its penetrating power.
6. Identify which types of radiation are capable of causing ionization in body tissues.
7. Identify two ways dental x-rays interact with matter.

THE PHYSICS OF RADIATION

The scientist conceives the world to consist of matter and energy. **Matter** is defined as anything that occupies space and has mass. Thus all things that we see and recognize are forms of matter. **Energy** is defined as the ability to do work and overcome resistance. Heat, light, electricity, and x-radiation are forms of energy. Matter and energy are closely related. Energy is produced whenever the state of matter is altered by either natural or artificial means. The difference between water, steam, or ice is the amount of energy associated with the molecules. Such an energy exchange is produced within the x-ray machine and will be discussed later.

11

To understand radiation we must understand atomic structure. Currently we know of 105 basic **elements** occurring either singly or in combination in natural forms. Typical elements of interest in radiography are aluminum, beryllium, copper, lead, oxygen, samarium, radium, and tungsten. Each of these elements is made up of atoms. An **atom** is the smallest particle of an element that still retains the properties of the element. If any given atom is split, the resulting components no longer retain the properties of the element. Atoms are generally combined with other atoms to form molecules. A **molecule** is the smallest particle of a substance that retains the properties of that substance. A simple molecule such as sodium chloride (table salt) contains only two atoms, whereas a complex molecule may contain hundreds of atoms.

Atoms are extremely minute and are made up of a number of subatomic particles. For our purpose we are concerned only with the electrons, protons, and neutrons. **Electrons** have little mass or weight, are electrically negatively charged, and are constantly in motion. **Protons** weigh about 1840 times as much as electrons and are electrically positively charged. **Neutrons** can be thought of as a combination of one proton and one electron and are electrically neutral, having a mass approximately equal to the proton.

The atom's arrangement in some ways resembles the solar system. The atom has a nucleus as its center or sun, and the electrons revolve around it like planets. The **nucleus** of all atoms except hydrogen contains at least one proton and one neutron (hydrogen in its simplest form has only a proton). Some atoms contain a very high number of each. The electrons and the nucleus normally remain in the same relative position to one another. To accommodate the electrons revolving about the nucleus, the larger atoms have several concentric orbits at various distances from the nucleus. These are referred to as "electron shells," which some chemists now call **energy levels.** (The number of electrons in each of these spherical layers of energy varies but is generally 2 in the first shell, a maximum of 8 in the second, 18 in the third, 32 in the fourth, 50 in the fifth, 72 in the sixth, and 98 in the seventh.) The innermost level is referred to

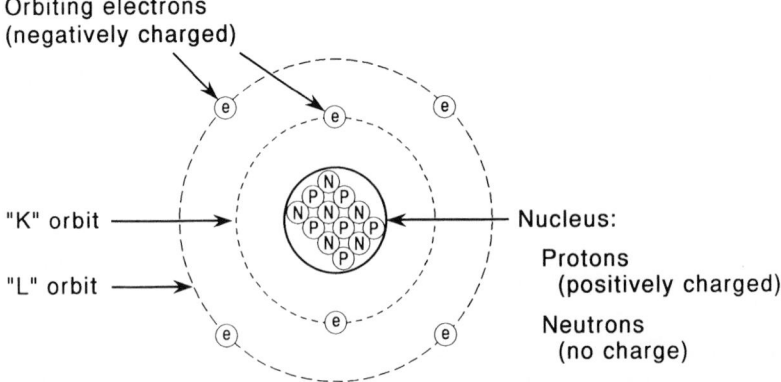

Figure 2–1. Diagrammatic representation of oxygen atom according to present fundamental concepts of matter. In the neutral atom, the number of positively charged protons in the nucleus is equal to the number of negatively charged orbiting electrons.

as the "K" shell, the next as the "L" shell, and so on (Fig. 2–1). No known atom contains more than seven shells.

BACKGROUND RADIATION AND RADIOACTIVITY

Radiation is briefly defined as the process by which energy in the form of heat, light, or rays is sent out of atoms and molecules as they undergo internal change. This energy is emitted and propelled outwardly from its source in all directions (unless the direction is controlled as in the x-ray machine). This may occur spontaneously, as with unstable elements such as radium or uranium or under man-made conditions.

The human race has always been subjected to exposure from natural **background radiations** originating from (1) cosmic radiations from outer space, (2) terrestrial radiations from the earth and its environments, and (3) background radiations from naturally occurring radionuclides (unstable atoms that emit radiations) that are deposited in our bodies by inhalation and ingestion.

Natural background radiation levels for the United States range from about 0.9 mSv (millisievert) or 90 mrem (millirem)* to 2 mSv or 200 mrem per year. The exact amount varies according to locality, the amount of radioactive material present, and the intensity of the cosmic rays—this intensity varies according to altitude and latitude. For example, persons living near sea level in Philadelphia receive about 0.9 mSv (90 mrem) per year whereas persons living in the mile-high city of Denver receive about 1.4 mSv (140 mrem) per year.

The whole body is exposed to background radiation, whereas in dental radiography only a small area of the head is directly exposed. For purposes of comparison, it is of interest that a typical single x-ray film subjects the average patient's body (reproductive organs) to no more than 0.002 mSv (0.2 mrem).

To understand radioactivity we must realize that while most elements are stable, a few undergo constant, spontaneous changes. As we have already seen, each atom of an element has an equal number of protons and electrons. Tungsten, the metal most involved in x-ray production, has 74 protons and 74 electrons and a constant number of neutrons. However, variations occur in some elements. For example, the majority of hydrogen atoms contain no neutrons, but two rarer forms exist. The first of these, deuterium, contains a neutron in its nucleus and is stable. The second and much rarer form, tritium, contains two neutrons and is unstable and radioactive. Such alternate forms are called **isotopes.** Each isotope of a specific atom has the same chemical properties. They differ only in mass and weight (Fig. 2–2).

Most elements are now believed to have one or more isotopes. Over 1500 have already been identified. Of these, more than half are unstable and radioactive. Instability in an atom can be natural or man-made; either type is important to medicine and dentistry. Many dental schools are conducting research with radioactive isotopes, and much is yet to be discovered about them.

---

* Radiation measurement terms are explained in Chapter 6. Beginning in 1985 the International System of unit measurements came into use. Thus, two sets of units are currently in use. The unit *rem* is now being replaced by *sievert*. The prefix *milli* indicates "one-thousandth of." The sievert and rem are the units used to express the dose equivalent for humans. One sievert is equivalent to 100 rem.

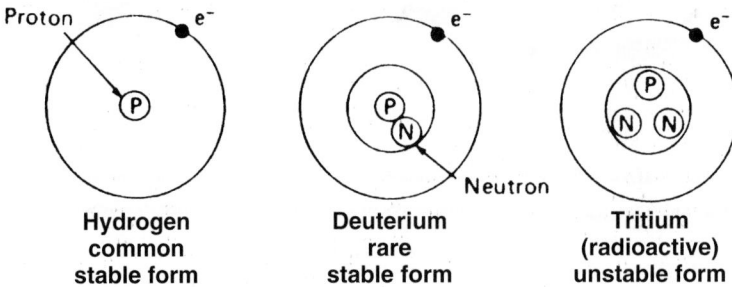

Figure 2–2. Isotopes of hydrogen. Approximately 1 in 14,000 hydrogen atoms contains one neutron in the nucleus (deuterium). Another rare hydrogen atom is tritium, which contains two neutrons in the nucleus. Each of these isotopes has the same chemical properties, but they differ in physical mass and weight. Unstable isotopes seek to become stable by a release of energy through a process known as decay. This process involves giving off two kinds of radiation: (1) corpuscular, or particulate, radiation and (2) electromagnetic radiation.

Unstable isotopes attempt to regain stability through the release of energy, by a process known as **decay,** in which the unstable nucleus of the isotope continues to decay (give off radiation) until stability of the nucleus is attained. This decay process involves the giving off of two distinct forms of radiation: **particulate radiation,** consisting of bits of matter traveling at high speeds (also called **corpuscular radiation**), and **electromagnetic radiation,** which is a combination of electric and magnetic energy and is emitted in the form of rays or waves.

Particulate radiation originates from naturally occurring isotopes and is given off in the form of alpha particles, beta particles, and neutrons. The alpha particles, which contain two protons and two neutrons, are positively charged and are much heavier than the beta particles, which are high-speed, negatively charged electrons. As already indicated, neutrons are uncharged.

Another form of naturally occurring radiation belongs to the family of electromagnetic radiation and is called **gamma radiation.** Gamma rays are very similar to x-rays but occur naturally, whereas x-rays are man-made. A further difference is that gamma rays originate from the nucleus, whereas x-rays result from the interaction of electrons with atomic materials inside the x-ray tube. Although radioactive isotopes are frequently used in hospitals and are also being used by dentists in some research and teaching centers, our concern is with the man-made forms of radiation; the information on natural radiation is included for the sake of completeness in presenting a proper background to the study of radiography.

Humans have learned to produce several types of radiations that are identical to natural radiations. Although our main concern deals with x-radiation, ultraviolet waves are also produced artificially for sunlamps or fluorescent lights and for numerous other uses. One of the most recent man-made radiations is the laser beam, whose potential is not fully known at this time. We can confidently await the development of further man-made radiations.

THE ELECTROMAGNETIC SPECTRUM

Electromagnetic radiations are forms of radiant energy, some natural and some man-made, that possess no mass or weight and are electrically neutral. They also share four other common characteristics: (1) all pass through space in wavelike motion; (2) all travel at the speed of light; (3) all give off an electrical field at right angles to their path of travel and a magnetic field at right angles to the electric field; and (4) all have energies that are measurable and different.

The basic differences between types of electromagnetic radiation are their **wavelengths** and **frequencies.** One determines wavelengths by measuring the distance from the crest of one wave to the crest of the following one and frequency by measuring the number of oscillations per second (Fig. 2–3). Each form of electromagnetic radiation has its own wavelength and frequency, which indicate its main property, source, or use. When wavelength and frequency change, the energy of the radiation also changes.

The **electromagnetic spectrum** consists of an orderly arrangement of all known radiant energies (Fig. 2–4). For convenience these are portrayed according to their wavelengths. The longest wavelengths, which are those used for low-frequency communications, are so long that they are best measured in kilometers (each kilometer is 1000 meters or about 5/8 mile), whereas the shortest cosmic rays are measured in **Angström units** (1 Å is about 1/250,000,000 in. or 1/100,000,000 centimeter). No clear-cut separation exists between the various radiations represented on the electromag-

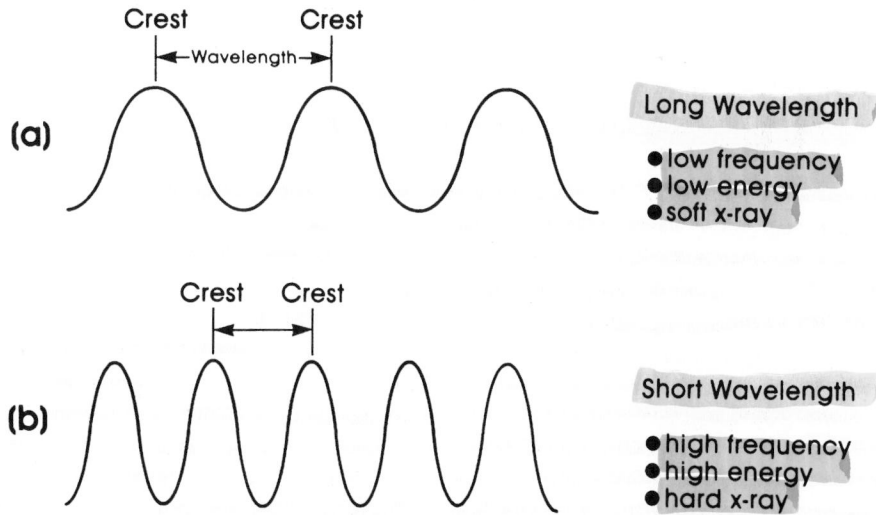

Figure 2–3. Differences in wavelengths and frequencies. Only the shortest wavelengths with extremely high frequency and energy are used to expose film in dental radiography. Wavelength is determined by the distances between the crests. Observe that this distance is much shorter in **(b)** than in **(a).** The photons that comprise the dental x-ray beam are estimated to have over 250 million such crests per inch. Frequency is the number of crests of a wavelength passing a given point per second.

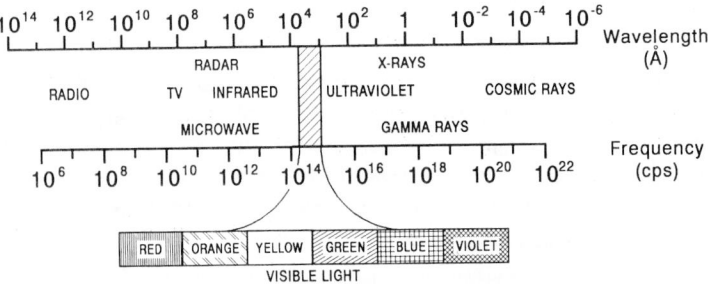

Figure 2–4. The electromagnetic spectrum. Å, angstrom; cps, cycles per second.

netic spectrum; consequently overlapping of the wavelengths is common. Each form of radiation has a range of frequencies; this accounts for some of the longer infrared waves being measured in meters while the shorter infrared waves are measured in Angström units. It therefore follows that all x-radiations are not the same wavelength. The longest of these are the **Grenz rays,** also called **soft radiation,** which have only limited penetrating power and are unsuitable for exposing dental radiographs. The wavelengths used in diagnostic dental radiography range from about 0.1 to 0.5 Å and are classified as **hard radiation,** a term meaning radiation with great penetrating power. Still shorter wavelengths are produced by super-voltage machines when still greater penetration is required, as in some forms of medical therapy and industrial radiography.

CHARACTERISTICS OF X-RADIATION

X-rays are believed to consist of minute bundles of pure energy called **photons** (or **quanta**). These have no mass or weight, are invisible, and cannot be sensed. Because they travel at the speed of light (186,000 mi/sec or 3×10^{10} cm/sec), these x-ray photons are often referred to as "bullets of energy."

Bodies in motion are believed to have **kinetic energy** (from the Greek word *kineticos,* "pertaining to motion"). As already discussed, the electrons of any atom are in continuous motion within their orbital shells, or energy levels, around the nucleus. The velocity of this motion is drastically increased as the temperature is raised; this happens within the x-ray tube when its components are heated and free electrons are propelled at extremely high speeds toward a tungsten target. The particular area of the target toward which these electrons are directed is the focal spot; it is here that the x-ray originates. The details of the x-ray tube, focal spot, and the methods by which the electrons cross the tube are explained in Chapters 3 and 4.

A form of energy transfer takes place within the x-ray tube as the electrons are either stopped or slowed down by impact with the tungsten target in which all or part of the kinetic energy is given up. However, because energy is always present in nature and can never be created or destroyed, the so-called "lost" kinetic energy is actually converted at the focal spot into heat and x-rays. Unfortunately, less than 1 percent of this converted energy is released in the form of useful x-ray photons; the other 99 percent is in the form of useless heat.

The amount and type of energy released during energy conversion depend on the manner in which the electrons strike the atoms of the target. At any given moment a slight difference in **potential** (the strength of the current) may alter the speed at which the free electrons are accelerated across the tube. All electrons hitting the target are not decelerated in the same degree. Some are absorbed by the target atoms, some are slowed down, and others are deviated from their path of travel (Fig. 2–5). Thus the x-ray beam formed at the focal spot is **polychromatic,** that is, it contains x-ray photons of various energies and penetrating power.

The degree of acceleration, the manner of impact at the focal spot, and the binding energy determine the type of wavelength that is produced. The term **binding energy** is used to describe the force that maintains the electrons in their relative positions around the nucleus. This binding energy increases, the closer the electron is to the nucleus. An electron from the inner K shell is more tightly held in position near the nucleus than an electron from the L shell or another of the outer shells; therefore it takes more energy to remove a K electron. The binding energy is not always the same from atom to atom, and the electrons of each shell have slightly different kinetic characteristics. In the event that the manner of impact forces a K electron into space, it is replaced by an electron from the L shell.

The conversion of kinetic energy into x-ray photons is accomplished in two ways within the dental x-ray tube. The first and most important for dental radiography is called **Bremsstrahlung** (German for "braking radiation"). Referring to Figure 2–5, ob-

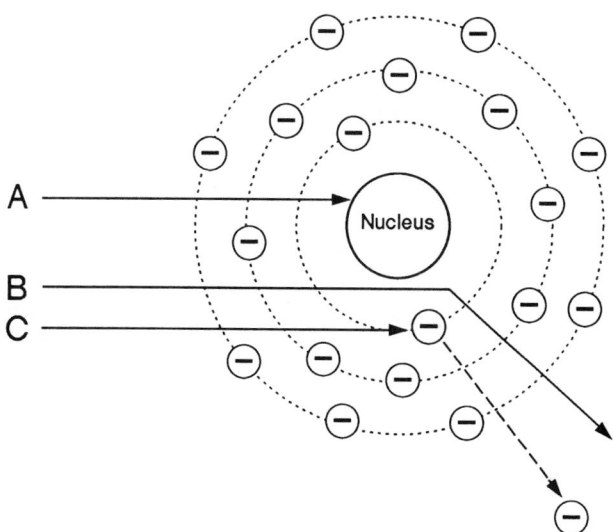

Figure 2–5. Electrons colliding with simulated atom: **A.** giving up all of its energy, **B.** relinquishing part of its energy, **C.** displacing a K shell (orbit) electron.

serve that the impact from both (A) and (B) produce Bremsstrahlung because when a free electron collides with the nucleus of an atom in the target metal and cannot travel further, as in (A), all of its energy is given off and converted to heat and very short x-ray waves; whereas if the impact is only a glancing one, as in (B), there will be a variation of wavelengths of the resulting x-rays because the angle of impact with the target atom will vary. The majority of x-rays produced by dental machines are formed by these types of collisions. The second way, **characteristic radiation,** is produced when the free electron collides with an orbiting K electron instead of the target atom, and the electron from the L shell replaces it and assumes K shell characteristics, as shown in (C). This can be accomplished only when the x-ray machine has the capability of being operated with an electric current of at least 70 kilovolts (kVp) because a minimum force of 69 kVp is required to dislodge a K electron from its energy level (voltage is explained in the next chapter). Because all dental x-ray machines do not have this capability, characteristic x-rays are not always produced.

Another important characteristic of x-ray photons is the ability to pass through gases, liquids, and solids. The ability to penetrate materials or tissues depends on the wavelength of the x-ray and the thickness and density of the object. The composition of the object or the tissues determines whether the x-rays will penetrate and pass through it or whether they will be absorbed in it. Materials that are extremely dense and have a high atomic number will absorb more x-rays than thin materials with low atomic numbers. This partially explains why dense structures such as bone and enamel appear **radiopaque** (white or light gray) on the radiograph, whereas the less dense pulp chamber, muscles, and skin appear **radiolucent** (dark gray or black). Some of the x-ray photons interact with the materials that they penetrate. This interaction is called **ionization,** or the formation of ions.

IONIZING RADIATION

Atoms that have gained or lost electrons are electrically unstable and are called **ions.** The formation of ions is easier to understand if we first review the normal structural arrangement of the atom. The atom normally has the same number of protons (positive charges) in the nucleus as it has electrons (negative charges) in the orbital levels. When one of these electrons is removed from its orbital level in a neutral atom, the remainder of the atom loses its electrical neutrality.

An atom from which an electron has been removed has more protons than electrons, is positively charged, and is called a **positive ion.** The negatively charged electron that has been separated from the atom and the resulting positively charged ion are called an **ion pair.** When an atom is struck by an x-ray photon, an electron may be dislodged and an ion pair created (Fig. 2–6). As high-energy electrons travel on, electrons from other atoms may be ejected in a chain reaction, creating additional ion pairs. These unstable ions attempt to regain electrical stability by combining with another oppositely charged ion.

Any radiation that produces ions is called **ionizing radiation.** Only a portion of the radiation portrayed on the electromagnetic spectrum—the x-rays and the gamma

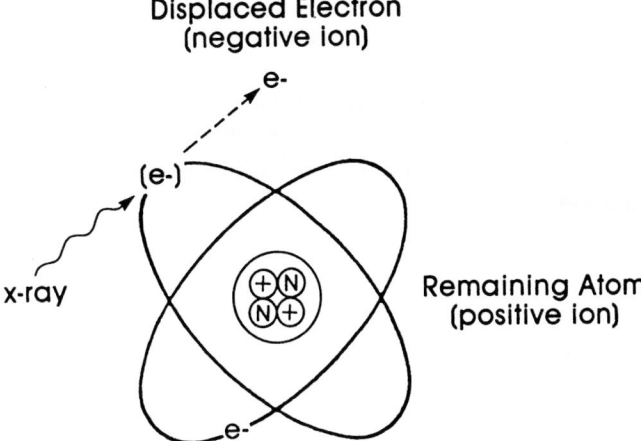

Figure 2–6. Ionization, showing the removal of an orbital electron (e⁻) by an x-ray. Thus, an ion pair results (+ represents a proton and N represents a neutron in the nucleus).

and cosmic rays—are of the ionizing type. In dental radiography our concern is limited to the possible changes that may occur in the cellular structures of the tissues as the ions are produced by the passage of x-rays through the cells. The mechanics of biologic tissue damage are explained in Chapter 5.

INTERACTION OF X-RAYS WITH MATTER

A beam of x-rays passing through matter is weakened and gradually disappears. Such a disappearance is referred to as **absorption** of x-rays. When so defined, *absorption* does not imply an occurrence such as a sponge soaking up water, but rather refers to the process of transferring the energy of the x-rays to the atoms of the material through which the x-ray beam passes. The chief method of absorption is ionization.

There are two important ways by which dental x-rays lose energy by interacting with matter—the **photoelectric effect** and the **Compton effect** (scattering).

The photoelectric effect is an all-or-nothing energy loss. The x-ray imparts all of its energy to an orbital electron of some atom. This dental x-ray, since it consisted only of energy in the first place, simply vanishes. The electromagnetic energy of the x-ray is imparted to the electron in the form of kinetic energy of motion and causes the electron to fly from its orbit with considerable speed. Thus, an ion pair results (Fig. 2–6). Remember, the basic method of the interaction of x-rays with matter is the formation of ion pairs. The high-speed electron (called a photoelectron) knocks other electrons from the orbits of other atoms (forming secondary ion pairs) until all of its energy is used up.

The Compton effect (often called Compton scattering) is similar to the photoelectric effect in that the dental x-ray interacts with an orbital electron and ejects it. But in the case of Compton interaction, only a part of the dental x-ray energy is transferred to the electron and a new, weaker x-ray is formed and scattered in some new direction. The new x-ray may even travel in a direction opposite to that of the original x-ray. Thus, it is important to remember that x-rays can be scattered in all directions and areas of the dental office. So we must protect ourselves from these scattered x-rays by standing at least 6 ft (1.8 m) from the head of our patient or, if that is not possible, by the use of lead shields.

CHAPTER SUMMARY

Some radiations occur in nature, and others are man-made. For convenience in identification, x-rays are arranged according to wavelength and occupy one segment of the electromagnetic spectrum. These x-rays travel at the speed of light. The length of the wave determines its penetrating power.

Only the shortest waves, measured in Angström units (Å), can be effectively used in dentistry. The length of the x-ray wave is determined by the manner in which the electrons impact on the target atoms within the x-ray tube. Since only the very shortest rays have sufficient penetrating power to pass through the bone and tooth structures, the majority of x-rays used to produce diagnostic radiographs range from 0.1 to 0.5 Å in length. Many forms of radiation, particularly x-rays and gamma rays, can ionize tissues and cause possible harm to patient or operator unless the exposure is controlled. This is why no one should be permitted to operate radiographic equipment without first understanding the characteristics of radiation.

KEY WORDS

Absorption

Angström unit (Å)

Atom

Background radiation

Bremsstrahlung

Characteristic radiation

Compton effect

Decay

Electromagnetic spectrum

Electron

Element

Energy levels

Frequency

Gamma rays

Hard radiation

Ionization

Isotope

Kinetic energy

Molecule

Neutron

Photoelectric effect

Photon

Polychromatic

Potential

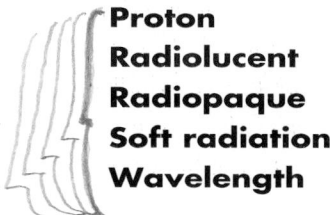

Proton

Radiolucent

Radiopaque

Soft radiation

Wavelength

REVIEW QUESTIONS

1. What term describes the smallest particle of a substance that retains the properties of that substance? (a) element, (b) molecule, (c) photon, (d) isotope.

2. Which of these subatomic particles carries a negative electric charge? (a) electron, (b) neutron, (c) nucleus, (d) proton.

3. What term describes an alternate form of an atom that does not contain the same number of neutrons? (a) ion, (b) neutron, (c) photon, (d) isotope.

4. Which of these has the shortest wavelength? (a) radar, (b) ultraviolet, (c) infrared, (d) x-rays.

5. Which of these forms of radiation has the greatest penetrating power? (a) x-ray, (b) infrared, (c) ultraviolet, (d) radio wave.

6. What percent of the kinetic energy inside the x-ray tube is converted into x-rays? (a) 1 percent, (b) 8 percent, (c) 69 percent, (d) 99 percent.

7. Which of these forms of radiation is least capable of causing ionization of body tissue cells? (a) cosmic rays, (b) x-rays, (c) gamma rays, (d) infrared.

8. Which x-ray wavelength has the most penetrating power? (a) 0.1 Å, (b) 0.5 Å, (c) 0.8 Å, (d) 1.0 Å.

9. Which form of radiation causes ionization of body tissue cells? (a) radar, (b) radio, (c) x-ray, (d) microwaves.

10. What term best describes the process of transferring the energy of the x-rays to the atoms of the material through which the x-ray beam passes? (a) Compton scattering, (b) photoelectric effect, (c) absorption, (d) Bremsstrahlung.

11. Draw and label a typical atom.

12. Define background radiation.

BIBLIOGRAPHY

Goaz PW, White SC: *Oral Radiology Principles and Interpretation*, 3rd ed. St. Louis, MO: CV Mosby, 1994

Langland OE, Sippy FH, Langlais RP: *Textbook of Dental Radiology*, 2nd ed. Springfield, IL: Charles C Thomas, 1984

Wuehrmann AH, Manson-Hing LR: *Dental Radiology*, 5th ed. St. Louis, MO: CV Mosby, 1981

CHAPTER 3

The Dental X-ray Machine—
Components and Functions

OBJECTIVES

By the end of this chapter the student should be able to

1. Identify the types of x-ray machines and their major parts and components.
2. Draw and label a typical dental x-ray tube.
3. Identify the functions of the electric circuits and the control devices.
4. Identify the factors involved in x-ray generation.
5. Differentiate between constant potential and varying potential x-ray machines.

TYPES OF DENTAL X-RAY MACHINES

The x-ray machine has undergone a long period of development. The unreliable gas tubes used in the early machines gave way to the vastly improved Coolidge hot cathode vacuum tube, a thermionic emission (the creation of ions by heat) tube invented by Dr. W. D. Coolidge, and the old machines with exposed high-tension wires are now museum relics. The first shock-proof machines were introduced in 1923. Few changes were made until the mid 1950s when the variable kilovoltage machines were introduced. At the suggestion of A. G. Richards, the recessed tube design was introduced in 1966. New technology employing miniaturized solid-state transformers and rare-earth materials for filtration of the x-ray beam has resulted in a modern dental x-ray machine that is safe, compact, easy to position, and simple to operate.

Many manufacturers, domestic and foreign, offer a variety of x-ray machine models and accessories. All x-ray machines—whether mobile or stationary, whether mounted on the wall, the floor, or the ceiling—operate on similar principles. The greatest differences among them are their size, their voltage range, their regulating controls, the position of the tube within the tube head, and whether the voltage varies or is constant.

The x-ray machines used in hospitals and industry are often much larger and more complicated. Only the conventional x-ray machines used in most dental offices are discussed in this chapter. The operation of the larger cephalometric and panoramic types of x-ray units are discussed in Chapters 20 and 21.

PARTS AND COMPONENTS

Dental x-ray machines vary in size and appearance but have similar structural components and electrical parts (Fig. 3–1). All these parts may vary in size, shape, and arrangement. The standard structural parts include (1) a **control panel,** which may be a cabinet, a panel mounted on the wall, or a portable control box; (2) a **tube head,** which houses the x-ray tube; and (3) a flexible **extension arm** from which the tube head is suspended. The extension arm is hollow to permit the passage of electrical wires to the tube. It folds up like a bracket and can be swiveled from side to side. The tube head is attached to the extension arm by means of a yoke that can revolve 360 degrees horizontally where it is connected. In addition, the tube head can be rotated vertically within the yoke. The tube head is made of cast metal (often aluminum) and protectively lined with lead to prevent the escape of radiation in any direction except toward the position indicating device (PID).

The fundamental electrical parts of the x-ray machine are (1) the **x-ray tube;** (2) the **electrical circuits** (the low-voltage or filament circuit and the high-voltage or cathode-anode circuit); and (3) the **timer.** The electric current enters the control panel either through a cord plugged into a grounded outlet in the wall or through a direct connection to a power line in the wall. It continues to and through the hollow extension arm and the **yoke,** entering the tube head from one or both sides at a point where the tube head attaches to the yoke. All areas are heavily insulated to protect the patient and the operator from electrical shock. More information on the circuits and wiring is provided later in this chapter.

THE X-RAY TUBE

The x-ray tube (Fig. 3–2) can be compared to the heart, and the control circuits to the arteries and veins; they are equally important, for without one the other could not achieve its purpose—the production of x-rays. These x-rays are produced when a stream of high-speed electrons strikes a target. Three conditions must exist for x-rays to be produced: (1) a source of free electrons; (2) high voltage to impart speed to them;

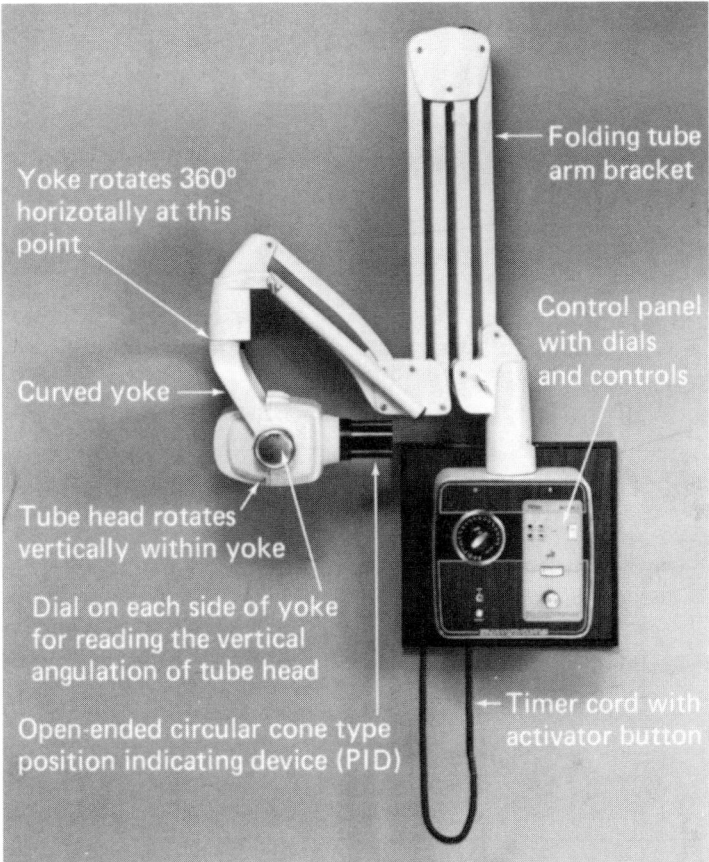

Figure 3–1. Typical wall-mounted dental x-ray machine. *(Courtesy of Ritter-Midwest Division of Sybron Corporation.)*

and (3) a target that is capable of stopping them. The x-ray tube and the circuits within the machine are designed to create these conditions.

The earliest tubes used in radiography were glass bulbs from which the air had been only partially evacuated and replaced with hydrogen or some other gas. An **anode** (the positive terminal or electrode in an electric circuit) and a **cathode** (the negative terminal or electrode in an electric circuit) were sealed within the tube, and the two protruding arms of the electrodes permitted the passage of the current through the tube. The electron supply was dependent on the ionization of gases within the tube when it was in operation. The current flowing between these electrodes from cathode to anode was called the **cathode stream.** Because the air evacuation was only partial, these early tubes were quite erratic in their operation, working well one day and not at all the next. A major breakthrough was the invention in 1913 of the Coolidge vacuum tube, an improved model that is still in use in today's x-ray machines.

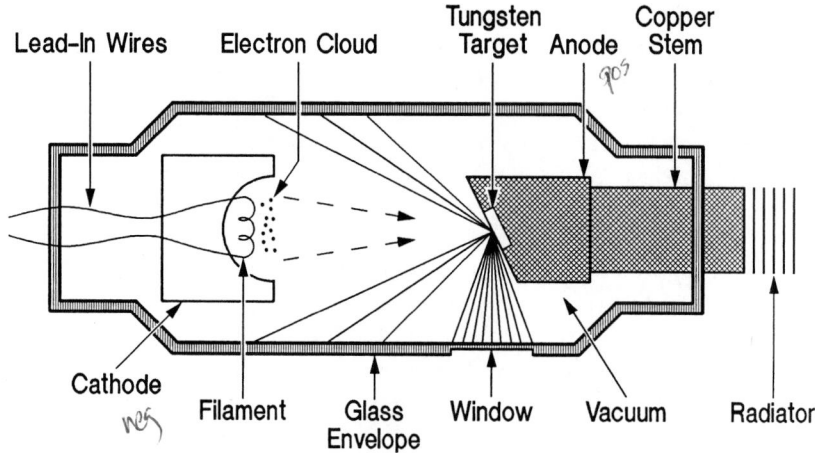

Figure 3–2. Typical dental x-ray tube.

The design of the Coolidge vacuum tube eliminated the need for gas to create electrons, replacing gas with an incandescent (glowing with heat) filament in the cathode. This process, known as **thermionic emission,** occurs whenever a wire is heated to incandescence. A familiar example of this phenomenon is the tungsten electric light bulb we all use. The operator, by adjusting the milliamperage, can accurately control the thermionic emission produced in the improved, highly evacuated Coolidge tube by determining how hot the filament in the cathode should be (Fig. 3–3).

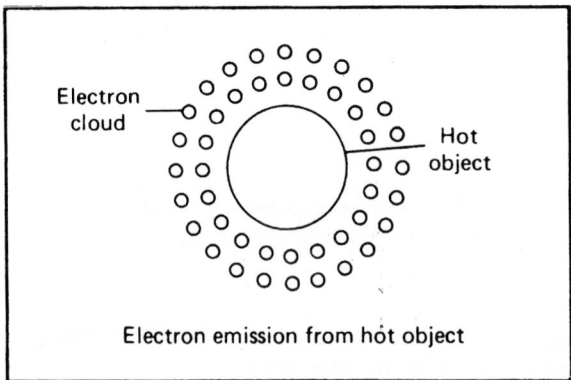

Figure 3–3. Cross section of a filament wire. When the filament wire in the x-ray tube is heated to incandescence (thermionic emission), some of the attached electrons are literally boiled out of the wire and become available as a source of free electrons, thus fulfilling the first requirement for x-ray production. The milliamperage selected by the operator will determine the size of the electron cloud and therefore the number of x-rays to be produced during any given exposure time.

The x-ray tube (Fig. 3–2), located inside the tube housing (Fig. 3–4), is a glass bulb from which the air has been pumped out to create a vacuum. The vacuum offers a minimum resistance to the stream of electrons flowing across the space between the two electrodes sealed in the tube and facing each other. In most x-ray machines used in the United States, the space between the electrodes is less than 1 in. (25.4 mm). The cathode and the anode are connected to the outside of the tube by massive copper wires, which permit a high-voltage current to flow across the tube when the x-ray machine is in operation. On x-ray machines of conventional design, the tube is located in front of the transformers (Fig. 3–4); on those employing the Richards design, the tube is recessed behind the transformers (see Fig. 4–5).

A metal housing surrounds the x-ray tube and performs several important functions: (1) it protects the tube from accidental damage; (2) it increases the safety of the x-ray machine by grounding its high-voltage components (the x-ray tube and the transformers) to prevent shock; (3) it prevents overheating and prolongs the useful life of the x-ray tube by providing a space filled with oil, gas, or air to absorb the heat created during the production of x-rays; and (4) it absorbs any x-rays produced except the primary beam that exits through the port.

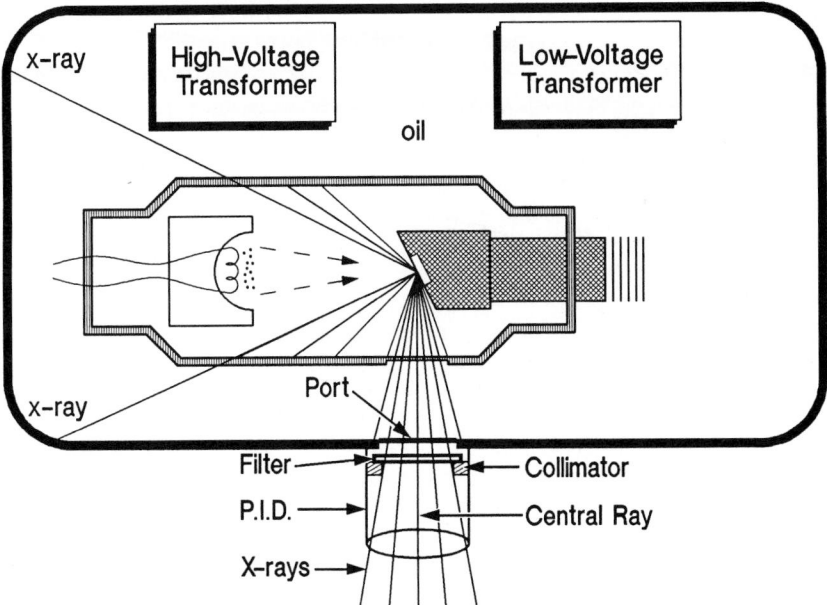

Figure 3–4. Dental x-ray tube housing, containing dental x-ray tube, transformers, and oil. When an electric current is applied to the high-voltage circuit (between the cathode and the anode), each electron is propelled from the cathode to the target on the anode, producing heat and x-rays. X-rays are emitted in all directions. Most of the x-rays travel toward the port because of the 20-degree angle of the anode target. These x-rays make up the primary x-ray beam and exit the housing via the port. The central ray is the x-ray in the center of the primary beam. PID, position indicating device.

The cathode assembly at the negative end of the tube consists of a thin, spiral filament of tungsten wire about 1/2 in. (12.7 mm) long. This filament, when heated to incandescence, produces the electrons. The wire filament is recessed into a molybdenum focusing cup, which directs the electrons toward the target on the anode (Fig. 3–5).

The anode assembly on the positive end of the tube consists of a copper bar with a tungsten button imbedded in the end that faces the focusing cup of the cathode. On dental x-ray machines this tungsten button, called the **target,** is set into the copper at an angle of 20 degrees to the cathode. The angle ensures that most of the x-rays (the primary beam) are produced in one direction.

Of major importance to the dental radiographer is a small area on the target that the electrons strike to produce x-rays. When the tube is in operation, a cloud of electrons first forms around the filament wire of the cathode as the tube warms. Later, when the high-voltage current is applied, these electrons are attracted and propelled toward a rectangular area on the surface of the target. This area is known as the **focal spot.** Its size is controlled by the manufacturer. A small focal spot not only improves the **definition** (sharpness) on the radiograph but also concentrates the electrons and creates enormous heat. To prevent damage to the tube, the size of the focal spot is effectively reduced by the application of the line–focus principle (Fig. 3–6). This involves focusing the electron stream and directing it into the narrow rectangle on the face of the target on the anode. If one were to stand directly beneath the x-ray tube and look up at it, the rectangular focal spot (actual focal spot) would appear square (effective focal spot). The purpose of the line–focus principle is to generate x-rays over a large area for better heat dissipation.

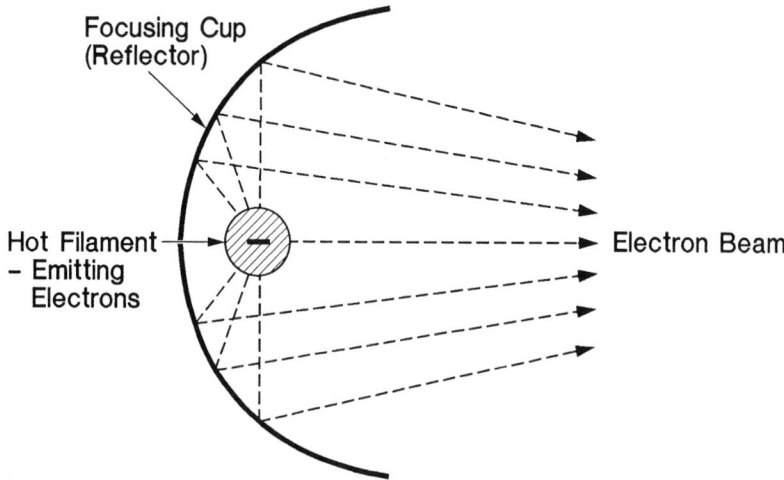

Figure 3–5. Formation of electron beam by focusing cup. A reflector, or focusing cup, within the cathode stucture, into which the filament is placed, focuses the electron beam similar to the way light is focused by a flashlight reflector. When the high-voltage circuit is activated, the free electrons are accelerated toward the focal spot on the anode target at approximately half the speed of light.

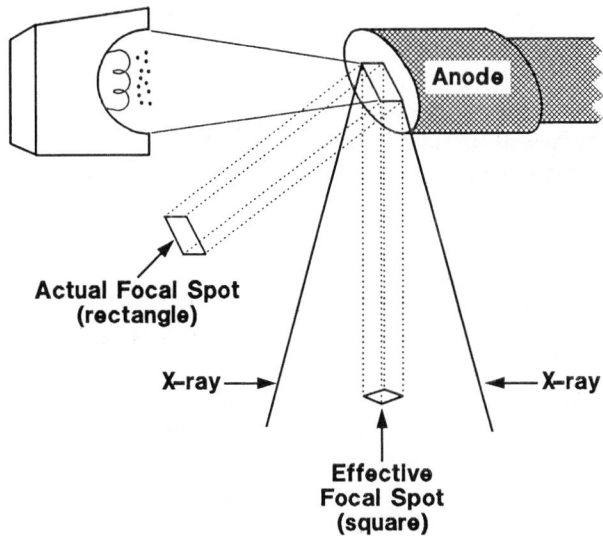

Figure 3–6. Representation of the anode, focal spot, and x-ray beam. As seen from points within the x-ray beam, the focal spot appears as a square of approximately 0.8 mm × 0.8 mm. This square is the source of radiation or **effective focal spot** for the beam of radiation. The **actual focal spot** is rectangular and has a considerably greater area (approximately 0.8 mm × 1.8 mm).

SIGNIFICANCE OF ELECTRON ACTIVITY

It is easier to understand x-ray production if one realizes how minute the powerful negatively charged electrons are. It has been estimated that 1 trillion electrons weigh less than a gram and occupy practically no space. It is not possible to accurately calculate the enormous number of electrons inside the energized x-ray tube. When accelerated by a high-voltage current of sufficient strength, these electrons become projectiles that can travel through the vacuum inside the x-ray tube at approximately half the speed of light. The resulting high-speed impact with the target atoms at the focal spot produces x-rays powerful enough to penetrate human tissues or many solid materials.

In simplified terms, an electric current is a movement of electrons through a conducting medium. Such a medium is normally a metal or a wire; however, as already mentioned, electrons can travel through a vacuum. Certain materials, such as aluminum, silver, and copper, are excellent conductors of current, whereas materials such as glass or plastics conduct poorly and are often used as insulators. The electrons within the electric current flow from a point of low voltage potential to a point of high voltage potential. Remember that the flow of the current is always from negative (minus) to positive (plus). Within the x-ray machine the direction of flow is from the filament of the cathode to the target of the anode.

PRINCIPLES OF X-RAY TUBE OPERATION

Before x-ray production can begin, the machine must be turned on and the necessary adjustments made on the control panel. The amperage selected determines the available number of free electrons at the cathode filament, and the kilovoltage selected determines their speed of travel toward the target on the anode. The total number of x-rays produced depends on the milliamperage selected multiplied by the duration of the exposure.

The process of x-ray production is initiated by firmly pressing the button on the hand switch. This permits the current to enter the filament circuit to form the electron cloud. After a **time delay** of less than 1/2 second the filament is fully heated, and the electron cloud is formed. The high voltage now automatically enters the cathode–anode circuit, speeding the free electrons across the tube to the focal spot on the target. These high-velocity electrons are stopped by the tungsten atoms in the target, and this energy is converted into 99 percent heat and 1 percent x-rays. The metal **tungsten** (symbol W and atomic weight 74—also known as Wolfram) is ideally suited for use in the filament and target because it can withstand extremely high temperatures (melting point 3370 degrees Celsius). Its high atomic number makes it possible to liberate electrons easily from their orbital shells when the metal is heated. Because it is subjected to such extreme heat and has low thermal conductivity, the tungsten button is always imbedded in a stem or core of copper. Copper is highly conductive and carries the heat off to the **radiator,** which is just outside the tube (refer to the tube diagram in Fig. 3–2). In an oil-cooled tube, the large mass of copper in which the tungsten is imbedded conducts the heat out of the tube into a radiator that transfers the heat to the oil surrounding the tube; in an air-cooled tube, the heat is transferred through the copper and the radiator into the air inside the tube head.

The x-rays produced by the energy exchange within the tube are emitted in all directions within the tube head. Many of these rays are absorbed by the oil, air, wires, transformers, or the tube head lining. A window (a thin area in the glass envelope) is located at a point where the emission of x-rays is most intense. In turn, this window is aligned with an opening in the tube head called the **port,** that is covered by a permanent seal of glass, beryllium, or aluminum. If the tube head is properly sealed, the port is the only place through which the x-rays can escape the tube head (Fig. 3–4). The PID fits over the port and can be moved to aim the central beam of radiation in the desired direction. Upon completion of the predetermined exposure, the high-voltage current is automatically shut off, and x-ray production stops.

AMPERAGE

The **ampere** (abbreviated **A**) is the unit of quantity of electric current. An increase in amperage results in an increase in the number of electrons that are available to travel from the cathode to anode when the tube is activated, and this results in a production of more x-rays. Only a small current is required to operate the x-ray machine; therefore, the term **milliampere,** denoting 1/1000 of an ampere, is used. This is abbreviated

mA. The majority of dental x-ray machines operate in ranges from 7 to 15 mA. On some x-ray units, the milliamperage can be selected by the operator; on others it is pre-set by the manufacturer.

VOLTAGE

Voltage is the electrical pressure or potential difference between two electrical charges. In radiography this difference in potential determines the electromotive force (the force that attracts the electrons to the anode) and the speed of the electrons when traveling from cathode to anode. This speed of the electrons, in turn, determines the energy (penetrating power) of the x-rays produced. When the voltage is increased, the electrons travel faster and produce the hardest type of radiation.

The **volt** (abbreviated **V**) is the unit of electromotive force used to measure the **electric potential.** It is defined as the electromotive force sufficient to cause 1 ampere of current to flow against a resistance of 1 ohm (the ampere is a measure of amount of current; the ohm is a measure of resistance). Because dental x-ray equipment operates at very high voltages, it is customary to express voltage in terms of **kilovolts.** The kilo-volt equals 1000 volts and is abbreviated **kV.** The voltage varies during an exposure, producing a polychromatic beam containing high-energy rays and also containing some rays that have barely enough energy to escape from the tube. The highest volt-age to which the current in the tube rises during an exposure is called the **kilovolt peak,** abbreviated **kVp.** Thus if the x-ray machine controls are set at 75,000 volts, the maximum x-ray energy that can be produced during this exposure is 75 kVp. Dental x-ray machines currently manufactured operate within a range from 50,000 to 100,000 volts.

ELECTRIC CURRENT

Electric current can flow in either direction along a wire or conductor; it can flow steadily in one direction or flow in pulses and change directions. **Direct current,** ab-breviated **DC,** flows continuously in one direction. Such a unidirectional current is used in flashlight batteries, for example, but cannot be used in the dental x-ray ma-chine unless modifications are made to the machine.

The ordinary household current used in most parts of the United States is a 110-volt and 60-cycle **alternating current,** abbreviated **AC,** which changes its direction of flow 60 times per second; thus the alternating current has two phases—one positive and the other negative—and alternates between these phases. Most dental x-ray ma-chines operate on 110- or 220-volt alternating current. Although it is customary to de-scribe the cathode as the negative electrode and the anode as the positive electrode, this is not quite the case during the time that the x-ray tube is producing x-rays be-cause the cathode and the anode each change from negative to positive 60 times per second. Since free electrons are available only at the cathode filament, x-rays can be produced only when the electrons flow across the gap from cathode to anode during the phase when the anode is positive. Theoretically, when the cycle reverses, any available electrons flow back to the cathode; however, x-rays cannot be produced

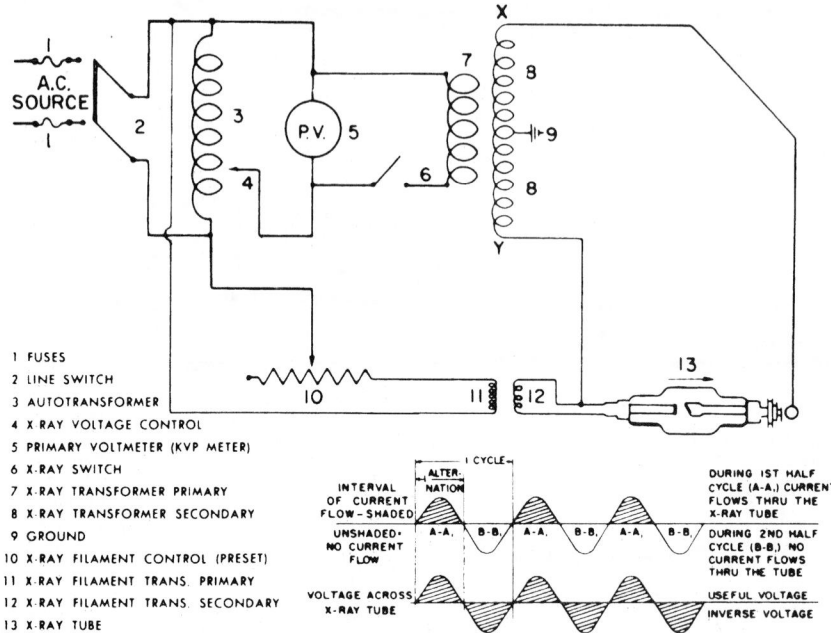

Figure 3–7. Basic x-ray unit consisting of three types of transformers, the x-ray tube, and several additional devices. For explanatory purposes, the basic circuit is divided into the filament (low-voltage) circuit and the anode–cathode (high-voltage) circuit. Ordinary household electric current is called 60-cycle alternating current because the current changes its direction of flow 60 times a second. Alternating current can be shown in wave form. The crest of the wave represents the maximum voltage when the current is moving in one direction, while the trough of the wave represents the maximum voltage when the current is moving in the other direction. The total cycle takes place in 1/60 second. *(Courtesy of General Electric Company, Medical Systems Division.)*

when the anode is in the negative phase because no free electrons are available at the target on the anode to be carried back across the gap to the cathode, and the current is thus blocked from traveling in that direction.

This alternation in current direction occurs every 1/120 second (twice during each full cycle) on x-ray machines of conventional design. It produces the x-rays in a series of bursts or pulses rather than in a continuous flow. The term **rectification** is used to describe the process in which the current is unidirectional. Because no special rectifying tubes or devices are used, x-ray equipment that operates only to produce x-rays during half of each cycle is known as **"self-rectifying"** (Fig. 3–7).

TRANSFORMERS

As already shown, each dental x-ray machine has a low-voltage filament circuit and a high-voltage cathode–anode circuit. A series of transformers is required to decrease (step down) or increase (step up) the ordinary 110-volt current that enters the x-ray machine. A **transformer** is an electromagnetic device for changing the alternating current and consists of two coils of electric wire wound on an iron core. The primary coil is connected to the alternating current supply, and the secondary coil is connected to the tube circuit. The wires in these coils are insulated from one another. When the current is flowing, a magnetic field around the primary coil induces an electric current in the secondary coil. The secondary voltage created can be accurately predicted. The number of wire turns in each coil determines whether the voltage is decreased or increased. For example, if there are ten times more turns on the primary than on the secondary coil, the voltage is decreased tenfold; if the ratio is reversed, the voltage increases tenfold.

A low-voltage (step-down) transformer (shown as items 11 and 12 in Fig. 3–7) decreases the potential of the current to approximately 8 volts, just enough to heat the filament and form the electron cloud. A primary preset resistor (item 10 in Fig. 3–7) further controls the voltage and stabilizes the milliamperage to compensate for sudden fluctuations in the current to ensure that the number of electrons available remains constant.

A high-voltage (step-up) transformer (items 7 and 8 in Fig. 3–7) increases the current as required by the technique the radiographer is using. The high-voltage current begins to flow through the cathode–anode circuit when the activator button on the line switch is depressed. X-rays are produced during the half of the cycle when the cathode is negative and the anode is positive.

An **autotransformer** is a voltage compensator that corrects minor fluctuations in the current flowing through the wires. Like the other transformers, it has an iron core but is wound with only a single coil that does the work of two (item 3 in Fig. 3–7). The action of the autotransformer is based on **self-induction** in a single coil rather than on mutual induction produced between two coils with different numbers of turns. By turning a knob on the control panel, the operator causes a selector switch to slide over a series of tabs that regulate the voltage by either decreasing or increasing it. This action is comparable to fine tuning on a radio.

Many transformers used in conventional x-ray machines are heavy and bulky. The trend is toward using lighter-weight and miniaturized solid-state components. This has the added advantage of reducing the size and the weight of the tube head, thus making it easier for the operator to position.

CONTROL DEVICES

The regulatory control devices vary greatly according to the manufacturer, with some even offering a choice of differently designed equipment control panels. There are four major controls that must be operated on most variable-type dental x-ray machines: the line switch to the electrical outlet, the milliampere selector, the kilovoltage selector, and the timer (Fig. 3–8).

The **line switch** may be a toggle switch that can be flicked on or off with light finger pressure, or it may be an ON-OFF push button. It is generally located on the side or face of the cabinet or control panel. On most machines a small red light turns on to warn that the machine is operational. In addition, all new x-ray machines are now re-

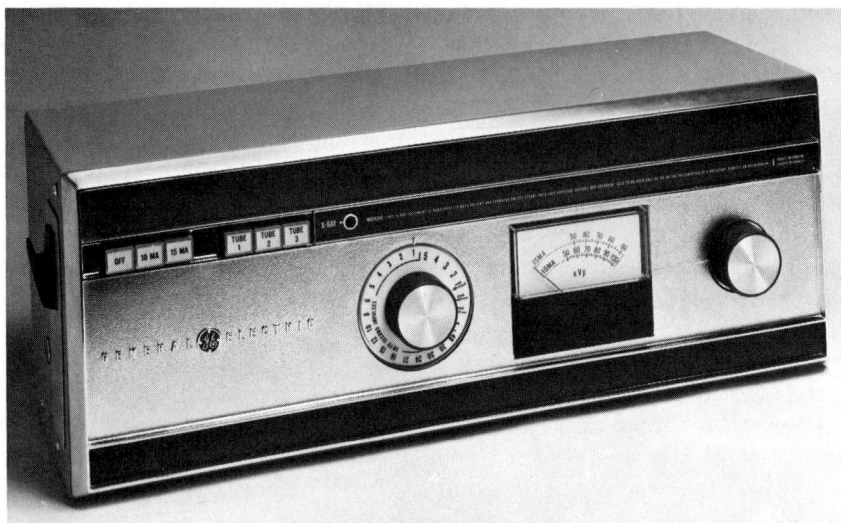

Figure 3–8. This basic master control unit accommodates three remote tube heads. Positive interlocks help assure operation of only one tube head at a time. This unit permits variable kVp and mA selection for settings of 50 kVp to 90 kVp at 15 mA and 50 kVP to 100 kVp at 10 mA. The solid-state timer permits 23 settings from 1 impulse (1/60 second) through 5 seconds. *(Courtesy of General Electric Company, Medical Systems Division.)*

quired by federal law to give off an audible signal when x-rays are produced. In the ON position, this switch energizes the circuits in the control panel but not the low- or high-voltage circuits. In the OFF position, the transformers are totally disconnected from the supply of electric current.

The milliampere selector may be a knob or push button. On a preset x-ray machine, it is connected directly to the ON-OFF switch. On some machines a needle on the control panel dial indicates that current is available for operation.

The **milliammeter** (or **ammeter,** as it is often called) measures the amount of current passing through the wires of the circuit. Mathematically, amperage is a linear factor expressed in the first power; this means that if amperage is doubled, the radiation produced is also doubled.

The **voltmeter** measures the electromotive force (the difference in potential or voltage across the x-ray tube). A kilovolt peak selector, in the form of push buttons, knobs, or dials, controls the tabs that slide over the turns of the wire in the autotransformer and enables the operator to change the peak kilovoltage. Mathematically, voltage is an exponential factor. For example, doubling the kilovoltage would result in far more than twice as much penetrating power. For practical purposes, an increase from 65 kVp to 80 kVp is sufficient to double the penetrating power of the x-rays that are produced.

The **timer** serves to regulate the duration of the interval that the current will pass through the x-ray tube. Some of the older x-ray machines that are still in use have mechanical or electric timers that are not sufficiently accurate for modern high-speed film and techniques. The newer units are equipped with a vacuum-type electronic timer, or timers, with a transistorized circuit that is accurate up to 1/60-second intervals. Time settings of less than a second may be indicated in fractions as 1/20 or 1/10 and in **impulses**—there being 60 impulses in a second. For example, the frequently used 1/10-second exposure lasts six impulses, 1/5 second for twelve impulses, and so forth. The timer is set by turning the selector knob or depressing the marked push botton. An activator button is located on the handle of the timer cord or the control panel. All dental x-ray machines are required to be equipped with an exposure switch of the **"dead-man"** type, which automatically terminates the exposure when the finger ceases to press the timer button. This makes it necessary to maintain firm pressure on the button during the entire exposure. Failure to do so results in the formation of an insufficient number of x-rays to properly expose the film. Ideally, the timer cord should be sufficiently long to enable the operator to step into an area of radiation safety (normally at least 6 feet—1.83 m—from the source of the x-ray beam). By observing the dial on the milliammeter and listening to the audible sound, it is possible to determine whether x-rays are being generated.

The present trend is toward simpler and automated controls. An example of this is the electrical timer that automatically resets itself and does not have to be altered unless a change in the exposure time is desired. This makes operation easier and results more consistent.

The operation of each x-ray machine is explained fully in the operating manual provided by the manufacturer. All persons operating an x-ray machine should study the manual until they are thoroughly familiar with the operational capability and maintenance requirements of the machine.

CHAPTER SUMMARY

All x-ray machines, regardless of size and voltage range, operate similarly and have the same components (control panel, cabinet, extension arm, and tube head) and electrical parts (x-ray tube, low- and high-voltage circuits, and a timing device). The advent of the Coolidge vacuum tube, operating on the principle of thermionic emission, has made the x-ray machine safe, compact, and easy to operate. Three conditions must exist within the energized vacuum x-ray tube: (1) a source of free electrons; (2) high voltage to accelerate them; and (3) a target to stop them. X-rays are produced only when the unit is turned on and a firm pressure is maintained on the activator button.

Electric current is a movement of electrons through a conducting medium. This flow may be in either direction along a wire but is always from negative to positive. The standard 110- or 220-volt alternating current is modified by low- and high-voltage transformers within the tube head. The current reverses direction from negative to positive 60 times per second as the voltage flows across the tube from cathode to anode. With most machines, x-rays are formed only during that phase of the cycle when the cathode is negatively charged; however, with some machines the potential is constant. Most dental x-ray units operate in ranges of 7 to 15 mA and between 50 and 100 kVp. The milliamperage determines the quantity of x-rays that can be produced in a predetermined time interval, and the kilovoltage determines the quantity and quality (penetrating power) of the rays. The operator can vary the mA and kVp settings on many machines, but some are preset by the manufacturer and only the time interval can be changed.

KEY WORDS

Alternating current

Ammeter

Amperage

Anode

Autotransformer

Cathode

Control panel

Dead-man switch

Definition

Electric potential

Electrode

Filament

Focal spot

Focusing cup

Impulse

Kilovolt (kV)

Kilovolt peak (kVp)

Milliampere (mA)

Port

Radiator

Rectification

Self-rectification

Target

Thermionic emission

Time delay

Timer

Transformer

Tube head

Tungsten

Voltage

Voltmeter

X-ray tube

Yoke

REVIEW QUESTIONS

1. Draw and label a typical dental x-ray tube.

2. Who invented the hot cathode tube? (a) Roentgen, (b) Rollins, (c) Coolidge, (d) Cieszynski.

3. List the three conditions that must exist for x-rays to be produced. (1) _Source free electrons_ (2) _high V to impart speed_, and (3) _target capeable stopping electrons_ _____.

4. Which of these must be charged negatively during the time that the x-ray tube is operating in order to produce x-rays? (a) the anode, (b) the radiator, (c) the cathode, (d) the aperture.

5. Which part of the x-ray tube is heated when the electric current is allowed to flow through the low-voltage circuit? (a) the focal spot, (b) the tube housing, (c) the anode target, (d) the cathode filament.

6. The process of heating the cathode wire filament until red hot and electrons "boil off" is called ___thermionic emission___

7. What metal is used for the target in the x-ray tube? (a) copper, (b) tungsten, (c) aluminum, (d) molybdenum.

8. What is the shape of the "effective" focal spot? ___Square___

9. Which term describes the opening in the tube head that allows the primary beam to escape? (a) focal spot, (b) port, (c) filament, (d) focusing cup.

10. Which term describes the electrical pressure or difference in potential between two electrical charges? (a) voltage, (b) amperage, (c) ionization, (d) rectification.

11. Why are x-rays not formed during the alternating phase when the anode is negative? (a) because there are no free electrons at the anode, (b) because the tube is evacuated, (c) because the voltage is too low, (d) because the radiator absorbs the electrons.

12. What should be done to increase the quantity of free electrons inside the tube so that more x-rays can be generated? (a) decrease the kilovoltage, (b) increase the milliamperage, (c) increase the kilovoltage, (d) decrease the milliamperage.

13. What happens to the penetrating power of x-radiation when the kilovoltage is increased from 65 kVp to 80 kVp? (a) no change, (b) is decreased by 12.5 percent, (c) is increased by 12.5 percent, (d) is almost doubled.

14. Which of these terms describes an electromagnetic device within the x-ray tube head for changing the voltage of alternating current? (a) rectifier, (b) transformer, (c) voltage regulator, (d) alternator.

15. If the x-ray machine timer is calibrated in impulses instead of fractions of a second, how many impulses are equivalent to 2/5 second? (a) 6, (b) 15, (c) 24, (d) 40.

60: 1

BIBLIOGRAPHY

Goaz PW, White SC: *Oral Radiology Principles and Interpretation,* 3rd ed. St. Louis, MO: CV Mosby, 1994

Langland OE, Sippy FH, Langlais RP: *Textbook of Dental Radiology,* 2nd ed. Springfield, IL: Charles C Thomas, 1984

Eastman Kodak: *Successful Intraoral Radiography,* Rochester, NY, 1990

Technical Aspects of Radiation Production

OPERATION OF THE DENTAL X-RAY MACHINE

A summation of the fundamentals of x-ray generation is in order before considering the technical aspects of radiation production. To review, when the line switch of the x-ray machine is turned on and the button at the end of the timer cord is held down until the exposure is completed, the line current enters the filament circuit of the x-ray machine. A step-down transformer reduces the voltage before it enters the circuit and heats the filament of the cathode to incandescence, separating electrons from their atoms. The degree to which the filament is heated depends on the milliamperage that is selected—the higher the mA, the more electrons in the electron cloud. These electrons are now in a state of excitation as they hover around the filament wire. After a time delay of about 1/2 second, the line current enters the cathode–anode circuit. A step-up transformer then increases the voltage to impart sufficient force to propel the free electrons to the focal spot on the anode where the energy conversion takes place, resulting in the production of x-rays. The x-ray beam formed at the focal spot is polychromatic, consisting of wavelengths of various energies. The higher the voltage, the greater the penetration power of the x-rays that are formed.

Whenever x-ray exposures are made on patients, it is assumed here and in all subsequent instructions that the patient is properly positioned, has received verbal instructions, and has been draped with a protective lead apron, that all equipment is sanitized, that the operator's hands have been washed and gloved, and that infection control procedures are followed (see Chapter 7).

To achieve consistent results, the x-ray machine operator should always follow an orderly procedure:

1. Turn on the line switch or depress the ON button. A red light will indicate that the machine is ready to operate.
2. Unless the machine is preset by the manufacturer, select the milliamperage and kilovoltage best suited for the exposure to be made. If the machine has a dial or dials, a needle will point to the mA and kVp that are available.
3. Set the timer for the desired exposure time.
4. Place the x-ray film packet in the patient's mouth. The film is usually held in place by a film-holding device.
5. Adjust the position indicating device (PID) so that the central beam of radiation is directed toward the center of the film at the proper horizontal and vertical angulations.
6. Pick up the timer cord and move to an area of safety at least 6 feet (1.83 m) away or behind the cover of structural shielding such as a lead-lined wall or partition. Press the release button and hold it down firmly until the exposure is completed. On new x-ray machines, an audible signal is heard for the duration of the exposure.
7. Watch the needle on the milliammeter while the exposure is being made. If it fails to move or go to the proper position, it indicates a malfunction caused either by a temporarily overloaded circuit or by failure to keep a firm pressure on the timer button.
8. On most machines the timer resets itself automatically and is ready for the next exposure unless a changed setting is desired. Although unlikely, it is possible to damage the x-ray tube through excessive repetition of prolonged exposures at short intervals, thus overheating the tube. To avoid abusing the equipment, consult the manufacturer's instructions regarding the tube ratings and duty cycle—the length of time that the tube may be energized in a given period.
9. Remove the film from the patient's mouth after each exposure. After the final exposure, turn off the line switch and fold the extension arm bracket up as far as it will go. The tube head is finely counterbalanced in its suspension from the extension arm. This balance can be disturbed if the tube

is left suspended for prolonged time periods with the extension arm stretched out.
10. As an additional precaution to prevent damage to the tube, turn off the machine at the end of each working day.

PRODUCING GOOD RADIOGRAPHS

The x-rays emerging from the tube head are of many energies. The weak ones lack sufficient energy to penetrate to the film and therefore do not contribute to the film image; instead they are absorbed in the patient's skin. This is undesirable, since it needlessly increases the radiation absorbed by the patient. Certain materials, especially aluminum, have the ability to absorb many of these "soft" undesired x-rays. This process is known as **filtration.**

The beam of radiation spreads out like the spokes of a wheel as it leaves the target and emerges from the tube head. This is undesirable because it spreads the radiation to parts of the body not being x-rayed. The ray in the middle of the beam is called the **central ray (CR).** Only the central part of the beam is normally required to expose a radiograph; therefore it is important to restrict the size of the beam to the minimum size necessary to expose the film. This can be done by placing a lead diaphragm (washer) in the port just in front of the aluminum filter disk. This process is called **collimation.** Another method to restrict the size of the beam is to use a rectangular PID (see Fig. 1–2). Both filtration and collimation are further discussed in Chapter 6.

The quality of the finished radiograph, as well as the total exposure that the operator and the patient receive, is determined by several things: (1) the degree of filtration and collimation of the machine; (2) the distance of the film from the source of the radiation; (3) the speed of the film; (4) the milliamperage; (5) the kilovoltage; (6) the exposure time; and (7) the size of the patient. An additional influence is how the film is processed. Faulty processing diminishes the diagnostic value of the film and often makes reexposure necessary. This wastes time and exposes the patient to unnecessary radiation.

There are three basic requirements for an acceptable radiograph. First, all parts of the structures radiographed must be shown on the film as close to their natural shapes and sizes as the patient's oral anatomy will permit. Distortion and superimposition of structures should be at a minimum. Second, the area examined must be shown completely, with enough surrounding tissue for the dentist to distinguish between the structures shown. Third, the film itself must be high in quality with proper density, contrast, and definition.

Density, also known as **film blackening,** is the amount of light transmitted through the film. The radiograph is a film negative, and all photographic negatives appear darker when more light reaches the film. Thus the degree of darkening of the radiograph is increased when the milliamperage or the exposure time is increased and more x-rays reach the film emulsion. **Contrast** refers to how sharply dark and light areas are differentiated. A film with good contrast will contain black , white, and many shades of gray. **Definition** refers to the sharpness and clarity of outline of the structures shown on the film.

VARIABLE RADIATION CONTROL FACTORS

Numerous factors are involved in the exposure of radiographs. All of these factors affect the quality of the radiograph and the safety of the patient and operator. Coincidentally, most factors that improve safety also improve the quality of the radiograph. Factors related to radiation hazards and protection are presented in Chapters 5 and 6.

Variations in the character and composition of the radiation beam have tremendous influence on the quality of the radiograph. There are three variables on the x-ray machine that can easily be adjusted by manipulating the controls. These variables—the milliamperage, the exposure time, and the kilovoltage—are known either as the control factors, the exposure factors, or the radiation beam factors.

Distance, an additional variable factor, is explained later. Whenever one of the control factors is drastically altered, one or a combination of the other factors must be proportionally altered. For example, exposure time may be decreased when milliamperage or kilovoltage is increased.

EFFECTS OF VARIATIONS IN MILLIAMPERAGE

The amount of electric current used in the x-ray machine is expressed in milliamperes. The milliamperage selected by the operator determines the quantity or number of x-rays that are generated within the tube.

The density of the radiograph is affected whenever the operator changes the milliamperage. Increasing the milliamperage increases (darkens) the density of the radiograph, whereas decreasing the milliamperage decreases (lightens) the density of the radiograph.

EFFECTS OF VARIATIONS IN EXPOSURE TIME

Exposure time is the interval that the x-ray machine is fully activated and x-rays are produced. The principal effect of changes in exposure time is on the density of the radiograph. Increasing the exposure time darkens the radiograph, while decreasing exposure time lightens it. Opinions differ on optimum density and contrast because visual perception varies from person to person. Some dentists may prefer lighter radiographs and others may prefer darker radiographs. Thus, the operator should consult with the dentist concerning which factor to increase or decrease.

Since both milliamperage and exposure time are used to regulate the number of x-rays generated and have the same effect on radiographic density, it is common practice to combine them into a common factor **milliampere-seconds (mAs)**. Both milliamperes and exposure time are linear factors in that they are expressed in the first power only—hence, doubling either factor also doubles the quantity of radiation produced. Combining the milliamperage with the exposure time is the only effective way to determine the total radiation generated. A simple formula for determining this total is mA times exposure time (in seconds or impulses) equals mAs.

$$mA \times s = mAs$$

PROBLEM

The exposure factors in a dental office are: 10 mA, 0.6 second, 90 kVp, and 16-in. (41-cm) target–film distance. The dentist decides to increase the mA to 15 and leave the kVp and target–film distance constant. What is the new exposure time?

SOLUTION

$$10 \text{ mA} \times 0.6 \text{ sec} = 6 \text{ mAs}$$

$$15 \text{ mA} \times ? \text{ sec} = 6 \text{ mAs}$$

$$? \text{ sec} = \frac{6 \text{ mAs}}{15 \text{ mAs}}$$

$$? \text{ sec} = 0.4 \text{ sec}$$

Answer: The new exposure time is 0.4 second.

EFFECTS OF VARIATIONS IN KILOVOLTAGE

The quality of the radiation (wavelength or energy of the x-ray photons) generated by the x-ray machine is determined by the kilovoltage peak (kVp). As already stated, the more the kVp is increased, the shorter the wavelength and the higher the energy and penetrating power of the x-ray photons thus produced. Although the main result of increasing the kVp is to increase the energy of the photons, a collateral effect is that the number of photons that enter the emulsion coating of the x-ray film is also increased. Thus, each exposure factor—milliamperage, exposure time, and kilovoltage—is related, and each contributes to the number of x-ray photons produced. Unlike milliamperage and exposure time, kilovoltage is an exponential factor; that is, it is expressed in powers other than 1. For practical purposes, the exposure time should be cut in half whenever an increase of 15 kVp is made and doubled when decreased by 15 kVp.

Because the use of higher kVp creates high-energy photons, it is advantageous to increase the kVp whenever the area to be examined is thick or has great density. With experience, the radiographer can evaluate the thickness of the patient's facial or dental structures and determine the optimum kVp. There is no standard kVp technique that is used in all dental offices, dental radiographs being exposed in ranges from 50 to 100 kVp. Most dental offices use 70 to 90 kVp.

RADIOGRAPHIC CONTRAST

The difference between density and contrast is that **density** refers to overall film blackening—the amount of light transmitted through a film—whereas **contrast** refers to the difference in the amount of light transmitted through two or more adjacent film areas.

The term **short-scale contrast** (Fig. 4–1) describes a radiograph in which the differences between adjacent areas are large. The contrast is high because there are few shades of gray, more black against white. The gray tones indicate the differences in absorption of the x-ray photons by the various tissues of the oral cavity or the head. The film is **radiolucent** (dark) where the tissues are soft or thin and **radiopaque** (white) where the tissues are hard or thick. Such radiographs result when low (60–70) kVp is applied. Some dentists prefer films with short-scale contrast, thinking that dental caries are easier to recognize; however, fine detail may be difficult to distinguish.

The term **long-scale contrast** (Fig. 4–1) describes a radiograph in which the density differences between adjacent areas are small. The contrast is low and very gradual because there are many shades of gray. Such radiographs result when high (80–90) kVp is applied. Much more detailed information can be obtained from such radiographs, provided that a view box with variable light control is used. The proper kVp to use is strictly a matter of individual preference.

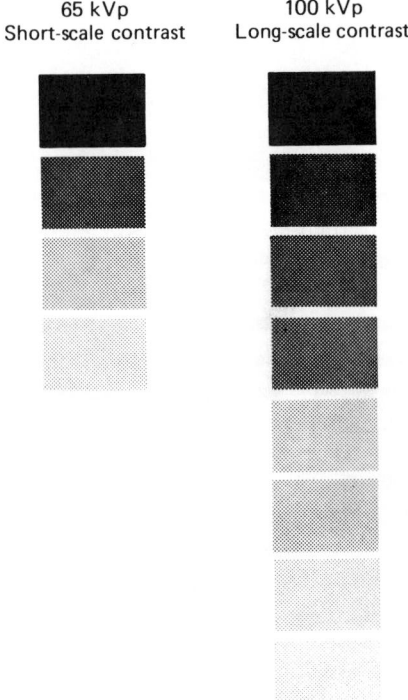

65 kVp
Short-scale contrast

100 kVp
Long-scale contrast

Figure 4–1. Penetrometer tests demonstrate radiographically that a much longer contrast scale results from the use of 100-kilovolt techniques. Dental radiographs at 100 kVp have longer-scale contrasts than radiographs at 65 kVp. (*Courtesy of General Electric Company, Medical Systems Division.*)

The customary procedure required to maintain film density is either to reduce the milliampere/seconds when higher kilovoltage is applied or to increase the milliampere/seconds when lower kilovoltage is applied. Thus one factor balances the other.

EFFECTS OF VARIATIONS IN DISTANCES

The operator must take into account several distances in making x-ray exposures: (1) the distance between the x-ray source (at the focal spot on the target anode) and the surface of the patient's skin, (2) the distance between the x-ray source and the recording plane of the film, and (3) the distance between the object to be x-rayed (usually the tooth) and the film. Various terms are used in dental literature to describe these distances. The terms **target–surface, anode–surface, focus–surface, tube–surface,** and **source–surface** are synonymous, as are **target–film, anode–film, focus–film,** and **source–film.** In this text the terms **target–surface distance, target–film distance,** and **object–film distance** are used (Fig. 4–2).

Generally, whenever the film is positioned intraorally (within the mouth), the length of the target–surface distance depends on the length of the position indicating device used. PIDs are classified as being short or long. All intraoral techniques require that the end of the PID should almost touch the skin—this is necessary to standardize measurements. The *National Bureau of Standards Handbook 76* sets the minimum target–surface distance at 7 in. (18 cm) for x-ray machines operating at above 50 kVp and at 4 in. (10 cm) for those that operate at 50 kVp or lower. There are no maximum dis-

18cm above 50 KVp

10 cm operat ≤ 50 KVp

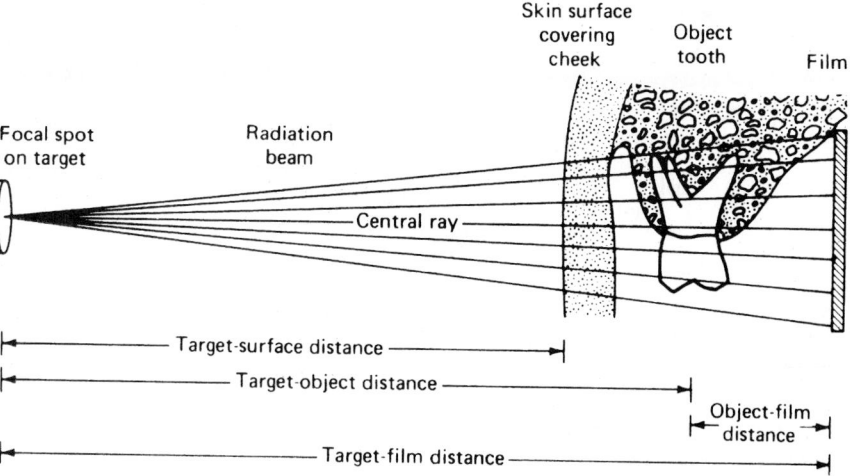

Figure 4–2. Relationship among target, skin surface, object (tooth), and x-ray film. Observe that the central ray passes through the roots of the tooth.

tances. These are governed to a certain extent by the energy of the beam. In extraoral radiography, where larger films are positioned outside the face, target–film distances of up to 72 in. (183 cm) are occasionally used.

The object–film distance depends largely on the method that is employed to hold the film in position behind the teeth. When the digital method in which the patient holds the film is used, the film is pressed against the lingual tissues as close as the oral anatomy will permit. This results in the object–film distance being shorter in the area of the crown, where the tooth and film may touch, than in the area opposite the root, where the thickness of the bone and gingiva may cause a divergence between the long axis of the tooth and the film. The least divergence occurs in the mandibular molar areas, whereas the greatest divergence is in the maxillary anterior areas where the palatal structures may curve sharply. With a few exceptions, most film holders are designed so that the film is held parallel to the average long axes of the teeth being x-rayed. This necessitates positioning the film sufficiently to the lingual of the teeth to avoid impinging on the supporting bone and gingival structures. This technique results in object–film distances that are often more than 1 in. (25 mm).

The target–film distance is the sum of the target–object and the object–film distance (Fig. 4–2). In most intraoral procedures, either an 8-in. (20-cm) or a 16-in. (41-cm) distance is used. In the 8-in. (20-cm) technique, a short PID is used and the film may be positioned in direct contact with the lingual tissues, while in the 16-in. (41-cm) technique, a longer PID is used and the film is positioned far enough from the teeth to enable it to be held parallel. These techniques are described in detail in Chapter 15.

The target–film distance is very important and has an effect on the intensity of the radiation, the amount of radiation that a patient receives, and the dimensional accuracy of the image produced on the radiograph (the latter is also affected by the object–film distance).

The intensity of the radiation beam varies inversely with the square of the target–film distance (Fig. 4–3). The x-ray beam spreads out as it moves away from the source (target) and decreases in intensity. This is based on the **inverse square law,** which states that the intensity of radiation varies inversely as the square of the distance from its source.

The inverse square law may be written as:

$$\frac{I_1}{I_2} = \frac{(D_2)^2}{(D_1)^2}$$

where I_1 is the original intensity, I_2 is the new intensity, D_1 is the original distance, and D_2 is the new distance.

PROBLEM

A dental radiographer stands 3 feet (0.9 meter) from the source of radiation where the measured intensity is 100 milliroentgens (mR) per minute. The radiographer is asked to move to a new location 6 feet (1.8 meters) from the source of radiation. What is the intensity at the new location?

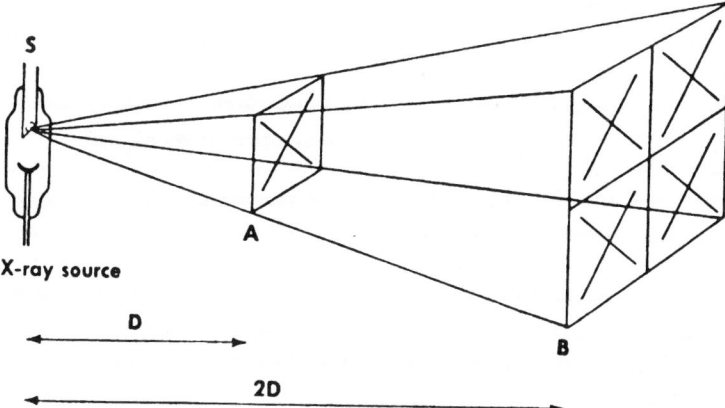

Figure 4–3. Relationship of distance (D) to the area covered by x-rays emanating from an x-ray tube. Photons emerging from the tube travel in straight lines and diverge from each other. The areas covered by the photons at any two points are proportional to each other as the square of the distances measured from the source of radiation. *(Reproduced with permission from Wuehrmann AH, Manson-Hing LR: Dental Radiology, 5th ed. St. Louis, MO: CV Mosby, 1981.)*

SOLUTION

$$I_1 = 100 \text{ mR per minute}$$

$$D_1 = 3 \text{ feet}$$

$$D_2 = 6 \text{ feet}$$

find I_2

$$\frac{100}{I_2} = \frac{6^2}{3^2} \quad I_2 \times 6^2 = 100 \times 3^2 \quad I_2 = \frac{100 \times 9}{36} = 25 \text{ mR per minute}$$

Answer: The intensity at the new location is 25 mR per minute.

Since the x-ray photons emerging from the tube travel in straight lines and diverge from one another, it follows that the intensity of the beam is reduced unless a corresponding increase is made in one or a combination of the exposure factors. Such changes in exposure factors are essential to maintaining optimum film density. Because milliamperage and time are the main factors influencing film density, the following formula can be used to determine the mAs–distance relationship:

$$\frac{\text{Original mAs}}{\text{New mAs}} = \frac{\text{Original distance}^2}{\text{New distance}^2}$$

For example, if a film of the same speed is used in two exposures and the mA and the kVp are left unchanged, it would only be necessary to increase the exposure time when the target–film distance is doubled. In that event, by applying the formula given, the exposure time must be increased fourfold. Tripling the distance would require a ninefold increase (Note: Usually time is the easiest exposure factor to change. This formula is useful for obtaining a multiplying factor for changing the exposure time when only the target–film distance is altered).

The quality of the radiograph image improves whenever the target–film distance is increased. Dimensional distortion and magnification are reduced, and sharpness of detail (definition) is increased. The decrease in dimensional distortion is largely attributable to the use of film holders that keep the film parallel with the teeth. Film holders form an integral part of the 16-in. (41-cm) target–film technique. When the 8-in. (20-cm) target–film distance is used, the outer, more divergent rays tend to magnify the image. The closer the target is to the teeth, the greater the magnification. As the distance from the target is lengthened, the image is produced by the more central rays of the beam, which are more parallel to one another and consequently decrease the magnification (Fig. 4–4). Image sharpness is also affected by movement of the patient, the size of the grains in the film emulsion, the size of the focal spot, and the object–film distance. Increasing the target–film distance reduces the fuzzy outline (called a **penumbra**) that is seen around all radiographic images.

More dentists are using the longer target–film distances than ever before. The acceptance of the 16-in. (41-cm) target–film distance was delayed until film manufacturers started to produce films so sensitive that they could be exposed in a mere fraction of the time required by the older films. At greater target–film distances the patient receives less radiation, but so does the film. The quadrupled exposure time required when the distance was doubled resulted in such long exposures that patient move-

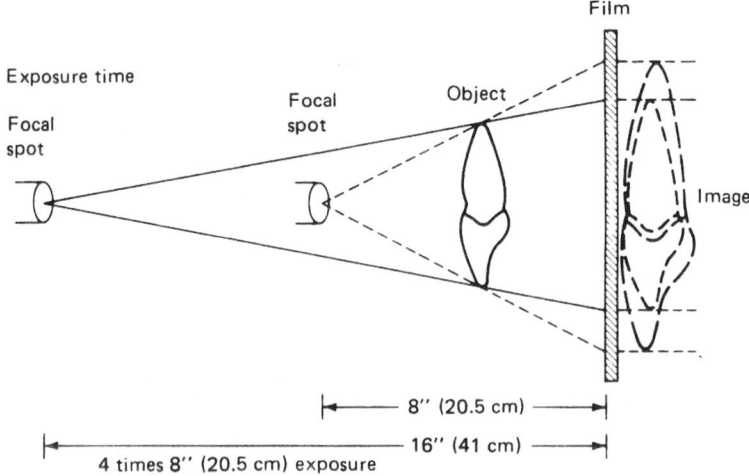

Figure 4–4. Comparison of 8-in. (20-cm) and 16-in. (41-cm) target–film (T-F) distance. The image is enlarged when the T-F distance is shortened and the object (tooth)-to-film distance is held constant. Ideally, the distance from the target to the object should be as long as possible and the object (tooth)-to-film distance should be as short as possible. When using the 16-in. (41-cm) T-F distance, the exposure time must be lengthened to four times that required at 8-in. (20-cm) T-F distance. *(Courtesy of Rinn Corporation, Elgin, IL.)*

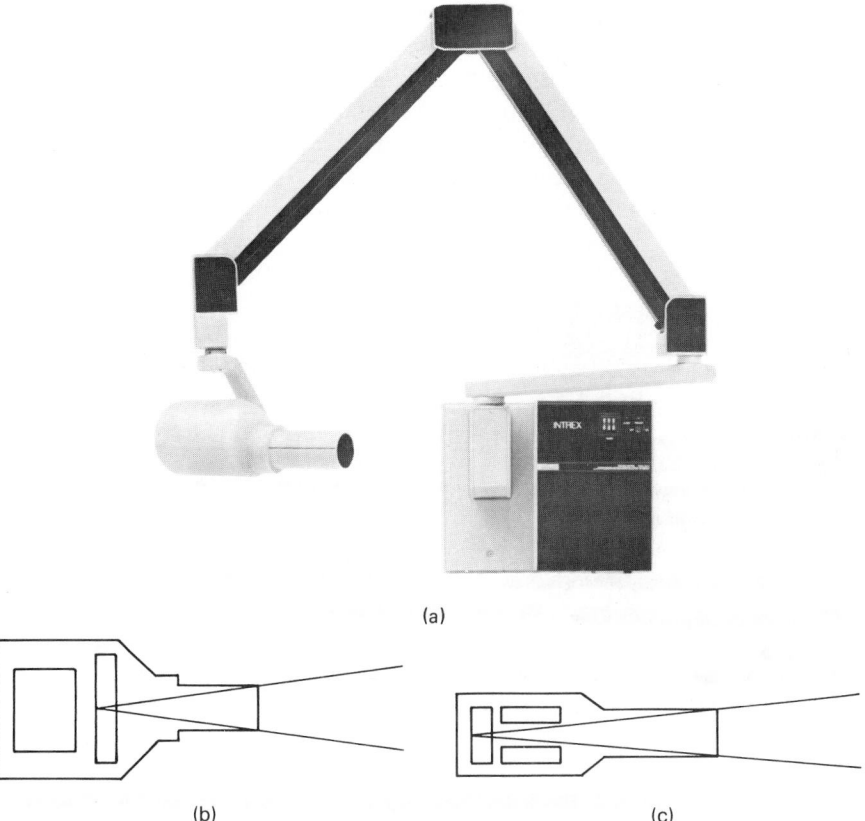

(a)

(b)   (c)

Figure 4–5. Comparison of conventional and recessed tube position within tube head. **(a)** Intrex recessed tube x-ray machine. **(b)** Conventional position with tube in front of transformer. Because x-ray source is in front, the beam pattern quickly flares out. **(c)** Recessed tube of Intrex machine with miniaturized transformers. Because x-ray source is at the rear, a relatively more parallel x-ray beam is produced. *(Courtesy of S.S. White Dental Products International.)*

ment or film slippage was likely to occur. Another factor that made longer target–film distances practical was the development of more powerful (higher kVp) x-ray machines with accurate electronic timers.

The location of the x-ray tube within the tube housing makes a big difference in the target–film distance when the aiming device (PID) is attached. On the conventional x-ray machine, either a short or long PID can be attached. When the tube is recessed, enough space is gained within the tube head so that a long target–film distance is achieved with a short PID (Fig. 4–5).

Many operators readily memorize the exposure factors they need to know for the particular technique they are using. Several excellent charts or conversion tables are available through the manufacturers of the films or the x-ray equipment. These show at a glance how much exposure time is required for a film of any given film speed when used with all possible combinations of exposure time, milliamperage, and peak kilovoltage. Many operators fasten these charts beside the control panel. Many health departments require that exposure charts be posted by the control panel. Some recent x-ray machine models incorporate the most commonly used film speeds and other exposure factors into the dial of the control panel. In that case the operator only has to set the pointer to the desired combination for a film of a given speed; all the rest is done automatically when the timer release button is depressed.

CHAPTER SUMMARY

For maximum effectiveness in exposing radiographs, the patient is first positioned and draped with a protective lead apron, and all controls on the x-ray unit are set as desired before the film is positioned. Following an orderly sequence in positioning the film packets reduces the likelihood of errors and retakes.

An acceptable radiograph must show the areas of interest—the designated teeth and surrounding bone structures—completely and with minimum distortion and maximum definition. The degree of density and contrast is optional. On many x-ray units it is possible to vary the four exposure factors: milliamperage, exposure time, kilovoltage, and target–film distance. Some units are preset, and only one or two factors can be altered. Each of these possible variations has an effect on the other exposure factors. If the interaction of these four factors is clearly understood, the operator can take advantage of them to produce radiographs that have the desired definition, density, and contrast.

KEY WORDS

Central ray (CR)

Collimation

Contrast

Definition

Density

Duty cycle

Filtration

Inverse square law

Long-scale contrast

Milliampere-seconds (mAs)

Object–film distance

Penumbra

Radiolucent

Radiopaque

Short-scale contrast

Target–film distance

Target–surface distance

REVIEW QUESTIONS

1. What target–film distance would produce a radiograph with the least image magnification? (a) 4 in. (10 cm), (b) 7 in. (18 cm), (c), 8 in. (20 cm), (d) 16 in. (41 cm).

2. Which term describes the white areas on the processed radiograph? (a) density, (b) penumbra, (c) radiolucent, (d) radiopaque.

3. Which term best describes an x-ray beam that is composed of a variety of wavelengths? (a) collimated, (b) short-scale, (c) filtered, (d) polychromatic.

4. Based on the inverse square law, what happens to the intensity of the x-ray beam when the target–film distance is doubled? (a) intensity is doubled, (b) intensity not affected, (c) intensity is half as great, (d) intensity is one quarter as great.

5. What term best describes the amount of light transmitted through a film? (a) definition, (b) contrast, (c) density, (d) penetration.

6. What factor has the greatest effect on film definition? (a) movement, (b) filtration, (c) kilovoltage (d) amperage.

7. What term best describes a fuzzy shadow around the outline of the radiographic image? (a) magnification, (b) penumbra, (c) detail, (d) distortion.

8. Which is most likely to produce a radiograph with long-scale contrast? (a) when kVp is increased, (b) when kVp is decreased, (c) when mAs is increased, (d) when mAs is decreased.

9. Which of these radiographs would show the largest degree of contrast between two adjacent areas? (a) exposed at 60 kVp, (b) exposed at 70 kVp, (c) exposed at 80 kVp, (d) exposed at 90kVp.

10. The dental radiograph will appear lighter if one increases the: (a) mA, (b) kVp, (c) exposure time, (d) target–film distance.

11. In order to increase the contrast on a radiograph, it is necessary to: (a) lengthen the target–film distance and increase the exposure time, (b) increase the kVp and decrease the exposure time, (c) increase the exposure time and decrease the developing time, (d) decrease the kVp and increase the mA.

12. Selection of proper kVp is influenced most by which two of the following? (a) size of film, (b) size of patient, (c) developing temperature, (d) density of the tissues, (e) diameter of the primary beam, (f) amount of decay of teeth.

13. The ray in the middle of the x-ray beam is called the _Central Ray_ .

14. The differences in density appearing on a radiograph is called _Contrast_ .

BIBLIOGRAPHY

Goaz PW, White SC: *Oral Radiology Principles and Interpretation*, 3rd ed. St. Louis, MO: CV Mosby, 1994

Langland OE, Sippy FH, Langlais RP: *Textbook of Dental Radiology*, 2nd ed. Springfield, IL: Charles C Thomas, 1984

Wuehrmann AH, Manson-Hing LR: *Dental Radiology*, 5th ed. St. Louis, MO: CV Mosby, 1981

Eastman Kodak: *X-Rays in Dentistry*. Rochester, NY, 1985

CHAPTER 5

Effects of
Radiation Exposure

OBJECTIVES

By the end of this chapter the student should be able to

1. Compare the theories of biological damage and the possible effect of radiation on somatic and genetic cells.
2. Identify the body cells in the order of their radiosensitivity.
3. Identify the factors that determine radiation injuries.
4. List the sequence of events that may follow exposure to radiation.
5. Identify the three areas in the head and neck that are most affected by radiation.
6. List the possible short- and long-term effects of irradiation.
7. Identify the effects of oral radiation therapy.

INTRODUCTION

The fact that ionizing radiation produces biological damage has been known for many years. The first x-ray burn was reported just a few months following Roentgen's discovery of x-rays in 1895. As early as 1902 the first case of x-ray–induced skin cancer was reported in the literature.

Evidence of harmful effects as a result of exposure to large amounts of radiation accumulated in the 1920s and 1930s. This was based upon injuries of early radiation workers, including dentists and radiologists. The potential, long-term effects of

wzp3 4

smaller, repeated exposures to radiation have only relatively recently been realized (since the 1940s).

As we have seen in Chapter 2, x-rays belong to the ionizing portion of the electro-magnetic spectrum. X-rays have the ability to detach and remove certain subatomic electric charges from the complex atoms that make up the molecules of body tissues. This process, known as **ionization,** creates an electrical imbalance within the normally stable cells. Because disturbed cellular atoms or molecules generally attempt to regain electrical stability, they often accept the first available opposite electrical charge. In such cases, the undesirable chemical changes become incompatible with the surround-ing body tissues. During ionization, the delicate balance of the cell structure is altered, and the cell may be damaged or destroyed.

CONCERNS WITH POTENTIAL RADIATION EFFECTS

Many dental patients are concerned with the safety of x-ray procedures. Such concerns are shared by the dentist and radiologists. Public concern has been further intensified by the testing of atomic weapons and by the accident at the nuclear power plant at Three Mile Island. These events have generated unfavorable attitudes toward the use of x-rays in dentistry and medicine and have resulted in the passage of several new laws including the Consumer-Patient Radiation Health and Safety Act of 1981. The subsequent nuclear disaster at Chernobyl, The Ukraine, in 1986 intensified this con-cern.

Some of the public concern is warranted, but much is the result of sensational and unsubstantiated newspaper or magazine articles. The trained professionals in the field of radiation are doing everything that is possible to avoid repeated exposures and to keep radiation to a minimum by following all possible safety procedures.

It should be understood that radiation may occur naturally or be man-made. Nat-urally caused radiation includes cosmic rays and those rays given off by radioactive el-ements in the earth. This is called **background radiation** and varies from place to place, generally being lowest at sea level and highest in the mountains. Background radiations are of small concern to us because apparently we can live with them and certainly can do very little about them.

What concerns us more are the man-made radiations—emissions from industrial atomic waste, from military testing of atomic weapons, and from certain commercial products. Of special concern are radiations used in industry, medicine, and dentistry. These account for some 90 percent of the man-made radiations to which the general public is exposed.

Any exposure to radiation is believed to have at least a little biological effect on the exposed person. Unfortunately, we do not yet fully understand all these effects or their future consequences. Scientists believe that some of these effects are cumulative, especially if exposure is too great and the intervals between exposures too frequent for the body cells to repair themselves. Unless the damage is too severe or the subject is in extremely poor health, many body cells **(somatic cells)** have a recovery rate of almost 75 percent during the first 24 hours; after that, repair continues at the same rate.

In determining whether or not an exposure is potentially harmful, the radiographer should consider the quantity and the duration of the exposure and which body area is to be irradiated. Continued exposure over prolonged periods alters the ability of the genetic cells (eggs and sperm) to reproduce normally. Present evidence indicates that chromosome damage is cumulative, increasing in effect by each successive additional radiation exposure, and genetic cells cannot repair themselves. Radiation may alter the genetic material in the reproductive cells so that mutations (abnormalities) may be produced in future generations. The use of lead aprons, thyroid collars, and proper safety techniques protect the patient from any conceivable damage.

There have been no reports of radiation injuries caused by normal dental procedures since safety rules have been adopted. The benefits of dental radiographs far outweigh the minor risks to the patient.

THEORIES OF BIOLOGICAL EFFECTS MECHANISMS

There are two generally accepted theories on how radiation damages biological tissues: (1) the **direct-hit** or **target theory** and (2) the **indirect-action** or **poison-water theory.**

According to the **direct-hit theory,** x-ray photons collide with important cell chemicals and break them apart, causing critical damage to large molecules (Fig. 5–1). Most x-ray photons, however, probably pass through the cell with little or no damage. A healthy cell can repair any minor damage that might occur. Moreover, the body contains so many cells that the destruction of a single cell or a small group of cells will have no observable effect.

The **indirect-action theory** is based on the assumption that radiation can cause chemical damage to the cell by ionizing the water within it. Since about 80 percent of body weight is water and ionization can dissociate water into hydrogen and hydroxyl radicals, the theory proposes that new chemicals such as hydrogen peroxide could be formed under certain conditions.

These chemicals act as a poison to the body, causing cellular dysfunction. Fortunately, when the water is broken down during **irradiation,** the ions have a strong tendency to recombine immediately to form water again instead of seeking out new combinations. This tendency holds cellular damage to a minimum. Under ordinary circumstances, even when a new chemical is formed, other cells that are not affected can take over the functions of the damaged cells until recovery takes place. Only in extreme instances, where massive irradiation has taken place, will entire body areas be destroyed or death result. However, it should be remembered that cellular destruction is not the only biological effect; the potential exists for the cell to become malignant.

Much about radiation effects remains to be discovered. Moreover, much of our radiation research is conducted with experimental animals. Not all species have the same radiosensitivity. Much of what we know about human's sensitivity to radiation is derived from studies of survivors who received large doses of whole-body radiation from atomic bombs at the end of World War II or from certain nuclear accidents. Conceivably, future research may demonstrate that human beings are not as sensitive to

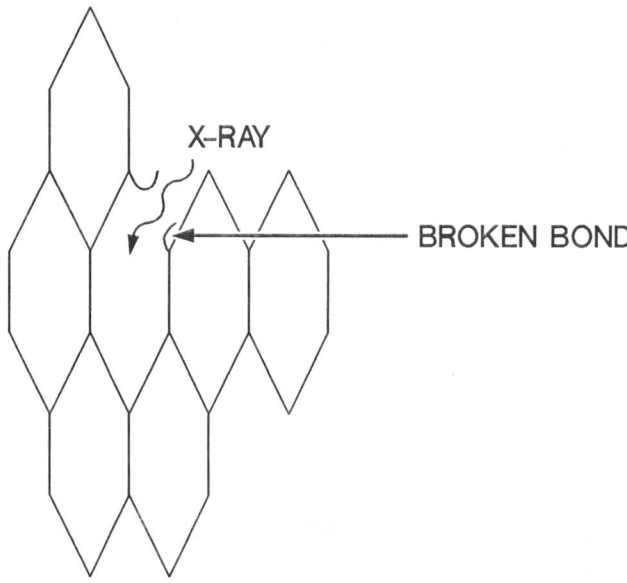

Figure 5–1. Radiation breaks the bonds connecting atoms in molecules, thus producing harmful effects. A living cell consists mostly of water. Ionization of water can form hydrogen and hydroxyl radicals forming chemicals such as hydrogen peroxide (HO), which can break down protein.

radiation damage as we now believe. But until we have such evidence, it is only common sense to improve radiographic safety techniques in every way possible.

CELL SENSITIVITY TO RADIATION EXPOSURE

The terms **radiosensitive** and **radioresistant** are used to describe the degree of susceptibility of various cells and body tissues to radiation. The cell is most susceptible to radiation injury during mitosis (cell division). All cells are not equally sensitive to radiation. The relative sensitivity of cells to radiation was first described in 1906 by two French scientists, Bergonie and Tribondeau, and is known as the Law of B and T. The law states that "the radiosensitivity of cells and tissues is directly proportional to their reproductive capacity and inversely proportional to their degree of differentiation."

The first half of the Law of B and T means that actively dividing cells, such as white blood cells, are more sensitive than slowly dividing cells. Embryonic and immature cells are more sensitive than mature cells of the same tissue. The second half of the Law of B and T means the more specialized a cell is, the more radioresistant the cell.

Based on these factors, it is possible to rank various kinds of cells in descending order of radiosensitivity: (1) white blood cells (lymphocytes); (2) red blood cells (erythrocytes); (3) immature reproductive cells; (4) epithelial cells; (5) endothelial cells; (6) connective tissue cells; (7) bone cells; (8) nerve cells; (9) brain cells; and (10) muscle cells.

The facial and oral structures, composed largely of bone, nerve, and muscle tissue, are fairly radioresistant. In dental radiography, exposure is limited to a very small area, and the amount of radiation is minimal. Specific measures for making radiation safe for both patient and operator are described in Chapter 6.

THE DOSE–RESPONSE CURVE

For drugs, radiation, or any other biologically harmful agent, it is useful to plot the dosage administered with the response or damage produced, in order to establish acceptable levels of exposure. In plotting these two variables, a dose–response curve is produced. With radiation, it is important to consider the nature and shape of this curve. Two possibilities are illustrated in Figure 5–2.

Unfortunately, radiobiologists have been unable to determine radiation effects at very low levels of exposure (for instance, below 10 roentgens) and cannot be certain whether or not a threshold effect exists. It is felt that somatic effects (changes in the irradiated individual) could be threshold, whereas genetic effects (changes in hereditary material affecting future generations) could be considered nonthreshold effects. This is as yet highly controversial and may need to be revised later.

To be on the safe side, radiation protection groups take the conservative approach and consider all radiation effects as being nonthreshold. This assumption has been made in the establishment of radiation protection guides and in radiation control activities. The concept that every dose of radiation produces damage and should be kept to the minimum necessary to meet diagnostic requirements is known as the **ALARA** concept, where ALARA stands for "as low as reasonably achievable."

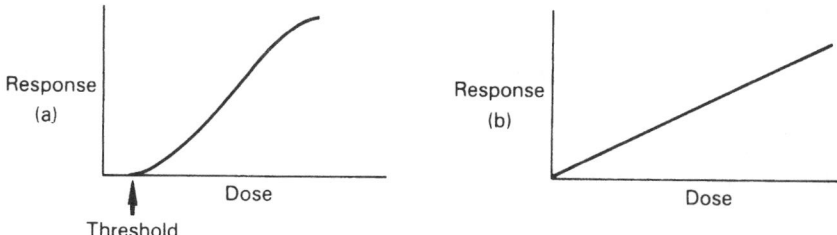

Figure 5–2. Diagram of dose–response curve. **(a)** A typical threshold curve. The point at which the curve intersects the base line (horizontal line) is the threshold dose, that is, the dose below which there is no response. If an easily observable radiation effect, such as erythema (reddening of the skin) is taken as "response," then this type of curve is applicable. **(b)** A linear nonthreshold curve, in which the curve intersects the base line at its origin. Here it is assumed that any dose, no matter how small, causes some response.

FACTORS THAT DETERMINE RADIATION INJURY

The factors that determine the amount of radiation injury are (1) total dose, (2) dose rate, (3) area exposed, (4) variation in species and individual sensitivity, (5) variation in cell sensitivity, and (6) age. The total dose of radiation depends on the type, energy, and duration of the radiation. The greater the dose, the more severe the probable biological effect.

The rate at which the radiation is administered or absorbed is very important in the determination of what effects will occur. Since a considerable degree of recovery occurs from the radiation damage, a given dose will produce less effect if it is divided (thus allowing time for recovery between dose increments) than if it is given in a single exposure. For instance, an exposure of 1 roentgen per week for 100 weeks would result in far less injury than a single exposure of 100 roentgens. This principle is utilized in determining doses for radiation therapy.

The amount of injury to the individual depends on the area or volume irradiated. The larger the area exposed, other factors being equal, the greater the injury to the organism. This is why it is recommended to expose as small an area as practical. In dentistry we use a very small (2 3/4-in. [7-cm]) beam diameter to limit the beam of radiation to the area of diagnostic concern, and this area can be further limited by the use of rectangular collimation (see Fig. 1–2).

There is a wide variation in the radiosensitivity of various species. Lethal doses for plants and microorganisms are usually hundreds of times higher than those for mammals.

Individuals vary in sensitivity within the same species. For this reason the **lethal dose (LD)** for each species is expressed in statistical terms, usually as the LD 50/30 for that species, or the dose required to kill 50 percent of the individuals in a large population in a 30-day period. For humans, the LD 50/30 is estimated to be 4.5 grays (Gy) or 450 rads (grays and rads are units of absorbed dose, more completely described in Chapter 6) of whole-body radiation. The following estimates are approximate, and they vary with different investigators:

LD 50/30

		Dose (Whole Body)	
	Species	Grays	Rads
	Guinea pig	2.5	250
	Dog	3.4	340
	Goat	3.5	350
	Monkey	5.0	500
	Humans	4.5	450
	Mouse	5.0	500
	Swine	5.5	550
	Rat	6.0	600

Within the same individual, a wide variation in susceptibility to radiation damage exists among different types of cells and tissues. As the Law of B and T pointed out, the cells that rapidly divide or have a potential for rapid division are more sensitive to radiation than those that do not divide. Furthermore, primitive or nonspecialized cells are more sensitive than those that are highly specialized. Within the same cell families, then, the immature forms, which are generally primitive and rapidly dividing, are more radiosensitive than the older, mature cells, which have specialized in function and have ceased to divide.

Some tissues (organs) of the body are more radiosensitive than others. For instance, blood-forming organs such as the spleen and red bone marrow are more sensitive than the highly specialized heart muscle.

In dental radiology, the most critical areas in the head and neck are the mandible (red bone marrow), the lens of the eye, and the thyroid gland. The mandible contains an estimated 15 grams of red bone marrow. This is only about 1 percent of the total amount of red bone marrow in the adult body. The lens of the eye is of interest because it is occasionally in the primary beam during some maxillary exposures. The thyroid gland is relatively radiosensitive. However, during dental radiographic procedures it is generally out of the range of the primary beam and is only exposed by scatter radiation. The risk can be further reduced by the use of a thyroid collar or shield (see Fig. 6–7).

Younger, more rapidly dividing cells are more radiosensitive than older, mature cells so it follows that children may be more susceptible to injury than adults from an equal dose of radiation. Also, in children the distance from the oral cavity to the reproductive and other sensitive organs is less than for adults. Therefore the dental doses to the critical organs may be higher than they would be for an adult. This is why it is wise to use leaded aprons and thyroid collars to protect all patients.

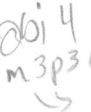

SEQUENCE OF EVENTS FOLLOWING RADIATION EXPOSURE

The sequence of events following radiation exposure are (1) a latent period; (2) a period of injury; and (3) a recovery period, of course, assuming that the dose received was nonlethal. Following the initial radiation exposure, and before the first detectable effect occurs, there is a time lag called the **latent period.** The latent period may be very short or extremely long. Effects that appear within a matter of minutes, days, or weeks are called short-term effects and those that appear years, decades, and even generations later are called long-term effects. Again, this relates to the types of cells involved and their corresponding rates of mitosis (cell division).

Following the latent period, certain effects can be observed. One of the effects that is seen most frequently in growing tissues exposed to radiation is the stoppage of mitosis, or cell division. This may be temporary or permanent, depending upon the radiation dosage. Other effects include breaking or clumping of chromosomes, abnormal mitosis, and formation of giant cells.

Following exposure to radiation, some recovery can take place. This is particularly apparent in the case of the short-term effects. Nevertheless, there may be a certain amount of damage from which no recovery occurs, and it is this irreparable injury that can give rise to later long-term effects.

SHORT- AND LONG-TERM EFFECTS OF IRRADIATION

When a very large dose of radiation is delivered in a very short period of time, the latent period is short. If the dose of radiation is large enough (generally over 1.0 gray or 100 rads, whole-body), the resultant signs and symptoms that comprise these short-term effects are collectively known as the **acute radiation syndrome.** The acute radiation syndrome is not a concern in dentistry, because our x-ray machines could not produce the very large exposures necessary to cause it.

Long-term effects of radiation are those that are seen years after the original exposure. The latent period is much longer (years) than that associated with the acute radiation syndrome (hours or days). Delayed radiation effects may result from a previous acute, high exposure that the individual has survived or from chronic low-level exposures delivered over many years. In dentistry, we are potentially exposed to these chronic low levels of radiation. From the public health point of view, the possibility of long-term effects on the large number of people receiving low, chronic exposures is cause for greater concern than the short-term radiation effects from acute exposures that involve only a few individuals.

There is no unique disease associated with the long-term effects of radiation. There is only a statistical increase in the incidence of certain already existing conditions. Because of the low normal incidence of these conditions, one must observe large numbers of exposed persons in order to evaluate this kind of an increase.

The long-term effects observed have been somatic damage, which may result in an increased incidence of cancer, embryological defects, cataracts, life-span shortening, and genetic mutations. The first four conditions are somatic effects and only involve the individual exposed. Genetic mutations involve hereditary material and may have an adverse effect for many generations after the original exposure.

Anything that is capable of causing cancer is called a carcinogen. X-rays, like certain drugs, chemicals, and viruses, have been shown to have carcinogenic effects. Carcinogenic mechanisms are not clearly understood. Moreover, cancer is probably "caused" by the simultaneous interaction of several factors, and the presence of some of these factors without the others may not be sufficient to cause the disease.

Some explanations for the carcinogenic action of x-rays include the following: x-rays activate viruses already present in cells; x-rays damage chromosomes, and certain diseases (such as leukemia) are associated with chromosomal injury; x-rays cause mutations in somatic cells, which may result in uncontrolled growth of cells; and x-rays ionize water, which results in chemical "free radicals" that may cause cancer.

Any one or a combination of these theories may explain how cancer is caused. X-radiation is only one of a number of possible carcinogens involved, and the precise mechanism is not yet understood. Much of the evidence that x-radiation is carcinogenic comes from studies of early radiation workers, including dentists, who were exposed to large amounts of radiation.

The immature, undifferentiated, rapidly growing cells of the embryo are highly sensitive to radiation. The first trimester of a pregnancy, when the fetus undergoes the period of major organogenesis (formation of organs), is especially critical. High doses of radiation may cause birth abnormalities, stunting of growth, and mental retardation. It is fortunate for dentistry that the dose from a dental x-ray examination is no more than 0.0003 to 0.003 milligrays (0.03 to 0.3 millirads). Of course, the use of a leaded apron reduces this potential dose to zero.

When the lens of the eye becomes opaque, it is called a **cataract.** Various agents, including x-rays, have been known to cause cataracts. It takes at least 2 grays (200 rads) of x-radiation to cause cataract formation. The dose to the eye from dental radiographic procedures is in the order of **milligrays (millirads).** Dental x-rays have never been reported to cause cataracts.

Life-span–shortening effects caused by x-radiation have been demonstrated in animal experiments. The effect seems to be due to premature aging. However, life-span shortening has never been demonstrated in humans.

X-radiation is known to sometimes cause changes in the genetic material of cells. These changes are referred to as **genetic mutations.** The genetic material is the means by which hereditary traits are passed from one generation to another. Drugs, chemicals, and even elevated body temperatures are also capable of causing mutations. Genetic effects are especially important, because there may be no level of radiation that will not produce at least some effect.

While humans might not have evolved if it were not for genetic mutations partly induced by naturally occurring radiations, most geneticists agree that the majority of genetic mutations are harmful. Because of their damaging effects, they are gradually eliminated from the population by natural means, since individuals with this damage are less likely to reproduce themselves successfully than are normal individuals. The more severe the condition produced by the mutation, the more rapidly it will be eliminated. As a balance to this natural elimination of harmful mutations, new ones are constantly occurring. Natural background radiation probably accounts for a small proportion of naturally occurring mutations.

Since the scattered radiation reaching the gonads from dental radiography is less than 1/10,000 that of the exposure to the surface of the face, the dental contribution to genetic mutations is extremely small, ranging from 0.0 to about 0.002 milligrays (0.2 millirad) per radiograph. With the use of a lead apron and thyroid collar, the dose is essentially reduced to zero.

EFFECTS OF ORAL RADIATION THERAPY

So much has been said and written about radiation hazards that, for the peace of mind of both patient and operator, it must be emphasized that the exposures used in dental radiation are so minimal that, unless repeated hundreds of times in rapid succession, it would be virtually impossible to create the conditions described in the previous section.

This, however, is not the case when radiation is applied therapeutically to treat cancer lesions. After 6 or more weeks of treatment, during which the patient may receive doses of 2 grays (200 rads) daily for 5 days a week at the site of the malignancy, the total localized dose is in the range of 60 grays (6000 rads). Remember that this is a local and not a whole-body dose. A person could not survive such a dose to the entire body.

Such tremendous doses over a short time period cause many adverse responses in the normal tissues surrounding the lesion being treated. Since oral radiation therapy has assumed an ever increasingly prominent role in cancer treatment, all members of the dental team—particularly the dental assistant or hygienist who frequently is the first one to see the patient in a professional capacity—should be aware of the complications and discomforts that are common with the irradiated patient.

Complications can appear soon after initiation of radiation therapy and continue at unspecified intervals over a period of years. During the 5 years following the initiation of treatment, the patient goes through three clinical stages: (1) an acute clinical period during the first 6 months; (2) a subacute clinical period during the second 6 months; and (3) a chronic clinical period that lasts from the second through the fifth year. Hopefully, recovery is complete by this time, but there may be a recurrence of the malignancy or a radiation-induced growth at a later time.

Obviously, the patient undergoes the greater degree of discomfort and emotional stress during the acute stage. Not only is the cancer irradiated but also the highly radiosensitive tissues of the mucosa that line the oral vestibule, pharynx, larynx, salivary glands, and tongue. If such patients require dental treatment, they must be handled with great care. The mouth is painful and sensitive to touch, and the danger of complications arising from trauma or infection must be considered. Patients lose their appetite and sense of taste. The saliva becomes thick and ropy, and the mouth feels dry **(xerostomia).** Swallowing becomes difficult **(dysphagia),** the tongue may be swollen, and the throat feels congested. Mucositis, an inflammation and sluffing of the mucous membranes, is common.

The dryness of the mouth continues through most of the subacute stage. The oral mucosa becomes blanched and takes on a spider-web appearance with red markings, and ulcers may appear. More serious, from a dental view, is that radiation caries may develop around the cervical portions of the teeth.

Salivary gland function and taste response generally return during the chronic stage. However, ulcers may continue, and a necrosis (cellular death) of the alveolar bone—a condition called osteoradionecrosis (bone death)—may occur. This is often accompanied by an inflamed appearance of the gingiva, looseness of the teeth, and extreme pain.

Obviously, there is a major concern whenever the necessity arises to expose additional radiographs on any patient who is currently receiving or has already undergone radiation therapy. The patient is extremely reluctant to receive additional radiation, no matter how minimal, and the dentist may be hesitant to order any additional radiographs. Likewise, the auxiliary making the exposure may feel apprehensive about the procedure.

The dental staff must communicate with the patient that the concerns for radiation safety are shared. Although the irradiated patient may already have received large therapeutic doses of radiation, there should be no hesitation in exposing additional radiographs provided that they are deemed to be necessary to make a diagnosis. The additional radiation that the patient receives is minimal, and its use is justified if the patient benefits.

CHAPTER SUMMARY

Ionizing radiation has the potential to produce biological damage because x-rays can detach subatomic particles from larger molecules and create an electrical imbalance within a normally stable cell. This potential for cellular damage is of great concern to everyone—the general public and those who work with radiation.

Everyone is exposed to some background and man-made radiations. Our concern is to keep dental radiation as low as possible, consistent with obtaining the desired diagnostic information. Genetic and somatic cell reaction to the ionization that occurs during radiation exposure depends on the age, size, and health of the patient, the output of the x-ray machine, the duration of the exposure, the degree of tissue radiosensitivity, and the area of exposure, local or whole-body.

There are two generally accepted theories on how radiation may cause damage to cellular tissues: (1) the direct-hit or target theory, and (2) the indirect-action or poison-water theory.

Whether cell damage from radiation is physical or chemical, it has been established that minor damage is soon repaired by a healthy body. Our main concern is that damage to genetic cells may result in altering the chromosomes and creating mutations in future generations. This can be avoided by draping the patient with a protective lead apron.

The terms **radiosensitive** and **radioresistant** are used to describe the degree of susceptibility of various cells and body tissues to radiation. Most facial tissues are fairly radioresistant.

The dose–response curve is a method used to plot the dosage of radiation administered with the response produced in order to establish responsible levels of radiation exposure. The conservative view that every dose of radiation potentially produces damage and should be kept to a minimum is expressed by the **ALARA** concept—"as low as reasonably achievable."

The factors that determine the amount of radiation injury include (1) total dose, (2) dose rate, (3) area exposed, (4) variation in species, (5) variation in cell sensitivity, and (6) age. The lethal dose for each species is expressed in statistical terms: the LD 50/30 for that species. In dental radiology, the most critical areas in the head and neck are (1) the red bone marrow in the mandible, (2) the lens of the eye, and (3) the thyroid gland.

Assuming that the dose received is not lethal, the sequence of events following radiation exposure are (1) a latent period, (2) a period of injury, and (3) a recovery period.

The effects of radiation exposure may be short- or long-term. Short-term effects often include erythema and general discomfort. Long-term effects may result in an increased incidence of cancer, embryological defects, cataracts, life-span shortening, and genetic mutations. Since dental exposures are very minimal, there is little danger if radiation safety techniques are followed.

Many patients receive large amounts of radiation during treatment for cancer. Such therapy produces many complications and discomforts, which may include dryness of the mouth, swollen tongue, difficulty in swallowing, looseness of teeth, and pain. Radiographs should be taken on irradiated patients only if deemed necessary for the patient's welfare. The auxiliary must exercise extreme care in film placement, as the patient's mouth may have many unhealed lesions.

KEY WORDS

Acute radiation syndrome
ALARA
Background radiation
Direct-hit theory
Dysphagia
Genetic mutations
Indirect-action theory
Ionization

Irradiation
Latent period
Lethal dose (LD)
Radioresistant
Radiosensitive
Somatic cell
Threshold dose
Xerostomia

REVIEW QUESTIONS

1. Which term best describes radiations of natural origin? (a) background radiations, (b) scatter radiations, (c) ionizing radiations, (d) leakage radiations.

2. Which of these cells is most radiosensitive? (a) muscle cells, (b) nerve cells, (c) red blood cells, (d) mature bone cells.

3. Which of these cells is most radioresistant? (a) red blood cells, (b) muscle cells, (c) epithelial cells, (d) white blood cells.

4. Which of the tissues that may be in the path of dental radiation is most radioresistant? (a) lens of the eye, (b) thyroid gland, (c) red bone marrow in mandible, (d) the enamel of the teeth.

5. The tissue that is most sensitive to radiation is: (a) skin, (b) muscle, (c) bone, (d) lymphoid.

6. Which of these factors has no effect on determining the extent of radiation injury? (a) the area exposed, (b) the age of the patient, (c) the type of film used, (d) the dose rate.

7. According to the Law of B and T, cells with a high reproductive rate are described as (a) radiopaque, (b) radiolucent, (c) radioresistant, (d) radiosensitive.

8. Which of these is not an event that follows major exposure to radiation? (a) a dose-response period, (b) a latent period, (c) a period of injury, (d) a recovery period.

9. Which of these is the earliest detectable symptom of excessive radiation exposure? (a) erythema, (b) xerostomia, (c) alopecia, (d) dysphagia.

10. Which of these is not considered to be a possible long-term effect of exposure to radiation? (a) cataracts, (b) arthritis, (c) embryological defects, (d) genetic mutations.

11. Approximately how much smaller is the radiation exposure in the area of the gonads than at the surface of the face? (a) 1/10, (b) 1/100, (c) 1/1000, (d) 1/10,000.

12. The LD 50/30 for humans is ___ grays (___ rads).

13. The two theories explaining how radiation damages biological tissues are _____ and _____.

14. ALARA stands for _____

BIBLIOGRAPHY

Carl W: Local and systemic chemotherapy: Preventing and managing oral complications. *J Am Dent Assoc.* **124:**119–123, 1993

Farman AG, Grammer S, Hunter N, et al: Survey of radiographic requirements and techniques in U.S. dental assisting programs, 1982. *Oral Surg, Oral Medi, and Oral Pathol.* 430–436, 1983

National Academy of Sciences, National Research Council: *The Effects on Populations of Exposure to Low Levels of Ionizing Radiation.* (BEIR III report) Washington, DC, 1980

National Cancer Institute. *Consensus Development Conference on Oral Complications of Cancer Therapies: Diagnosis, Prevention and Treatment.* Bethesda, MD: National Institutes of Health, 1990. National Cancer Institute Monographs no. 9

National Council on Radiation Protection and Measurements. *Implementation of the Principle of as Low as Reasonably Achievable (ALARA) for Medical and Dental Personnel.* Washington, DC: 1991 NCRP Report no. 107

Eastman Kodak: *Radiation Safety in Dental Radiography.* Rochester, NY, 1993

CHAPTER 6

Radiation Protection

OBJECTIVES

By the end of this chapter the student should be able to

1. Identify the areas of professional responsibility and concern for radiation safety.
2. Identify the terms used to measure radiation.
3. Differentiate among the various terms used in radiation safety procedures.
4. Identify the procedures for maintaining radiation safety for operator and patient.
5. Differentiate among the various radiation monitoring devices.

PROFESSIONAL CONCERN AND RESPONSIBILITY

As partially explained in Chapter 5, any radiation exposure carries a potential for biological damage to the patient and operator, however slight. The dentist shares the public's concern over the effects of needless or unnecessary radiation. Since the hazard increases with the amount of radiation, everything must be done to keep radiation exposures as low as possible.

The use of outdated and malfunctioning equipment, the absence of protective shielding, and carelessness or ignorance on the part of the operator all contribute to unnecessary radiation. Dentists have the obligation to safeguard everyone in their practice by eliminating these sources of trouble. If necessary, they must make structural changes in the walls of the operatories and replace or modify their equipment. They must also instruct or supervise all who have access to the x-ray units. In fact, dentists are legally responsible for all acts or services performed in their office. For this reason, x-ray films should be exposed only under the direct supervision of the dentist or a qualified instructor.

RADIATION SAFETY LEGISLATION

The Tenth Amendment gives the states the constitutional authority to regulate health. Because many federal agencies are involved in the development and use of atomic energy, the federal government has preempted the control of radiation. Certain provisions of the Constitution and Public Law 86-373 have enabled the states to assume this preempted power and pass laws that spell out radiation safety measures to protect the patient, the operator, or anyone (the general public) near the source of radiation. In fact, even counties and cities have passed ordinances to protect their citizens from radiation hazards. Most states and a few localities require periodic inspection or monitoring of the equipment and its surroundings. Many are considering laws to provide for monitoring and to set minimum standards for x-ray operators.

The entry of the federal government into the regulation of x-ray machines began in 1968 with the enactment of the Radiation Control for Health and Safety Act, which standardizes the performance of x-ray equipment. Subsequently the Consumer-Patient Radiation Health and Safety Act of 1981 was passed, requiring the various states to develop minimum standards for operators of dental x-ray equipment.

Since the laws concerning radiation control vary greatly, individuals working with x-rays are urged to become familiar with the major provisions of their own state or local radiation code and observe its requirements. Regardless of laws, failure to observe safety procedures cannot be justified morally. Many excellent booklets and articles on radiation safety and radiation hygiene methods are available. Especially recommended are National Council on Radiation Protection and Measurements (NCRP) Reports nos. 35, 39, and 43, which are available at nominal cost. These are listed in the bibliography.

RADIATION MEASUREMENT TERMINOLOGY

The terms used to measure x-radiation are based on the ability of the x-ray to deposit its energy in air, soft tissues, bone, or other substances. These terms can be quite confusing to anyone lacking a strong background of mathematics and physics. Keeping in mind that the main reason for studying radiation measurement terminology is to protect the health of the patient and operator whenever x-ray equipment is used and that the requirements for in-depth studies of these terms will vary depending on the educational level of the student, the authors have made every attempt to simplify the definitions and explanations that follow. Those desiring additional information are urged to refer to the glossary for more complete explanations.

The International Commission on Radiation Units and Measurements (ICRU) has established standards that clearly define **radiation units** and **radiation quantities.**

At the present time, there are two sets of terms used for **units of radiation.** The older terms—roentgen, rad, and rem—are being phased out. Gaining greater acceptance is the International System in which **coulombs per kilogram (C/kg)** replaces the **roentgen,** the **gray (Gy)** replaces the **rad,** and the **sievert (Sv)** replaces the **rem** (Table 6–1). In this book we will use the new units first, followed by the old units.

A "quantity" may be thought of as a description of a physical concept such as time, distance, or weight. The measure of the quantity is a "unit" such as minutes, miles (kilometers), or pounds (kilograms).

For practical x-ray protection measurement three quantities are used: (1) **exposure,** (2) **absorbed dose,** and (3) **dose equivalent.**

Exposure: Exposure can be defined as the measurement of ionization in air produced by x- or gamma rays. The units of exposure are **coulombs per kilogram (C/kg)** and the **roentgen (R):**

- **Coulomb per kilogram (C/kg):** A coulomb is a unit of electrical charge. Therefore, the unit C/kg measures electrical charges (ion pairs) in a kilogram of air.

- **Roentgen (R):** One roentgen is the amount of radiation that will produce 2.08×10^9 ion pairs (about 2 billion) in 1 cc of air at standard conditions of pressure and temperature (Fig. 6–1).

Absorbed Dose: The amount of energy deposited in any form of matter (such as wood, bracket table, air, teeth, muscles, and so on), by any type of radiation (alpha or beta particles, gamma or x-rays) is defined as the absorbed dose. The units for measuring the absorbed dose are the **gray (Gy)** and the **rad** (radiation absorbed dose):

- **Gray (Gy):** A new unit for measuring absorbed dose that is replacing the rad. One gray equals 1 joule (J) (which is a unit of energy) per kilogram of tissue. One gray equals 100 rads.

- **Rad (radiation absorbed dose):** A special unit of absorbed dose equal to 0.01 joule per kilogram of tissue. For x-rays absorbed in the soft tissues, the rad is approximately numerically equivalent to the roentgen.

Dose Equivalent: A term used for radiation protection purposes to compare the biological effects of the various types of radiation. Dose equivalent is defined as the product of the absorbed dose times a biological-effect modifying factor. Because the modifying factor (see glossary) for x-rays is one, the absorbed dose and the dose equivalent are equal. The units for measuring the dose equivalent are the **sievert (Sv)** and the **rem (roentgen equivalent man).**

TABLE 6–1. RADIATION MEASUREMENT TERMINOLOGY

	Unit	
Quantity	**New**	**Old**
Exposure	coulombs per kilogram (C/kg)	roentgen (R)
Absorbed dose	gray (Gy)	rad
Dose equivalent	sievert (Sv)	rem

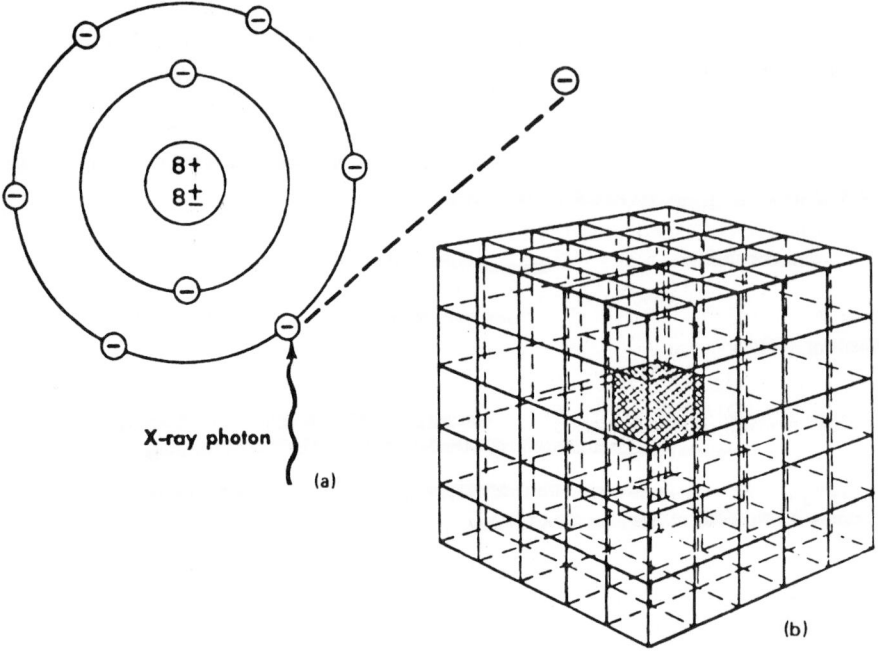

Figure 6–1. Schematic representation. **(a)** Ionization of an oxygen atom. **(b)** A 1-cm cube of air surrounded by an infinite amount of air. *(Reproduced with permission from Wuehrmann AH, Manson-Hing LR: Dental Radiology, 5th ed. St. Louis, MO: CV Mosby, 1981.)*

- **Sievert (Sv):** A unit used to measure the dose equivalent. One sievert equals 1 gray times a biological-effect modifying factor. Because the modifying factor for x- and gamma radiation equals one, the number of sieverts is identical to the absorbed dose in grays for these radiations. One sievert equals 100 rems.

- **Rem** (roentgen equivalent [in] man): A unit used to measure the dose equivalent. One rem equals 1 rad times a biological-effect modifying factor. Because the modifying factor for x- and gamma radiation equals one, the number of rems is identical to the absorbed dose in rads for these radiations. One rem equals 0.01 sievert.

The terms just defined can be quite confusing. Fortunately, in dental radiology, grays and sieverts are equal while roentgens, rads, and rems are considered to be numerically equal; however, it should be pointed out that only x-rays and gamma rays are measured in coulombs per kilogram or roentgens. Grays or rads and sieverts or rems are used to measure all radiations: gamma and x-rays, alpha and beta particles, neutrons, and high-energy protons.

A simplified comparison of the terms explains the coulomb per kilogram or roentgen as a measurement of x-ray exposure in air; the gray or rad represents the amount of energy the tissues absorb; and the sievert or rem represents the relative biological effect of radiation absorbed in the body tissues.

Because units of measurement in dental radiology are fairly large, smaller multiples of these units are commonly used. For example, the word *milli* means "one-thousandth of" and we express a smaller dose of a gray as a **milligray (mGy).**

An internationally accepted system of writing and abbreviating units has been accepted. To avoid confusion with the name of the person for whom a unit may be named, the word is capitalized when referring to the person (Roentgen) but when referring to the unit, the word is written in lower case (roentgen). The abbreviation for the unit is, however, capitalized (R).

Maximum Permissible Dose (MPD): For radiation protection purposes, the maximum dose that a person or body part is allowed to receive in a stated period of time. For whole-body radiation, this is currently set at 0.05 Sv (5 rems) per year for radiation workers.

Exposure Rate: The exposure per unit of time.

Radiation (Ionizing): Radiation capable of producing ions directly or indirectly by interaction with matter.

Threshold Exposure: The minimum exposure that will produce a detectable degree of any given effect.

Erythema Exposure: The amount of radiation required to produce temporary redness of the skin.

Latent Period: The period of time between exposure to radiation and clinically observable symptoms.

RADIATION MEASUREMENT AND MEASURING DEVICES

The problem of radiation measurement is complicated because radiation measuring instruments can measure only radiation received at the skin surface but not that within the body. One may attach a measuring device to the skin surface at one side of the face to determine the **entrance dose** (also called **skin exposure)** and attach another meter to the other side of the face to determine the exit dose. However, one may only estimate the **depth dose,** or amount of dose between entrance and exit, by considering such factors as the distance from the point of entrance or exit, the quality of the radiation, and the types of intervening tissues. The same holds true when attempting to estimate radiation to genetic tissues. The size and sex of the patient make a difference, the gonads of a child being closer to the source of radiation than those of an adult and the female organs being better protected by the abdominal structures than those of the male.

Figures dealing with exposure and dosage can be very misleading. It makes a difference whether all of the body is exposed or only a small area of the face. Obviously the dose received in an internal organ is less than that received by the skin, because the strength of the radiation beam diminishes inversely proportional to the square of the distance from the source; also some of the radiation is absorbed by the intervening tissue. Another variable is the density of the structures through which the rays are directed. Also to be considered is the **output** of the x-ray machine used. This is the amount of radiation produced, calculated in C/kg/sec (R/sec), measured at the open end of the position indicating device (PID). A typical modern dental unit, depending on the milliamperage and kilovoltage, has an output between 1.81×10^{-4} C/kg/sec and 2.58×10^{-4} C/kg/sec (0.7 R/sec and 1.0 R/sec). Thus most figures are mere estimates and subject to many variables.

Although effects of radiation on patients are difficult to determine and depth doses difficult to measure, it is possible to measure accurately the amount of radiation on a monitoring badge or similar device. These will be described later in this chapter.

RADIATION SAFETY TERMINOLOGY

The following terms are important in radiation control:

Primary Beam (Primary Radiation): The original radiation that emanates from the focal spot on the tube of the x-ray unit. It leaves the tube head through an opening (port) behind the PID and travels in a cone-shaped path, becoming constantly larger as the distance from the focal spot (on the target) increases. This beam is composed of x-ray photons of various wavelengths.

Useful Beam (Useful Radiation): That part of the primary beam that is permitted to emerge from the housing of the tube and is limited by the aperture, lead diaphragm (collimator), or other collimating device such as a lead-lined PID. The size of the useful beam of x-radiation can be determined by the size of the opening in the collimator. This opening should not be any larger than necessary to produce a beam big enough to expose all parts of the film. According to the recommendations of the American Dental Association, the diameter of the useful beam should not exceed 2 3/4 in. (7 cm) at the tip of the PID.

Secondary Radiation: The radiation given off (scattered) by any matter being irradiated with x-rays. This new form of radiation is created the moment the primary beam comes into contact with matter. During dental x-ray procedures it originates mainly in the soft tissues of the face, the soft and hard tissues of the patient's head, the plastic materials of the cone (PID), and the filters. During this reaction, the energy of the primary radiation is diminished and transformed into energy of longer wavelength.

Scatter Radiation: The radiation that has been deflected from its path by impact during its passage through matter. This form of secondary radiation (the terms **secondary** and **scatter radiation** are often used interchangeably) is scattered in all directions by the tissues of the patient's head during radiation. It then travels to all parts of the body and to adjacent areas of the room. That is why the operator should stand at least 6 ft (1.8 m) from the head of the patient when exposing x-ray film and why the patient should be draped with a lead apron. The possibility of biological damage from secondary or scatter radiation must not be taken lightly. Although seldom in the path of the primary beam, the operator can be exposed by scattered rays unless protected by adequate distance or, if necessary, structural shielding or movable lead-lined screens. Scatter radiation presents the most serious danger to the operator.

Leakage Radiation: A form of radiation that originates at the target inside the tube and escapes in all directions through the protective shielding of the tube and tube head. Most modern x-ray units have well-protected tube heads, but occasionally leakage occurs, especially at the points where the electrical connections enter.

Filter: An absorbing material (usually aluminum) placed in the path of the beam of radiation in order to remove a high percentage of the soft x-rays (the longer wavelengths).

Filtration: The absorption of the less penetrating x-rays of the polychromatic x-ray beam by passage of the beam through a sheet of material called a **filter.** In the dental x-ray machine, these filters are disks of pure aluminum that vary in thickness. These filters may be sealed into the tube head or inserted into the port where the PID attaches. Pure aluminum or its equivalent will not hinder the passage of high-energy photons but will absorb a high percentage of the low-energy photons. The latter do not contribute to the radiographic image. However, they are harmful to the patient because they are absorbed by the skin and increase the dose (Fig. 6–2).

Inherent Filtration: Filtration produced by the internal barriers to the passage of the x-rays from the focal spot to the external surface of the tube housing. These barriers include the glass tube window, the insulating oil surrounding the tube, and the port seal. All x-ray units have some built-in filtration.

Added Filtration: Filtration placed outside the tube head. When the inherent filtration is not sufficient to meet present safety standards, a disk of aluminum of the appropriate thickness can be inserted between the port of the tube head and the PID. Several manufacturers have introduced x-ray units in which the traditional aluminum filter is replaced with samarium, a rare-earth metal.

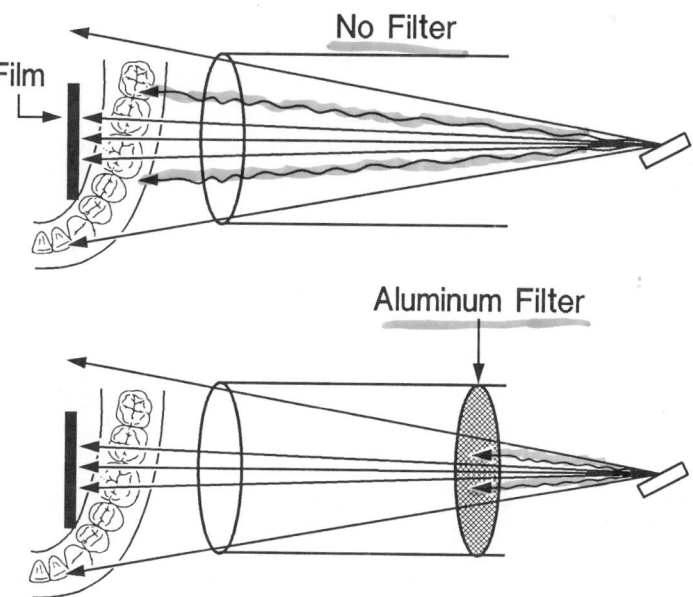

Figure 6–2. Effect of filtration on skin exposure. Aluminum filters selectively absorb the long-wavelength x-rays.

Total Filtration: The sum of the inherent and added filtration expressed in millimeters of aluminum equivalent. Present safety standards require an equivalent of 1.5 mm aluminum for x-ray machines operating in ranges below 70 kVp and a minimum of 2.5 mm aluminum for machines operating at or above 70 kVp.

Collimator: A diaphragm or tubular device made of dense material (usually lead) designed to restrict the dimensions of the useful beam.

Collimation: The control of the size and shape of the useful beam. The most common method of collimation in dental radiography is to insert a lead diaphragm or washer at the base of the PID (Fig. 6–3).

Controlled Area: A defined area in which the occupational exposure of personnel to radiation is under the supervision of the radiation protection supervisor. The dental office is designated as a controlled area; a public hallway or traffic corridor through a dental office is not so considered if used by the public.

Half-Value Layer (HVL): The thickness of a specified substance that, when introduced into the path of a given beam of radiation, reduces the exposure rate by one half (Fig. 6–4).

Protective Barrier: A barrier of radiation-absorbing materials, used to reduce radiation exposure.

Primary Protective Barrier: A barrier sufficient to attenuate the useful beam to the required degree.

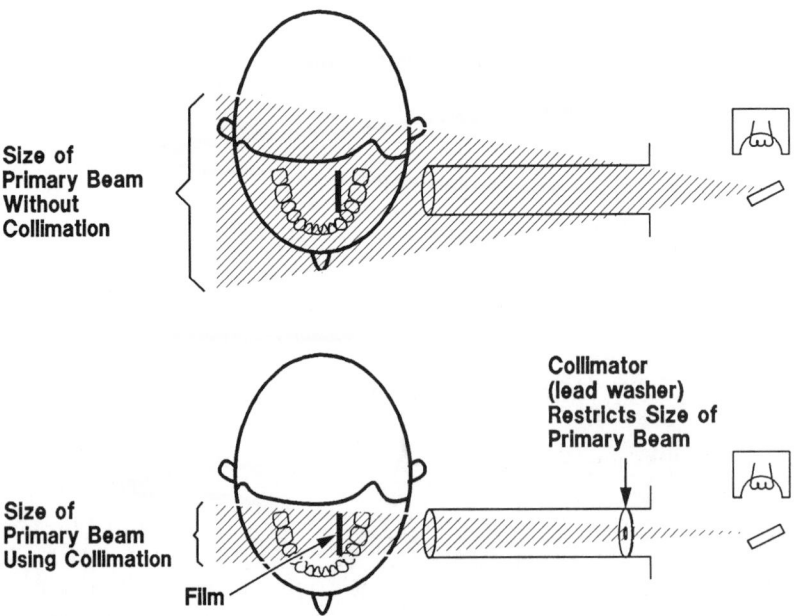

Figure 6–3. Effect of collimation on primary beam. Lead collimators control the shape and size of the primary beam. The beam is limited to the aproximate size of the film.

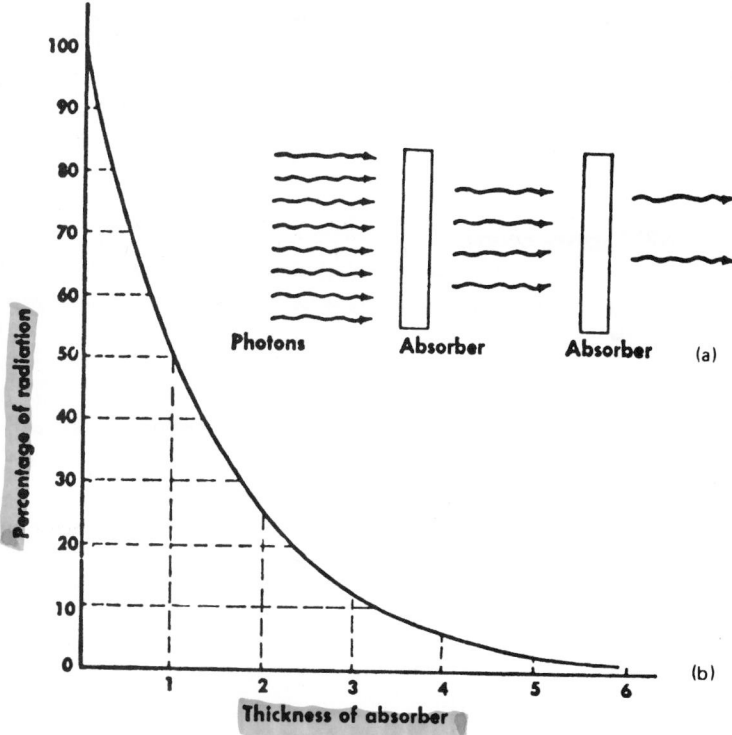

Figure 6–4. (a) Diagram showing the effect of two half-value layers of absorbing material on a monochromatic beam of x-ray photons. (b) Graph showing the exponential curve of x-ray absorption. *(Reproduced with permission from Wuehrmann AH, Manson-Hing LR:* Dental Radiology, *5th ed. St. Louis, MO: CV Mosby, 1981.)*

Radiation Protection Supervisor: The person directly responsible for radiation protection. In the dental office it is usually the dentist.

Secondary Protective Barrier: Barrier sufficient to attenuate stray radiation to the required degree.

Structural Shielding: The protection afforded by structural materials.

RADIATION PROTECTION MEASURES FOR OPERATOR AND PATIENT

Since the dangers of overexposure to radiation were first recognized, many safeguards have been devised. Some of these safeguards, such as filtration, collimation, and protective shielding, are mechanical; others are technical. Some of these radiation safety techniques protect primarily the patient; others protect primarily the operator. Generally, both patient and operator benefit by them.

One of the cardinal principles in radiography is to use the least radiation needed to perform the task. This is called the **ALARA** concept—As Low As Reasonably Achievable—economic and social factors being taken into account.

Another important rule is never to hold the film for the patient or stabilize the tube head or the PID. Holding the tube head subjects the operator to possible exposure from leakage radiation, and holding the PID places the hand right in the path of the primary beam.

Distance is an important factor for operator protection. The operator should always stand as far away as practical—at least 6 ft (1.8 m)—from the source of the radiation unless protected by shielding. The intensity of the x-radiation diminishes the farther the x-rays travel (Fig. 6–5). A careless operator who stands close to the patient while making an exposure can receive unnecessary secondary or scatter radiation.

Although rarely necessary, lead-lined walls, thick or specially constructed partitions between the rooms, or specially constructed lead screens or shields afford ex-

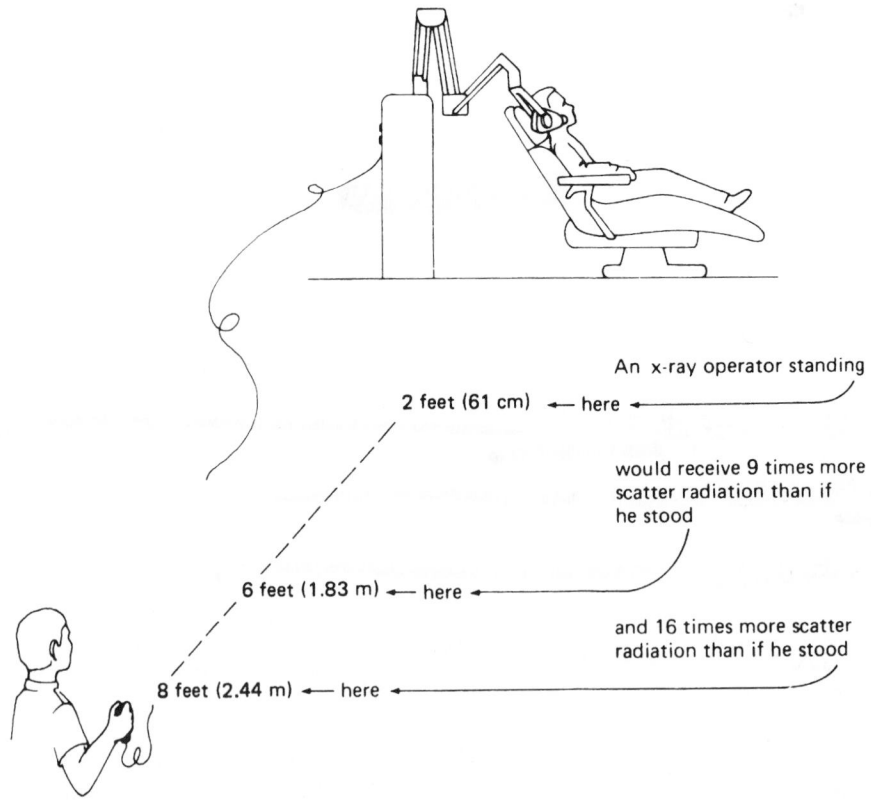

An x-ray operator standing

2 feet (61 cm) ← here ←

would receive 9 times more scatter radiation than if he stood

6 feet (1.83 m) ← here ←

and 16 times more scatter radiation than if he stood

8 feet (2.44 m) ← here ←

Figure 6–5. Distance is an effective means of reducing exposure from scatter radiation. *(Reproduced with permission from Bureau of Radiological Health: Radiation Protection in Dental Practices. Sacramento: State of California, Department of Public Health, 1977.)*

cellent protection for the operator. The lead screens or shields contain a radiation-resistant glass through which the operator looks at the patient during the exposure. When the dental office is not equipped with such shielding, an extra-long timer cord can be used to enable the operator to stand at least 6 ft (1.8 m) from the head of the patient while making the exposure.

The safest place for the operator to stand is from 45 to 90 degrees out of the primary beam, behind the bulkiest part of the patient's head. The head thus absorbs most of the primary beam and much of the scatter radiation. All persons not directly concerned with the x-ray exposure should leave the room.

Several states have laws requiring the use of a lead apron over the abdominal area. Even if it is not legally required, the use of a lead apron is important, especially for women in the reproductive age and for children. Additional protection can be derived from the use of a thyroid collar (Fig. 6–6). The thyroid collar protects a radiosensitive area in the neck region; however, its use is not convenient when using rotational panoramic equipment because the collar or the upper part of the apron to which it is attached may interfere with the rotation of the panoramic unit.

Another radiation safeguard is the use of the largest film that can be placed comfortably in the patient's mouth, so that fewer films and exposures are needed. However, this is not always practical. Sometimes smaller films are needed to avoid bending, which distorts the image.

Use of high-speed film with an ASA speed of D or E means shorter exposure times. And shorter exposure times mean less radiation to the patient and operator. To-

protective aprons

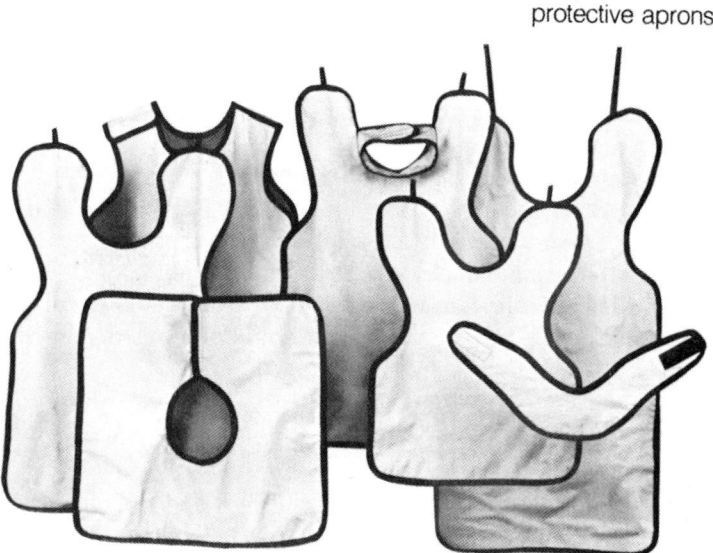

Figure 6–6. Lead aprons and thyroid collars. This assortment shows aprons and collars in child and adult sizes. The thyroid collar may be separate or be a part of the larger lead apron. *(Courtesy of Rinn Corporation, Elgin, IL.)*

TABLE 6–2. GUIDELINES FOR PRESCRIBING DENTAL RADIOGRAPHS

Patient category	Child	
	Primary dentition (prior to eruption of first permanent tooth)	Transitional dentition (following eruption of first permanent tooth)
New patient		
All new patients to assess dental diseases and growth and development	Posterior bitewing examination if proximal surfaces of primary teeth cannot be visualized or probed posterior bitewings or panoramic	Individualized radiographic examination consisting of periapical/occlusal views and examination and posterior bitewings
Recall patient		
Clinical caries or high-risk factors for caries	Posterior bitewing examination at 6-mo intervals or until no carious lesions are evident	
No clinical caries and no high-risk factors for caries	Posterior bitewing examination at 12- to 14-mo intervals if proximal surfaces of primary teeth cannot be visualized or probed	Posterior bitewing examination at 12- to 24-mo intervals
Periodontal disease or a history of periodontal treatment	Individualized radiographic examination consisting of selected periapica and or bitewing radiographs for areas where periodontal disease (other than nonspecific gingivitis) can be demonstrated clinically	
Growth and development assessment	Usually not indicated	Individualized radiographic examination consisting of a periapical occlusal or panoramic examination

Courtesy of the US Department of Health and Human Services.

day, radiographers using speed group E film can expose 16 films for each speed group A film exposed 30 years ago. Fast film has been the single most important factor in reducing unnecessary radiation.

Proper darkroom procedures should be followed (see Chapter 9). Always process film using time–temperature techniques in an adequately equipped darkroom. Many dental offices overexpose and underdevelop the film in order to save time. This results in needless exposure to the patient and films of inferior quality.

The use of film holders affords the patient additional protection by reducing the number of retakes and avoids having the patient hold the film with the fingers.

GUIDELINES FOR PRESCRIBING DENTAL RADIOGRAPHS

The decision to use dental radiographs as diagnostic aids rests on the professional judgment of the dentist. Guidelines developed by an expert panel of dentists convened by the Public Health Service have been published to help the dentist decide when, what type, and how many radiographs should be taken (Table 6–2). The recommendations are subject to clinical judgment and may not apply to every patient. They are to be used by the dentist only after reviewing the patient's health history and completing a clinical examination. These guidelines do not need to be altered because of pregnancy.

Adolescent	Adult	
Permanent dentition (prior to eruption of third molars)	Dentulous	Edentulous
Individualized radiographic examination consisting of posterior bitewings and selected periapicals. A full mouth intraoral radiographic examination is appropriate when the patient presents with clinical evidence of generalized dental disease or a history of extensive dental treatment.		Full-mouth intraoral radiographic examination or panoramic examination
Posterior bitewing examination at 6- to 12-mo intervals or until no carious lesions are evident	Posterior bitewing examination at 12- to 18-mo intervals	Not applicable
Posterior bitewing examination at 18- to 36-mo intervals	Posterior bitewing examination at 24- to 36-mo intervals	Not applicable
Individualized radiographic examination consisting of selected periapical and bitewing radiographs for areas where periodontal disease (other than nonspecific gingivitis) can be demonstrated clinically.		Not applicable
Periapical or panoramic examination to assess developing third molars	Usually not indicated	Usually not indicated

The guidelines suggest that all new patients have a recent full-mouth radiographic examination before treatment begins. Recall patients should not have radiographs made as a "matter of routine," but only after determining their diagnostic needs. For instance, a decay-prone teenager may need radiographs more often than a middle-aged patient.

EQUIPMENT MODIFICATIONS FOR SAFETY

Some older x-ray machines lack adequate filtration and collimation. Their mechanical timers are not accurate enough to measure the short exposure times used with high-speed films. Thus, they often fail to meet recommended safety standards. Some of these machines should be replaced, whereas others can be modified to make them safer.

The addition of aluminum disks of the proper thickness to meet the recommended standards will increase the filtration and reduce harmful low-energy radiation; proper collimation will restrict the size of the primary beam; replacing the closed plastic cone with an open-ended PID (especially one with lead lining) further reduces scatter radiation; and replacing the mechanical timer with an electronic one will permit shorter exposure times. These modifications can be made at a modest expense and improve both safety and the diagnostic quality of the radiograph.

STRUCTURAL MODIFICATIONS

In many states it is required that dental rooms containing x-ray machines be provided with primary barriers at all areas struck by the useful beam, that protective barriers be provided between the x-ray rooms and nearby operatories or hallways, and that each installation be provided with a protective barrier for the operator or be so arranged that the operator can stand at least 6 ft (1.8 m) from the patient and away from the useful beam of radiation.

When these conditions cannot be met by relocating the x-ray machines or equipment in adjacent operatories, structural modifications must be made. In many cases structural materials of ordinary walls will suffice as a protective barrier without additional special shielding material. A wall made of two thicknesses of 5/8-in. (16-mm) gypsum board (1 1/4 in. or 32 mm total) can be assumed to provide minimum protection from scattered radiation only if the following conditions are met: (1) the occupiable areas protected by the wall are at least 6 ft (1.8 m) from the dental x-ray chair; and (2) the use of the x-ray equipment does not exceed 60 seconds per week of "on time" at 90 kVp or 100 seconds per week of "on time" at 65 kVp.

The average dental installation can usually meet the above conditions by proper layout and planning, and gypsum board or plastered walls will then provide adequate protection. For example, the primary beam can be directed toward an outside wall or into an unoccupied area. When these conditions cannot be met, as when two x-ray chairs are side by side or when a receptionist sits immediately adjacent to the wall receiving the primary beam, additional structural shielding in the form of lead sheathing with a thickness of 1/32 in. (0.8 mm) may be needed. When properly located, such lead shielding is almost always adequate in the dental office. The thickness and locations of these barriers should be determined by an individual qualified in x-ray shielding design.

In addition to this, darkroom modifications to prevent light leaks and the use of better processing equipment and chemicals—coupled with standardized exposure and processing techniques—increase radiation safety and produce better radiographs. Most of the "unnecessary" radiation in the dental office today is due to overexposure and underdevelopment of the film.

RADIATION MONITORING

The only way to make sure that x-ray equipment is not emitting too much radiation and people are not receiving more than the maximum permissible dose is to use monitoring devices. In radiography, **monitoring** is defined as periodic or continuing measurement to determine the dose rate in a given area or the dose received by a person.

Radiation has four qualities that make accurate measurements possible: it affects photographic emulsions, produces ionization in air, produces a rise in temperature, and causes certain salts to fluoresce. All measuring devices make use of one of these qualities.

Area monitoring involves making an on-site survey to measure the output of the dental x-ray unit, to check for possible radiation leakage and danger areas in the room (hot spots), and to determine if any radiation is passing through walls. Special equipment is needed to detect the exact amount of ionizing radiation at any given area. Numerous firms specialize in monitoring. In some regions this service may be performed at the dentist's request by qualified state personnel.

Personnel monitoring requires office staff members to wear a device that measures how much radiation they are receiving. Monitoring devices vary in cost and effectiveness. Some merely indicate that radiation has been received; others show the amount, and still others measure the amount and type of radiation. In hospitals, industrial plants, and some dental offices, everyone working around radiation is required to wear a monitoring device at all times while on duty. The **monitoring badge** (discussed later in this chapter) is sufficiently accurate and economical to be worn in the dental office. More and more dentists are providing monitoring devices and services for themselves and their employees. Legislation is pending to make this mandatory in several states.

MONITORING DEVICES

The major problem with radiation measurements is that what we actually measure is the effect of radiation on photographic emulsion, on gas or air, and on certain crystals of fluorescent salts rather than making a direct measurement of radiation itself, and for this we need monitoring devices.

The more complex devices, such as the Geiger counter and the scintillation counter, are not practical in the dental office and are mentioned here only for the sake of completeness. The Geiger counter contains a needlelike electrode inside a hollow metallic cylinder that is filled with gas that sets up a current in an electric field when it is ionized by radiation. The scintillation counter contains a photoelectric cell that helps to measure the flashes of visible light emitted when the radiation that bombards certain salt crystals within the instrument causes them to fluoresce.

Our major interest is in the personnel monitoring devices. The forerunner of these devices used in the dental office was an unexposed film to which a paper clip was attached. One wore it in a pocket with the clip and the exposure side of the film facing toward the outside. The film was developed at intervals ranging from 1 to 3 months. Although extremely simple and economical, the shortcoming was that this homemade film badge showed only that radiation had been received and failed to record the amount of radiation.

A more sophisticated device is the pocket dosimeter, also called an ionization chamber. The **dosimeter** resembles a fountain pen and attaches to a garment with a clip. The dosimeter contains an ion chamber, a small sealed container of air designed so that the air can be ionized. The dosimeter can only be read when it is inserted into a more complex piece of equipment called a charger-reader. When the ionized air is exposed to radiation, changes within the ion chamber can be measured through the movements of a spring electroscope when the dosimeter is inserted in the charger-reader. Dosimeters are very useful in installations with a high work load because they can be recharged every morning and read at the end of the day; their disadvantages are that no permanent record of radiation is made and that they are not very practical in the dental office.

A more effective device is the **film badge,** a descendant of the paper clip device.

Firms provide a film badge service on a subscription basis. Each subscriber is supplied with a badge loaded with a radiosensitive film. The plastic or metal holder is lined with various thicknesses of filters of different materials that make it possible to measure the types of radiation received. Film badges are not accurate at very low exposures.

Film badges are now being replaced by a new radiation detection device called a **thermoluminescent dosimeter (TLD)** (from the Greek word therme, meaning "heat," and the Latin words *lumen,* meaning "light," and *escent,* meaning "any giving off of light caused by absorption of radiant or corpuscular energy") (Fig. 6–7). These devices have crystals—usually lithium flouride—that absorb energy when exposed to radiation. When the crystals are heated, after being exposed to radiation, energy in the form of visible light is given off. The total light emitted is proportional to the amount of radiation (energy) absorbed by the crystals. TLDs are extremely accurate.

Several manufacturers make **TLD badges** and offer a monitoring service that includes periodic reports to the subscriber. The typical TLD badge is small, lightweight, has a clip for attachment to the clothes or uniform, and should be worn throughout the work day.

These badges are easy to load and have no dials to set or read. Each badge is identified by a number, the wearer's name, and the dates on which the badge will be used. All that is necessary is to periodically replace the packet of crystals and mail it in to be read. At agreed monitoring periods, generally 1 month, the subscriber receives an easy-to-read report that compares each person's exposure reading with the maximum allowable level. The monitoring firm updates the subscriber's records to keep the wearer in full compliance with all federal and state safety regulations.

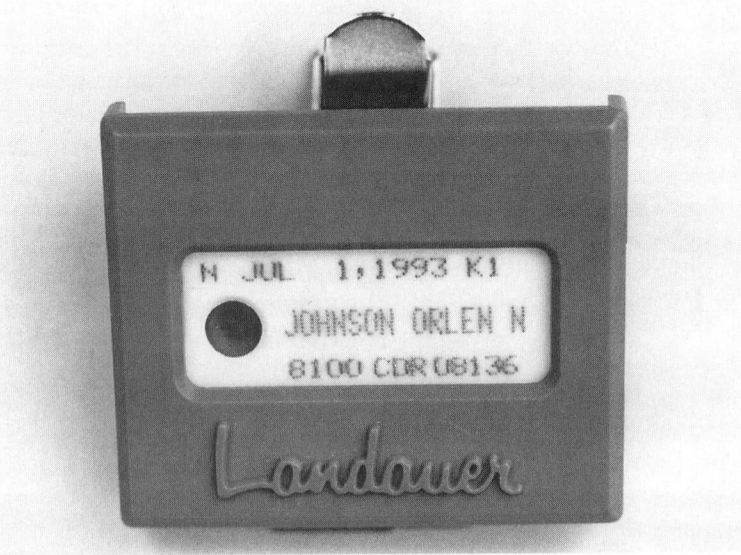

Figure 6–7. TLD badge. A container that can be attached to the uniform. Used for radiation detection and measurement in personnel monitoring.

The wearing of TLD badges is not mandatory in every state; however, for maximum protection, a TLD badge is recommended for each person working directly with radiation or other personnel subject to radiation exposure.

STUDIES ON RADIATION EXPOSURE PROTECTION

As early as 1902 some studies were undertaken to determine the effect of radiation exposure on the body and to consider setting limits on radiation exposure. The International Commission on Radiation Protection was formed in 1928, and in 1929 the National Council on Radiation Protection and Measurements (NCRP) was created in the United States. The American Dental Association (ADA), through its various committees and affiliated organizations, works closely with all organizations interested in radiation safety. It will send its publications to those who write for them.

Research on the effects of radiation and on radiation hygiene procedures sped forward when scientists and the public became alarmed in the early 1950s about possible radiation effects produced by atomic testing. Many organizations studied the various aspects of radiation safety simultaneously but not necessarily from the same viewpoint. All known forms of radiation were studied, but the major effort was directed toward finding out what levels of radiation could safely be tolerated.

The NCRP has proposed two sets of limits, one for occupationally exposed persons working in radiography or with radioactive materials (dentists, dental assistants, dental hygienists, radiography technicians) and the other for the general population. These limits do not apply to medical or dental radiation used for diagnostic or therapeutic purposes. The NCRP suggests that patient exposures be kept to a minimum consistent with clinical requirements but leaves the amount of exposure up to the professional judgment of the dentist. The maximum limits were set higher for workers than for the public, but the suggested limits of the maximum permissible accumulated dose for both groups were purposely set far lower than it was believed the body could safely accept.

Over the years there has been a constant downward revision of the acceptable limits, which are now about 700 times smaller than those originally proposed in 1902. Many aspects of tissue damage from radiation are still not clearly understood.

Although the NCRP and similar organizations have no legal status, their suggestions and recommendations are highly regarded. Many regulatory bodies have used them to formulate legislation controlling the use of radiation in the dental office. Three publications are recommended for obtaining additional information concerning radiation protection: (1) NCRP Report no. 35 [*Dental X-ray Protection*, Washington, DC, 1970]; (2) NCRP Report no. 39 [*Basic Radiation Protection Criteria*, Washington, DC, 1971]; and NCRP Report no. 91 [*Recommendations on Limits for Exposure to Ionizing Radiation*, Washington, DC, 1987]. (See this chapter's Bibliography for further listings.)

GUIDES FOR MAINTAINING SAFE RADIATION LEVELS

The NCRP developed **radiation protection guides (RPG)** (also referred to as the **maximum permissible dose [MPD]**) for the protection of radiation workers and the general public. The guides represent doses far below those at which any effects have ever been observed. The general public is permitted one tenth the exposure permitted radiation workers. This was done because workers represent only a small fraction of the total population, and it was believed that if they suffer greater genetic damage than the general population, the damaged hereditary material will be so diluted in the general population that it will not result in a disastrous mutation level. Radiation necessary for medical or dental diagnostic purposes is not counted in the permissible amounts of radiation.

Permissible exposure limits for dentists and dental personnel are the same as for other radiation workers. According to these guidelines, the dose may not exceed 50 mSv (5 rem) per year.

There is no established weekly limit, but the average weekly exposure should be limited to 1.0 mSv (0.1 rem). There are some exceptions to these guidelines; the skin of the whole body, the hands and forearms, and the feet and ankles may receive larger doses.

The reports from any monitoring service are the most reliable permanent records of accumulated doses. If a worker's monitoring device indicates that the average weekly levels are frequently exceeded, there is justifiable cause for concern. All techniques should be reviewed for errors, and the x-ray machine should be tested for leakage.

The 50 mSv (5 rem) yearly limit for radiation workers has two very important exceptions. It does not apply to persons under 18 years or to any female members of the dental team—whether dentist, assistant, or hygienist—who are known to be pregnant. Persons under 18 years are classified as part of the general public and can accumulate only 5 mSv (0.5 rem) per year. In the case of pregnant women, it is recommended the fetus be limited to 5 mSv (0.5 rem), not to be received at a rate greater than 0.5 mSv (0.05 rem) per month. The wearing of a monitoring device, while not mandatory, is a good procedure in these circumstances.

Guides are also established for students. Until the student gains some degree of proficiency, all radiographic exposures must be made on a skull, dummy, or **phantom** known as **DXTTR**—dental x-ray teaching training replica—pronounced "dexter" (Fig. 6–8). In learning to expose radiographs, students should not expose more than one full-mouth series on one another. These radiographs must serve a diagnostic purpose and be interpreted by a dentist. Additional practice on patients (if permissible by state law) can be accomplished by the use of referred patients, provided that the radiographs are sent to their dentist for diagnostic interpretation.

All those using dental x-ray equipment must be aware of the rigid standards and regulations established by city, county, state, and federal agencies and must be prepared to observe them. Several states require that dental workers must pass a radiation safety examination before they can expose radiographs; similar legislation is considered in other states. In some instances, city and county regulations are stricter than those imposed by the states.

Some patients have heard highly exaggerated stories concerning radiation—a few based on facts now outdated and many on misinformation and rumor. Occasionally, patients are reluctant to submit to any form of x-radiation. Their objections can gener-

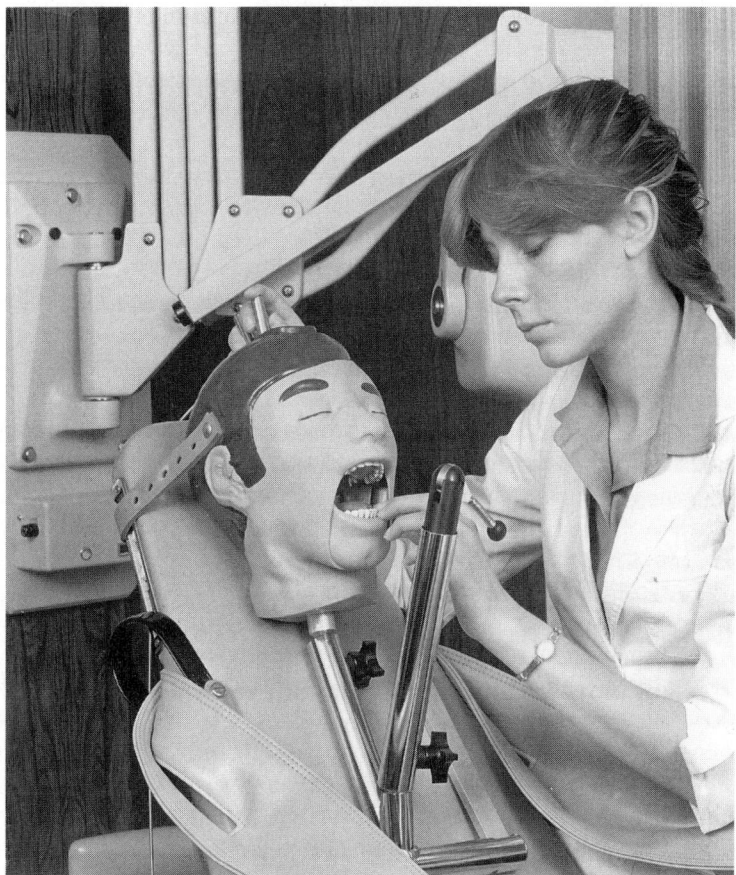

Figure 6-8. Dental x-ray teaching and training replica (DXTTR). The phantom (pronounced "dexter") is used by students to gain proficiency in making dental radiographs before exposing patients. *(Courtesy of Rinn Corporation, Elgin, IL.)*

ally be overcome if the dentist, dental hygienist, or dental assistant takes the time to educate them. Thus, it is doubly important that anyone who practices radiography be thoroughly informed.

CHAPTER SUMMARY

Everyone working with radiation in dental offices shares in the responsibility of keeping all radiation levels as low as possible, consistent with acceptable diagnostic results.

The concern is for the safety of the patient, the radiographer, and anyone working or passing by within the range of the radiation beam.

In response to public and professional concern, the federal government entered into the regulation of x-ray machines. States and cities have enacted radiation safety legislation.

Radiation measurement terminology includes terms such as exposure, absorbed dose, and dose equivalent. These terms are complex and essential for understanding radiation safety. The units coulombs per kilogram (C/kg), gray (Gy), and sievert (Sv) are used to measure radiation.

The output of the x-ray machine is the exposure in air measured in coulombs per kilogram (roentgens). Radiation absorbed doses are measured in grays (rads) and radiation dose equivalents are measured in sieverts (rems). An exposure does not become a dose until the radiation is absorbed in the body.

The manufacturer assists by providing the x-ray machine with lead collimators to restrict the beam size and aluminum or samarium filters to remove undesirable wavelengths before they can be absorbed. The operator protects the patient by understanding the significance of the exposure factors and using proper techniques. This is done by draping the patient with a lead apron and thyroid collar whenever possible, setting and aiming the machine correctly, and proper film placement and development; all these combined reduce radiation and decrease the necessity to retake certain exposures. The operator at the same time achieves maximum protection by using only D- (or preferably E-)speed films, by being careful to aim the PID, by avoiding scatter radiation through distance and protective shielding, and by wearing a monitoring device. Personnel monitoring is accomplished through the use of thermoluminescent dosimeters.

Studies on radiation protection have been conducted by numerous organizations including the American Dental Association and the National Council on Radiation Protection and Measurements. As a result of these studies, a series of guides have been developed for the maintenance of safe radiation levels. The maximum permissible dose (MPD) is 50 mSv (5 rem) per year for radiation workers and 5 mSv (0.5 rem) for the general public, radiation workers who are pregnant, and children under 18 years of age.

KEY WORDS

Absorbed dose	Coulombs per kilogram (C/kg)
Added filtration	Dose equivalent
Collimation	Dosimeter
Collimator	DXTTR (phantom)
Controlled area	Erythema exposure

Exposure	**Protective barrier**
Exposure rate	**Rad**
Film badge	**Radiation**
Filter	**Radiation protection guides (RPG)**
Filtration	**Radiation protection supervisor**
Gray (Gy)	**Rem**
Half-value layer (HVL)	**Roentgen (R)**
Inherent filtration	**Scatter radiation**
Latent period	**Secondary protective barrier**
Leakage radiation	**Secondary radiation**
Maximum permissible dose (MPD)	**Sievert (Sv)**
Monitoring	**Structural shielding**
Monitoring badge	**Thermoluminescent dosimeter (TLD)**
Output	
Primary beam	**TLD badge**
Primary protective barrier	**Total filtration**
Primary radiation	**Useful beam**

REVIEW QUESTIONS

1. Who has the legal responsibility for all acts and services performed in the dental office? (a) the dental hygienist, (b) the dental technician, (c) the dental assistant, (d) the dentist.

2. Which of these terms best describes the x-rays that are coming directly from the focal spot on the target of the x-ray tube? (a) filtered beam, (b) central beam, (c) primary beam, (d) scatter beam.

3. Who is the only person who should be in the path of the useful beam? (a) the dentist, (b) the patient, (c) the dental assistant, (d) the receptionist.

4. In normal dental radiographic procedures, the principal hazard to the operator is produced by: (a) direct radiation, (b) scattered radiation, (c) gamma radiation, (d) alpha radiation.

5. What is a device that restricts the size of the radiation beam called? (a) a dosimeter, (b) a filter, (c) a collimator, (d) a primary barrier.

6. What material is the collimator made of? (a) copper, (b) tungsten, (c) samarium, (d) lead.

7. What is the minimum total filtration that is required by an x-ray machine that can operate in ranges above 70 kVp? (a) 1.5 mm of aluminum equivalent, (b) 5/8 in. (16 mm) of gypsum, (c) 2.5 mm of aluminum equivalent, (d) 1/32 in. (0.8 mm) of lead.

8. What is the recommended minimum distance that the operator should stand from the source of the radiation? (a) 16 in. (41 cm), (b) 3 ft (91 cm), (c) 6 ft (1.83 m), (d) 9 ft (2.74 m).

9. Which of these terms is the unit used to measure radiation exposure? (a) curie, (b) gray (rad), (c) sievert (rem), (d) coulombs per kilogram (roentgen).

10. What is the recommended size of the diameter of the primary beam at the end of the PID (at the skin of the patients face)? (a) 2 3/4 in. (7 cm), (b) 3 1/4 in. (8.2 cm), (c) 4 1/2 in. (11.4 cm), (d) 5 in. (12.7 cm).

11. Total filtration is the sum of the _inherent_ and _added_ filtration expressed in millimeters of _aluminum_

12. The collimator is used to control the _size_ and _shape_ of the useful beam.

13. The filter is an absorbing material usually made of _aluminum_.

14. The filter is placed in the path of the beam of radiation in order to remove a high percentage of the _longer_ wavelength x-rays.

BIBLIOGRAPHY

US Department of Health and Human Services: *The Selection of Patients for X-ray Examinations: Dental Radiographic Examinations.* Rockville, MD: US Department of Health and Human Services, 1987. HHS publication (FDA) 88-8273

National Council on Radiation Protection and Measurements: *Dental X-ray Protection.* Washington, DC, NCRP, 1970. NCRP Report no. 35

National Council on Radiation Protection and Measurements: *Basic Radiation Protection Criteria.* Washington, DC, NCRP, 1971. NCRP Report no. 39

National Council on Radiation Protection and Measurements: *Review of the Current State of Radiation Protection Philosophy.* Washington, DC, NCRP, 1975. NCRP Report no. 43

National Council on Radiation Protection and Measurements: *Review of NCRP Dose Limit for Embryo and Fetus in Occupationally Exposed Women.* Washington, DC, NCRP, 1977. NCRP Report no. 53

National Council on Radiation Protection and Measurements: *Recommendations on Limits for Exposure to Ionizing Radiation.* Washington, DC, NCRP, 1987. NCRP Report no. 91

National Council on Radiation Protection and Measurements: *Implementation of the Principle of As Low As Reasonably Achievable (ALARA) for Medical and Dental Personnel.* Washington, DC, NCRP, 1991. NCRP Report no. 107

Eastman Kodak: *Radiation Safety in Dental Radiography.* Rochester, NY, 1993

Council on Dental Materials, Instruments, and Equipment: *Recommendations in Radiographic Practices: An Update, 1988. J Am Dent Assoc* **118:**115–117, 1989

CHAPTER 7

Infection Control

By the end of this chapter the student should be able to

1. Identify the benefits of infection control.
2. Differentiate between disinfection and sterilization.
3. Describe measures to be taken to avoid cross-contamination.
4. Make a check list of procedures that are essential to minimizing the spread of disease in the dental office.

INCREASED NECESSITY FOR INFECTION CONTROL

As little as 20 years ago, face masks were seldom worn by the dentist or the auxillary personnel. Gloves were rarely used unless there was a suspicion that the patient had some infectious disease. At that time there was a minimum of thought given to infection control, and what there was consisted mainly of normal sanitation procedures and wiping off some parts of the equipment or work areas with alcohol or some other disinfectant.

But that was in the days before the advent of **hepatitis B, AIDS (acquired immune deficiency syndrome),** and numerous other recently discovered diseases. Blood is the most common transmission route of the **hepatitis B virus (HBV)** and the **human immunodeficiency virus (HIV).** Saliva can be considered to be contaminated by blood. Cross-contamination occurs when pathogenic microorganisms are transmitted from one patient to another or to dental personnel. Currently many procedures to control infections are being studied and guidelines are recommended for proposed infection control. Undoubtedly many changes will take place in future years.

One of the major problems is that most infectious organisms cannot be seen and become visible only when viewed through a microscope. This makes the task of infection control more difficult because there is a natural tendency to assume that there is nothing wrong because nothing unusual can be seen.

Although there will undoubtedly be some under-concern on the part of some personnel, there will also be some over-concern. In many instances there will be laws mandating various procedures. Some of these procedures will be very costly and time-consuming but essential to prevent cross-contamination.

GUIDELINES FOR INFECTION CONTROL

Practicing dental health care providers who have not attended continuing education programs may not be aware of current thinking regarding infection control. Previously, little thought was given to dental radiographic procedures. Also, many group practices have one or two individuals who are responsible for the darkroom and the exposure and processing of most radiographs. Because the responsibility for infection control has not been clearly understood by many, the need to set up guidelines to minimize the risk of infection has arisen. Currently there are publications available from the American Dental Association that provide detailed information about infection control and treatment of patients with infectious diseases. These include *Proceedings of the National Symposium on Hepatitis B and the Dental Profession,* and *Facts About AIDS for the Dental Team.* Also, the Centers for Disease Control (CDC) provides guidelines that recommend covering "surfaces that are difficult or impossible to clean" (see Bibliography). Current research activity explores ways of keeping the risk of infection as low as it can be reasonably achieved—the ALARA principle. The goal of these and future guidelines will be to set standards for controls that are simple enough to be practical. Since we cannot be certain, it must be assumed that each patient is potentially infected and that the development of a single standard of patient care is essential.

Each dental installation, whether a teaching institution, clinic, single or multiple practice, should have a written infection control policy, which should be practical and compatible with local or state regulations. The dentist (or designated personnel) has the authority and the responsibility see to it that it is correctly carried out.

BENEFIT OF INFECTION CONTROL

Everyone in the dental office—the patient, the auxilliaries, and the dentist—benefits when measures are implemented that decrease the likelihood of transmitting bacterial, fungal, or viral infections. A malpractice suit can be defended more easily if it can be proven that the office adheres to an approved infection control plan. Infection control, properly carried out, gives the entire professional staff a feeling of security or "peace of mind," for it is well known that some infected patients are reluctant to admit their condition. In situations where a double standard was used and protective measures only employed when the patient was known to be infectious, everyone was at risk. Thus, the failure to use a single standard for all patients provided inadequate protection because taking a thorough medical history and making a dental examination will not always identify potential infected patients.

Any risk, no matter how small, must be evaluated. It is far better to be safe than to be sorry. Therefore, all patients, whether known to be infected or not, are assumed to be potentially infected and the necessary precautions are applied.

INFECTION CONTROL TERMINOLOGY

Several terms are frequently used in infection control. They should be studied and understood.

Infection control is the prevention and reduction of disease-causing (pathogenic) microorganisms.

A **pathogen** is a microorganism that can cause disease (*pathos* means disease). Infection control procedures are used to prevent the cross-contamination of pathogens between patients and dental personnel.

The term **sepsis** means infection.

Asepsis means just the opposite (*a* means without) and describes an absence of septic matter, or freedom from infection. The term is sometimes applied to the prevention of infection of tissues by microorganisms.

Antiseptic refers to agents used on living tissues to destroy or stop the growth of bacteria. An example is antiseptic soaps used by dental personnel for washing hands.

The term **disinfection** is generally used to describe those efforts made to reduce the disease-producing microorganisms to an acceptable level on inanimate objects. This is done by wiping off those portions of the equipment that come into contact with the patient or operator with gauze saturated with iodophor or some form of chemical disinfectant such as an EPA-registered ADA-approved surface disinfectant. Spores are not necessarily destroyed. Therefore, microorganisms not causing disease may still be present. Disinfecting agents are usually only used on surfaces and instruments because they are too toxic for living tissues.

The term **sterilization** is used to describe the total destruction of spores and disease-producing microorganisms. This is accomplished by autoclaving or dry heat processes. Ideally, all equipment or instruments used should be sterilized. Unfortunately this is not feasible with most radiographic equipment because of its large size.

Disinfection and sterilization are just as important in dental radiography as in any other dental procedure. It is important to recognize the danger of cross-infection between patient and operator and from one patient to another.

Cold sterilization is a term that has been commonly misused in medicine and dentistry for many years. It has usually been applied to procedures resulting in disinfection, not sterilization.

Sanitation is a term used when microorganisms are reduced to a level of concentration considered to be safe. Food handling facilities are usually concerned about adequate sanitation.

The term **barrier** is used to describe any material that is used to prevent the transmission of infective microorganisms to the patient. Barriers include gloves, masks, protective eyewear, surface covers, and operating gowns.

Immunization is the process of making someone immune to a disease. All dental personnel should have the recommended immunizations, including that for the hepatitis B virus.

INFECTION CONTROL PROCEDURES

Hands should be washed thoroughly with an antiseptic skin cleanser at the beginning of each day and before gloving. Gloves should be worn at all times when taking x-rays (just as with any other dental procedure) to prevent skin contact with blood, saliva, or mucous membranes. Masks and protective eyewear may be worn as an additional precaution.

All personnel must be instructed to avoid touching areas such as doorknobs, unexposed film packets, or records with contaminated gloves. Care should be taken to avoid touching anything that is not essential to the procedure being carried out. Mirrors, explorers, or necessary biteblocks should be kept covered when not in use. Obviously standard sanitation procedures are followed in any correctly maintained dental installation. These include sanitizing the headrest, the armrests, the bracket table, and the handles of the operating light. When x-ray equipment is involved, the tube head, PID, cassettes, and any other item handled by the operator or contacted by the patient should be disinfected. Be sure to use the correct immersion time when using chemical disinfectant.

Protective barriers should be used whenever practical. Gloves, masks, and protective eyewear are worn by dental personnel (Fig. 7–1) and plastic wrap, plastic bags, paper towels, paper cups, aluminum foil, etc are used on appropriate surfaces, equipment, and supplies. Barrier material is commonly placed over surfaces likely to be contaminated (chair headrest and controls, PID, tube head yoke, control panel, exposure switch, counter surfaces, etc) (Figs. 7–2, 7–3, and 7–4). Surfaces not covered must be disinfected after the radiographic procedures are completed. Disinfectants have several drawbacks. They, like all liquids, have the potential to affect electrical connections. Also, disinfecting solutions may not reach all irregular surfaces.

Certain biteblocks and intraoral film holders, panoramic biteblocks, and beam aligning devices can be sterilized by autoclaving. Head positioners, chin rests, and ear rods that are not practical for sterilization may be disinfected with EPA-registered, ADA-approved surface disinfectants.

The film packet must be handled carefully to prevent cross-contamination. When the packet is removed from the mouth, it will be coated with saliva or, in rare instances, with blood (saliva should always be treated as though it were contaminated with blood). The film packet with its heat-sensitive emulsion cannot be disinfected or sterilized in the dental office. Therefore the operator should protect the packet by keeping it in the factory-sealed package or dispenser until ready to use. There are two

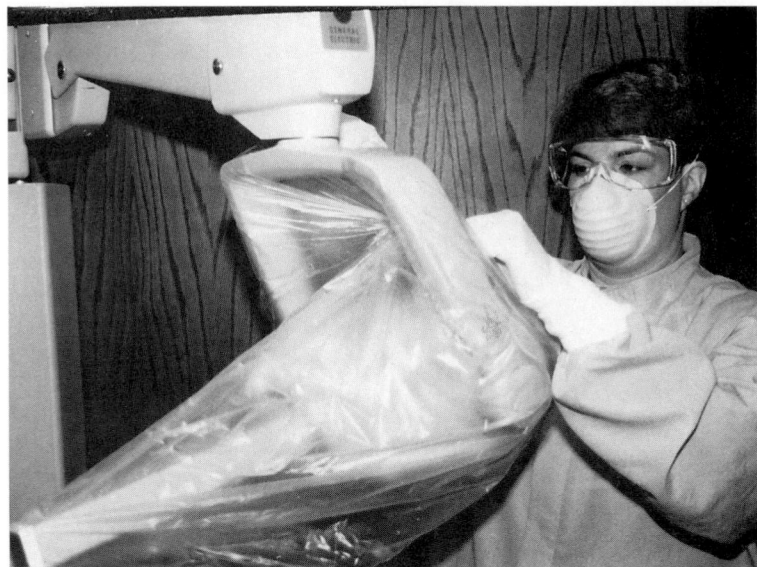

Figure 7-1. Operator wearing gloves, mask, and protective eyewear, placing barrier bag to cover PID, tube housing, and yoke.

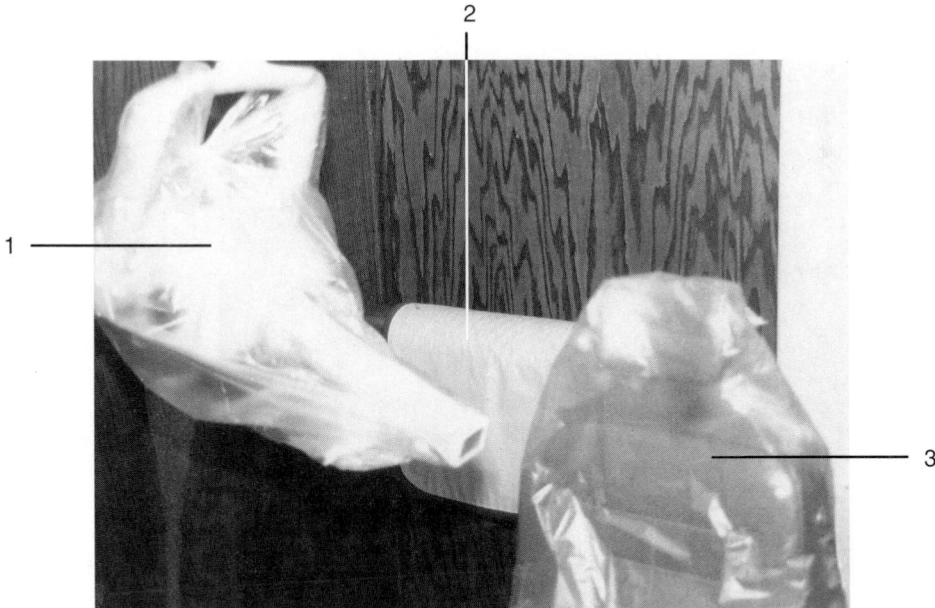

Figure 7-2. Picture of dental operatory showing **(1)** plastic barrier bag covering PID, tube housing, and yoke, **(2)** lead apron draped over storage rack, and **(3)** plastic barrier bag covering chair, headrest, and chair controls.

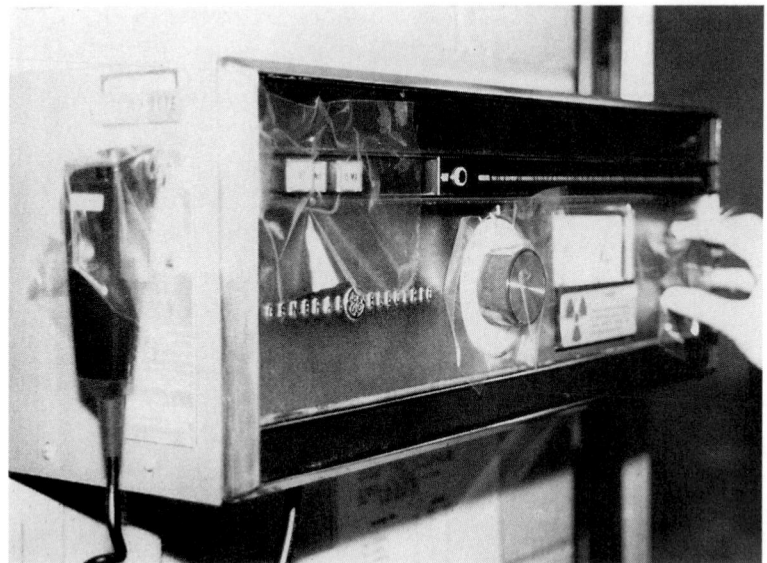

Figure 7-3. Plastic barrier wrap covering exposure switch and controls on control panel.

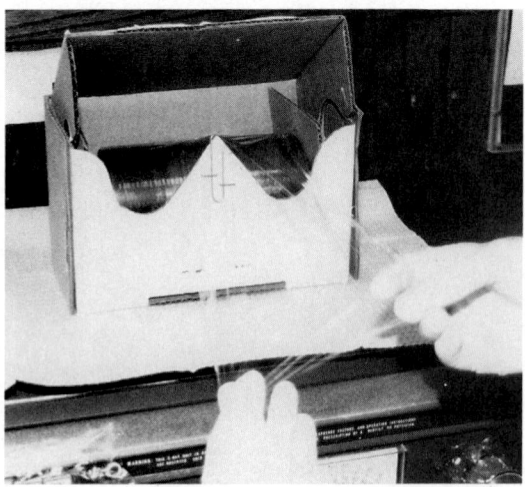

Figure 7-4. Operator dispensing plastic barrier wrap.

methods used to prevent the transmission of microorganisms by the film packet: (1) handling technique, and (2) barrier protection.

1. Exposed film packets should be placed in a container (usually a paper cup or towel) that is outside the radiographic operatory. When all the exposures have been made, the container is carried to the darkroom. In the darkroom, under safelight conditions, the film packets are opened. Take care not to touch the films as they drop onto a paper towel or clean, disinfected surface. Remove and discard the contaminated gloves. The films are then processed.

2. Barrier envelopes are commercially available for film sizes #0, 1, and 2. Film packets from the factory-sealed package are placed and sealed in the plastic envelopes (Fig. 7–5). Film packets sealed in barrier plastic envelopes at the factory are also available commercially (Fig. 7–6). The film packet in the barrier envelope is then exposed. In the darkroom, the barrier envelope is opened, allowing the film packet to drop on a clean surface (Fig. 7–7). Then with clean hands (or new gloves), the film packets are opened and the film is processed.

After the film packet is exposed, it should be wiped dry and carried to the darkroom in a disposable container such as a paper cup or towel. Gloves should always be worn while handling contaminated film packets. All darkroom surfaces that may be contaminated by the film packet should be regularly disinfected.

It has been suggested that exposed film packets be sprayed with disinfectant prior

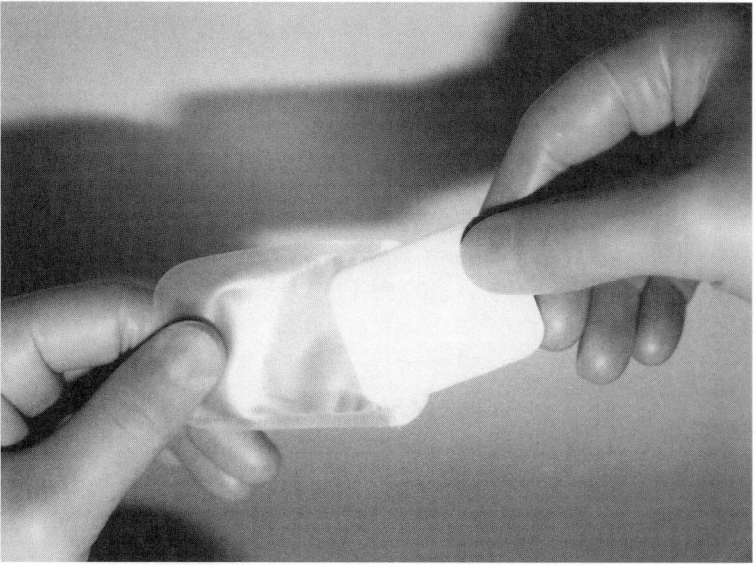

Figure 7–5. Film packet is placed (and then sealed) in a plastic barrier envelope.

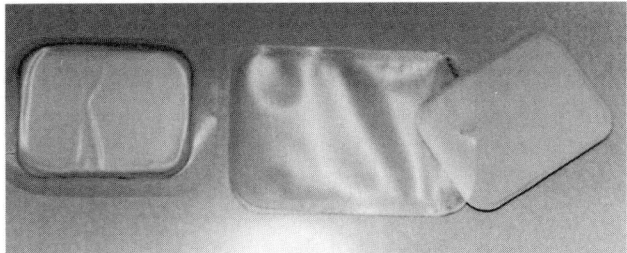

Figure 7–6. Film sealed in barrier packet ready to use from the manufacturer (**left**), and (**right**), barrier envelope with film packet partially inserted.

to processing. This may result in artifacts if moisture reaches the film. Paper film packets would be especially vulnerable.

The following are infection control procedures for the radiography operatory:

1. Surfaces likely to be contaminated should be covered with a barrier material (plastic wrap, aluminum foil, etc).
2. Those surfaces not covered shall be cleaned and disinfected with an EPA-registered, ADA-approved surface disinfectant.
3. Set out necessary supplies (film packets, film holding devices, paper cups, paper towels, etc).
4. Seat and drape patient with lead apron.

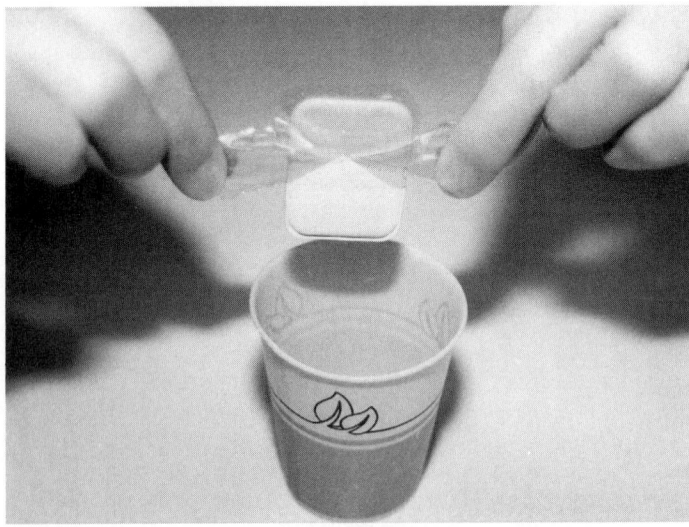

Figure 7–7. Opening the envelope of the barrier packet with a steady pull, allowing the film packet to drop into a clean cup.

5. Wash hands with an antimicrobial skin cleanser and put on gloves.
6. Expose required film packets.
7. Blot film packets dry and place in a film container (disposable paper cup, barrier-lined lead box, etc) outside the operatory.
8. Dismiss the patient (unless other dental procedures are necessary).
9. Dispose of all contaminated supplies and barriers.
10. Clean and disinfect all appropriate surfaces.
11. Remove gloves.
12. Carry film container to the darkroom.

NOTE: If work is interrupted for any reason and you have to leave the room, remove and dispose of your gloves. Wash hands and put on a new pair of gloves before resuming work.

The following are infection control procedures for the darkroom:

1. Put on clean gloves.
2. Work under darkroom conditions.
3. Remove films from film packets by allowing them to drop on a clean disinfected surface (or disposable paper towel). Be careful not to touch the film with your gloved hands because the gloves are contaminated as they touched the film packets.
4. Dispose of the film packet wrappers and film container (paper cup, etc).
5. Remove and dispose of gloves.
6. Process uncontaminated film manually or by automatic processor.
7. Mount radiographs. Gloves should not be worn while mounting radiographs.

NOTE: All contaminated supplies that cannot be disinfected or sterilized for reuse must be disposed of as required by local regulations to minimize health hazards to patients and employees.

The following are infection control procedures while using daylight loaders:
Daylight loaders require special consideration. Two methods are suggested.

1. Use of barrier bags.
   a. Remove film packets from barrier bags.
   b. Use the daylight loader.
2. Nonuse of barrier bags.
   a. Remove gloves and wash hands before using the loader.
   b. Place gloves and contaminated film packets inside the loader through the removable cover.
   c. Put hands into the loader and put on gloves.
   d. Unwrap film packets.
   e. Remove gloves before withdrawing hands.

NOTE: The use of daylight loaders should be discouraged because contamination is difficult to avoid.

CHAPTER SUMMARY

Recognizing the importance of infection control has been a very slow process. It is difficult to comprehend that there was a time when physicians did not consider it necessary to first wash the hands before delivering a child. The rapid spread of new diseases has changed these attitudes and has made infection control a necessity.

Infection control procedures are being studied and additional guidelines are being developed. The use of gloves by all personnel is now mandatory. Face masks and protective eyewear are frequently used. It is a safe assumption that further stringent measures will be proposed.

Unfortunately it is often not possible to determine whether the patient has a contagious disease. Since we cannot be certain, it must be assumed that every patient is potentially infectious. A single standard of patient care is therefore mandatory.

Ideally, all equipment and instruments should be sterilized, but the large size of many of these items makes this impractical.

Each step in the infection control procedures is of equal importance. When these steps are strictly adhered to, everyone benefits.

KEY WORDS

AIDS (acquired immune deficiency syndrome)

Antiseptic

Asepsis

Barrier

Disinfection

Hepatitis B

HIV (human immunodeficiency virus)

Immunization

Infection control

Pathogen

Sanitation

Sepsis

Sterilization

REVIEW QUESTIONS

1. Gloves should be worn when exposing dental radiographs to prevent skin contact with (a) blood, (b) saliva, (c) mucous membranes, (d) all of the above.

2. Which of these terms describes efforts made to reduce disease-producing microorganisms to an acceptable level? (a) sterilization, (b) asepsis, (c) disinfection, (d) sepsis.

3. Which of these items is not suitable for sterilization? (a) film packet, (b) explorer, c) forceps, (d) cutting instruments.

4. The best method for sterilizing instruments that come into contact with saliva or blood is by (a) autoclaving, (b) wiping with alcohol, (c) washing with soap and water, (d) immersing in an ADA-approved surface disinfectant.

5. The responsibility for carrying out infection control measures is the sole responsibility of (a) the patient, (b) the dental assistant, (c) the entire office staff, (d) the person that makes the exposure.

BIBLIOGRAPHY

American Dental Association: Infection control recommendations for the dental office and the dental laboratory. *J Am Dent Assoc* August 1992; pp. 1–8

Brand J, Benson B, Ciola B: American Academy of Oral and Maxillofacial Radiology: Infection control guidelines for dental radiographic procedures. *Oral Surg Oral Med Oral Path* 73:248–249, 1992

Centers for Disease Control: Recommendations for preventing transmission of human immunodeficiency virus and hepatitis B virus to patients during exposure-prone invasive procedures. *Morb Mortal Wkly Rep* **40:**1–9, 1991

Centers for Disease Control: Recommended infection-control practices for dentistry, 1993. *Morb Mortal Wkly Rep* **41:**1–12, 1993

Cottone JA, Terezhalmy GT, Molinari JA: *Practical Infection Control in Dentistry.* Philadelphia, PA: Lea & Febiger, 1991

Council on Dental Materials, Instruments, and Equipment, Council on Dental Practice, and Council on Dental Therapeutics: Infection control recommendations for the dental office and the dental laboratory. *J Am Dent Assoc* **16:**241–248, 1988

Eastman Kodak: *Infection Control in Modern Dental Practice.* Rochester, NY: 1992

Katz JO, Cottone JA, Hardman PK, et al: Infection control protocol for dental radiology. *Gen Dent* **38:**261–264, 1990

Proceedings of the national symposium on hepatitis B and the dental profession. *J Am Dent Assoc* **110:**613–650, 1985

Dental X-ray Films

INTRODUCTION

The quality of dental x-ray films and intensifying screens is continually improving as a result of research and advanced manufacturing techniques. This benefits the patient because exposure times are shortened. The recently introduced E-speed group films are approximately 50 times faster than the films used 40 years ago.

There are two basic types of dental x-ray films: (1) direct-exposure films that are exposed when x-radiation comes into direct contact with the film emulsion, and (2) indirect-exposure films, better known as **screen films,** that are exposed primarily by a fluorescent type of light given off by special emulsion-coated intensifying screens that are positioned between the film and the x-ray source. The great intensity of the fluorescent light permits a significant reduction in the required exposure time. A cassette, generally made of metal and plastic, is required to protect and hold screen film in position during exposure. This is explained in greater detail later in this chapter.

Depending on where the film is to be used—inside or outside the mouth—the film is classified as **intraoral** or **extraoral.** Unfortunately, space limitations seldom permit the use of a cassette inside the mouth. Therefore, the small intraoral films are direct-exposure films. With few exceptions, the majority of extraoral films are screen films—hence, are indirect-exposure films.

COMPOSITION OF DENTAL X-RAY FILMS

Dental x-ray films are very similar to those used in photography; in fact, the first dental radiograph was made on a photographic plate a few weeks after Roentgen announced the discovery of the x-ray. Dr. Otto Walkhoff, given credit for taking the first dental x-ray picture, inserted an ordinary glass photographic plate, protected against light and moisture by an inner wrapping of black paper and an outer wrapping of rubber dam, into his mouth and exposed it. Although film emulsions and film packaging have undergone many changes since that time, the fundamentals have not. The films used in dental radiography are photographic films that have been especially adapted in size, emulsion, film speed, and packaging to dental uses.

Most films used in dental radiography have a thin, flexible, clear or blue-tinted polyester base (Fig. 8–1). This base is about 0.008 in. (0.2 mm) thick—the thickness

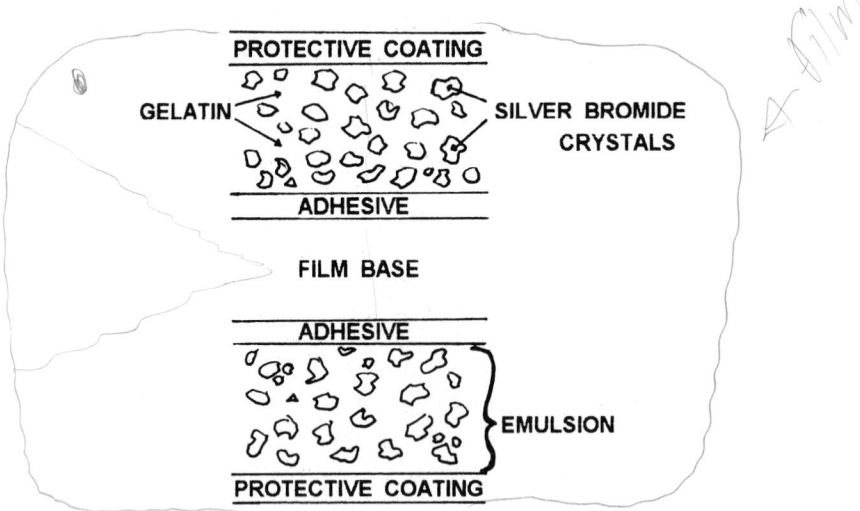

Figure 8–1. Schematic cross-sectional drawing of dental x-ray film. The rigid but still flexible **film base** is coated on both sides with an **emulsion** consisting of **silver bromide** (or other halide) **crystals** embedded in **gelatin.** Each emulsion layer is attached to the base by a thin layer of **adhesive.** The emulsion layers are covered by a supercoating of gelatin to protect the emulsion from scratching and rough handling.

deemed necessary for proper manipulation—and is covered with a photographic emulsion on both sides. This emulsion is composed of gelatin in which crystals of silver halide salts are suspended. **Halides** are compounds of a halogen (fluorine, chlorine, bromine, or iodine) with another element—in photography, silver. Silver is most frequently combined with bromine in dental films. Each emulsion layer is attached to the base by a thin layer of adhesive. The emulsion layers are covered by a supercoating of gelatin to protect the emulsion from scratching and rough handling.

This emulsion is sensitive to light, radiation, heat, chemical fumes, and bending. Great care must be taken not to expose the film accidentally to radiation, extreme heat, chemical fumes, or light. Minor bending can crack the surface of the emulsion, and major bending may loosen the protective wrapping and let in moisture or light.

During radiation exposure the emulsion covering the film base receives and stores energy. This energy is the basis for the film's **latent image,** which does not become visible until the film has been immersed in a sequence of chemicals at a given temperature for a given time. Film processing is explained in Chapter 9.

FILM COVERING AND PACKAGING

The film manufacturer cuts the films to the sizes required in dentistry. Smaller films suitable for intraoral (inside the mouth) radiography are made into what is called a **film packet.** Larger films used in extraoral (outside the mouth) radiography are packed differently.

All intraoral film packets are assembled similarly. The film is first surrounded by a black, lightproof paper; next, a thin sheet of lead foil backing to shield the film from "backscatter" is placed on the side of the film that will be away from the radiation source; an outer wrapping of moisture-resistant paper or plastic completes the assembly. The purpose of the lead foil backing is to absorb scattered radiation, preventing it from striking the film emulsion from the back side of the film (the side away from the tube), thus fogging the film. The lead is embossed with a pattern that becomes visible on the developed x-ray film in the event the packet is accidentally positioned backwards during the exposure.

In most dental offices the film packet is referred to simply as the film. Each film (packet) has two sides—a tube side that faces the tube (radiation source) and a back side away from the source of radiation. The tube side is solid white (either paper or plastic) that is either smooth or slightly pebbly to prevent slippage. It also has a small embossed identifying dot near one of the corners. In intraoral radiography, the tube side of the film faces the lingual surfaces of the teeth to be x-rayed. The dot is also embossed on each film and aids in positioning it on a film mount and in identification of the patient's right and left side.

The back side containing the tab is white or may be color coded. This makes it easy to identify the nontube side. To open the packet, one lifts the end of the flap on the tab and pulls it back gently. The following information is printed on the back side: manufacturer's name, film speed, the number of films in the packet (one or two), a circle or mark indicating the location of the identifying dot, and the legend "opposite side toward tube." When a packet containing two x-ray films is exposed, duplicate radiographs result. This is useful whenever a radiograph is to be sent to another practitioner to whom the patient is referred (the other radiograph remains a part of the patient's permanent record) or whenever a radiograph is needed for legal evidence.

Because several court rulings and a 1982 California law concerning the "patient's right of access to dental records" require the dentist to furnish records (including x-ray films) to the patient on demand, the use of the two-film packets is increasing rapidly.

Depending on the size, intraoral films are packaged 10, 25, 50, 144, or 150 to a box, the most popular being the 144- and 150-film packages. A layer of lead foil surrounds the films inside the box to protect them from damage by stray radiation or chemical fumes during storage.

FILM EMULSION SPEEDS (SENSITIVITY)

Because dental x-ray films are now coated with emulsion on both sides, the main factor that determines the **film speed (film sensitivity)** is the size of the silver halide crystals in the emulsion—the larger the grains, the faster the film speed.

Image definition (sharpness of details) is more distinct when the grains are small. The larger grains used in high-speed films results in a "graininess" that makes the radiograph difficult to interpret.

Film names like *super, ultra,* or *ekta* tell little or nothing about the actual film speed. The standards for film speeds have been outlined by the Council on Research of the American Dental Association. Dental films are given ASA (speed) ratings from A for the slowest through F for the fastest. Reduced demand and laws by some communities prohibiting the use of slower films have recently resulted in the discontinuation of the C film for the US market. Currently only the high-speed D (Kodak UltraSpeed) and the new E-speed films (Kodak Ektaspeed) are used. Although the latter require approximately half the exposure time, many dentists still hestiate to use them in situations where a maximum of diagnostic interpretation is required and because their eyes are accustomed to the D film. Similar problems with image definition occurred when the D films were first introduced. As emulsion technology progresses, these problems with the E-speed films will undoubtedly be resolved. Even faster films will probably be used in the future.

The use of high-speed film has made it possible to reduce exposures to a fraction of the time formerly deemed necessary. This has contributed more to radiation safety than any other factor. Obviously, faster film could not be effectively used until x-ray machines with high-voltage capability and split-second timing devices were available.

INTRAORAL FILMS

Intraoral films are designed principally for use inside the mouth. However, an intraoral film may be used to make an extraoral exposure. One may use any film whenever it can bring about the desired result.

Three types of intraoral films, each named after its most common use, are the periapical, the bitewing, and the occlusal (Fig. 8–2).

Periapical films are used to make a detailed examination of the entire tooth, the periodontal membrane, and the surrounding bone tissues. Four sizes are manufactured (#0, #1, #2, and #3)—the larger the number, the larger the film.

The #0 films are especially designed for small children and thus are often called

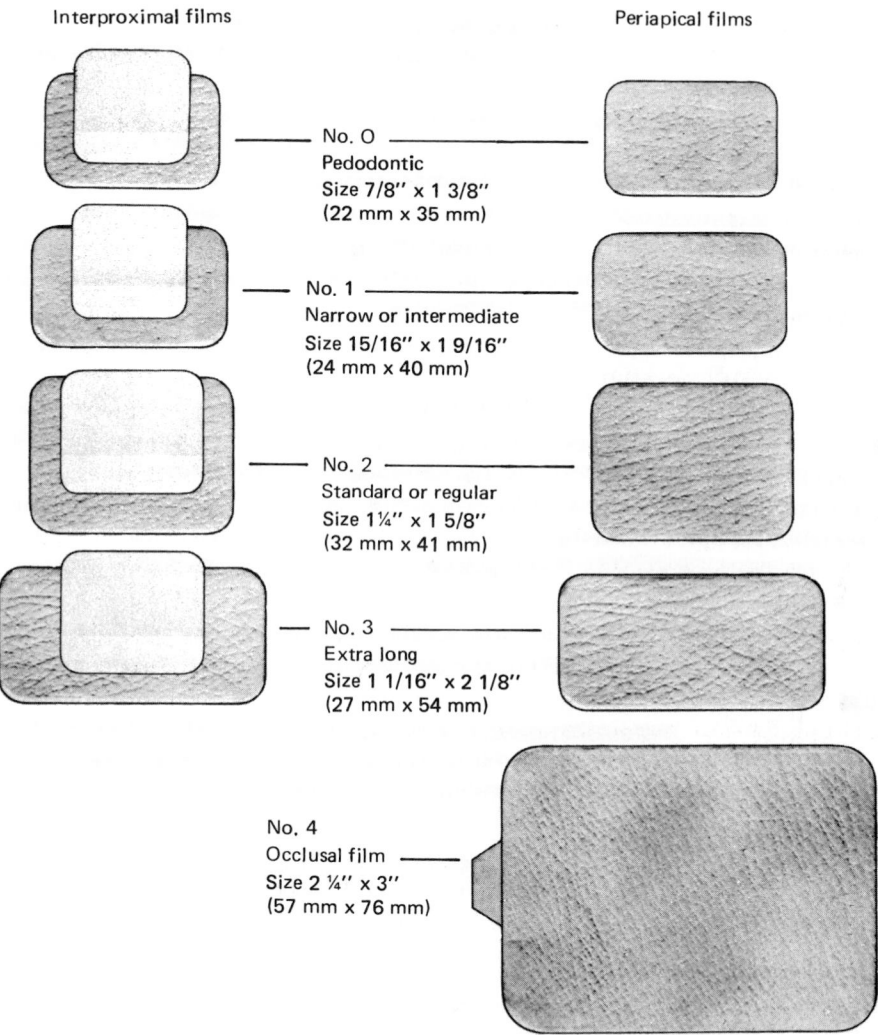

Interproximal films   Periapical films

No. O
Pedodontic
Size 7/8" x 1 3/8"
(22 mm x 35 mm)

No. 1
Narrow or intermediate
Size 15/16" x 1 9/16"
(24 mm x 40 mm)

No. 2
Standard or regular
Size 1¼" x 1 5/8"
(32 mm x 41 mm)

No. 3
Extra long
Size 1 1/16" x 2 1/8"
(27 mm x 54 mm)

No. 4
Occlusal film
Size 2 ¼" x 3"
(57 mm x 76 mm)

Figure 8–2. With the exception of the large occlusal films that are used occlusally or extraorally on occasion, all intraoral films are available in two forms: plain for periapical use or with an attached bite tab for bitewing use. *(Courtesy of Rinn Corporation, Elgin, IL.)*

pedo (from the Greek word *paidos*, "child") or **pedodontic** films. Both the #1 and #2 films are most commonly used on larger children and adults. Use of the narrow #1 film is normally limited to exposing radiographs of the anterior teeth. Although it shows only two or three teeth, this film is ideal for areas where the mouth is narrow and curves a great deal. Its narrowness also makes it the best choice when film holders and the 16-in. (41-cm) target-film technique are used in the anterior areas of the mouth. The wider #2 film is generally referred to as the **standard film**. This film is used in at least 75 percent of all intraoral radiography. The extra-long #3 film, also called the **long bitewing film**, is rarely used as a periapical film.

The **bitewing** films are used to examine the crowns of the teeth, the alveolar crests, and the surfaces of the teeth that touch each other. The exposures made with these films show the coronal portions of both the maxillary (upper) and mandibular (lower) teeth on the same film. They are particularly valuable when the dentist is trying to determine the extent of proximal caries between the teeth.

All bitewing films are available in the same sizes as the periapical films and have the same film numbers (Fig. 8–2). The chief difference is that each film has a flap or tab attached to it on which the patient must bite to hold it in place between the occlusal surfaces of the maxillary and mandibular teeth. These films may be purchased with tabs. A periapical film can be converted to a bitewing film by being slipped into a commercially made cardboard film loop (Fig. 8–3).

The **occlusal** films (#4) are the largest of the intraoral films. The patient normally holds them in position by biting directly on them. These films are ideal for making a rapid survey of a large area of the maxilla, mandible, and floor of the mouth. They can reveal gross pathological lesions, root fragments, bone and tooth fractures, and impacted or supernumerary teeth, and many other conditions. Occlusal films may be used to make a rapid survey of an edentulous (without teeth) mouth or of the mouth of a child who is afraid to hold one of the smaller periapical films tightly against the teeth. The #4 film is the only one for which a cassette is available. Even though the cassette is quite thin, its extra bulk makes it difficult to position inside the mouth and limits its use. Few dental offices use the occlusal film cassette.

Occlusal films are sometimes used extraorally for radiographs of the third molar areas when it is not practical to place a film far back in the mouth or when the patient's face is swollen and opening the mouth is difficult. This versatile film has many

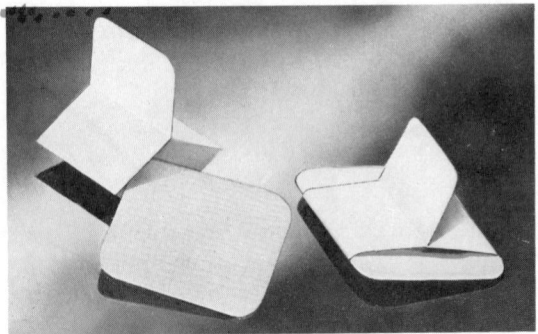

Figure 8–3. Bite loops for bitewing films. Bite loops offer an easy way to convert film from periapical to bitewing use. The loop is spread open, and the desired film is centered into the loop. The tube side of the film must face toward the bite tab and the source of radiation. Bite loops are available in various sizes. *(Courtesy of Rinn Corporation, Elgin, IL.)*

other uses that are considered later in the text. Although only the #4 film is called the occlusal film, periapical films of any size can be used to make occlusal exposures.

X-ray machines taking panoramic films (in which all the teeth are shown on a single exposure) are becoming more common. At present, however, at least 85 percent of all radiographs are intraoral, including only the teeth and the tissues immediately surrounding them. Extraoral films are generally used to examine larger areas and to provide the dentist with supplemental information. Occasionally, as in the case of accidents or fractures or for special situations, extraoral films may be used alone.

EXTRAORAL FILMS

The larger extraoral films are generally packaged 25, 50, or 100 to a box. With the exception of films sold in Ready-Pack envelopes, films are sometimes sandwiched between two pieces of protective paper, and the entire group is wrapped in lead foil for protection. Because these films are designed for extraoral use, they require neither individual lead backing nor moistureproof wrappings. The films vary in size depending on what area is to be radiographed. The most common sizes are 5 by 7 in. (13 by 18 cm), used mainly for lateral views of the jaw, 8 by 10 in. (21 by 26 cm), used for profiles and posteroanterior views, and 5 or 6 in. by 12 in. (13 or 15 cm by 30 cm), used for panoramic radiographs of the entire dentition.

The large extraoral films are used to examine gross structures such as the skull, the maxilla and mandible in relationship to each other, or specific areas of the facial bones or the temporomandibular joint. They can show the extent of a fracture, growth, or malignancy and can be used to study jaw development, tooth eruption, or any of a long list of normal and abnormal conditions. Except for the panoramic radiographs, which are rapidly gaining in popularity, extraoral films are not frequently used by general practitioners. Their major users are orthodontists, prosthodontists, and oral surgeons.

Orthodontists use facial profile radiographs (*cephalometric*, meaning "measuring the head") periodically to record, measure, and compare changes in growth of the bones and the teeth.

The prosthodontists use facial profile radiographs to record the contour of the lips and face and the relationship of the teeth before removal. This helps them to construct prosthetic appliances that look natural.

Oral surgeons use extraoral radiographs extensively to determine the location and extent of fractures and to locate impacted teeth, abnormalities, malignancies, and injuries to the temporomandibular joint.

The varieties of extraoral film are too numerous to discuss in detail. They vary in size and intended usage. Most extraoral films can be processed automatically, whereas others must be processed manually. The dentist must determine which type of film is most suitable to the needs of the patient and is compatible with the equipment in the office.

Advances in emulsion and processing technology are so rapid that the user must be extremely alert to use the correct combination of extraoral film, intensifying screen, darkroom illumination, and processing technique. Failure to do this will lead to very inferior results.

The large extraoral films are classified as screen and nonscreen films. The overwhelming majority of these are **screen films,** so called because they are used in a cassette with two intensifying screens. All screen films are more sensitive to blue, violet, and green fluorescent light—formed inside the cassette by the action of the x-rays on the crystals of the emulsion that coats the intensifying screens—than to x-radiation. This fluorescence increases enormously the amount of illumination inside the tightly closed cassette, thus drastically reducing the exposure time.

The **nonscreen film,** by way of contrast, is exposed directly to x-rays. It can be placed within a cardboard exposure holder or a cassette without intensifying screens. It is also available in a packaged form (Ready-Pack) that does not require loading under darkroom conditions. The use of nonscreen film should be discouraged because of the long exposure times required. Very little nonscreen film is being used today.

CASSETTES

Cassettes hold and protect the film for which they are designed. Most are rigid and flat, but the ones used to make panoramic radiographs may be rigid or flexible, flat or curved. Most cephalometric exposures use a cassette measuring 8 by 10 in. (20 by 25 cm) whereas a cassette measuring 5 by 12 in. (12.5 by 30 cm) is commonly used for panoramic exposures.

A typical cassette (Fig. 8–4) is constructed of two vinyl-covered aluminum panels

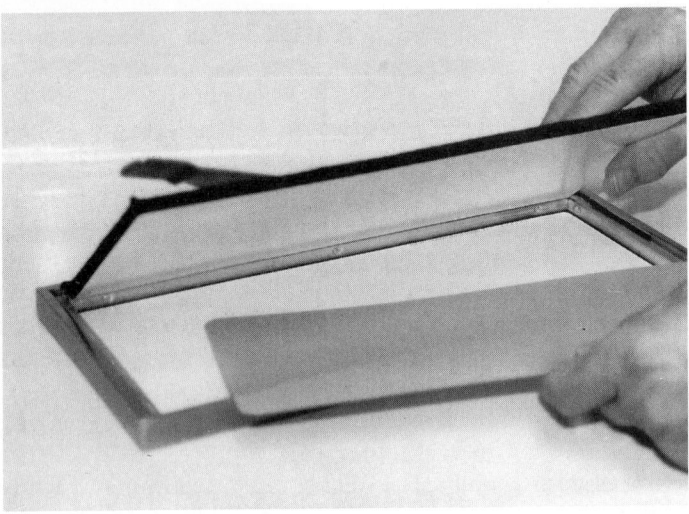

Figure 8–4. View of open extraoral cassette. The film is placed between the intensifying screens. The film must be loaded or unloaded in the darkroom with special subdued light.

mounted on a polyurethane frame and joined together with a hinge. The materials in the panel on the tube side (the source of the radiation) offer little resistance to the passage of the x-rays. Cassettes contain an intensifying screen in each panel. A thin layer of metal in the back panel absorbs radiation. A hinge or spring-type clasp is used to close the cassette and prevent light leaks.

The protective paper surrounding the film must be removed when the screen film is placed in the cassette; otherwise the blue, purple, or green light rays emanating from the screens cannot reach the film surface. Closing the cassette tightly is important to obtain screen-to-film contact. When the contact is not closed, it causes screen lag—an afterglow—which creates a blurry area on the film. It is also important to remember that the tube side of the cassette must face toward the head or face of the patient because in all extraoral procedures, the film is outside the mouth and the x-rays enter the patient from the opposite side.

An **intensifying screen** is a smooth cardboard or plastic sheet coated with minute fluorescent crystals mixed into a suitable binding medium. It produces the desired image in a shorter (1/15 to 1/40) exposure time than is possible with nonscreen film in a cardboard exposure holder. It is based on the principle that crystals of certain salts—in

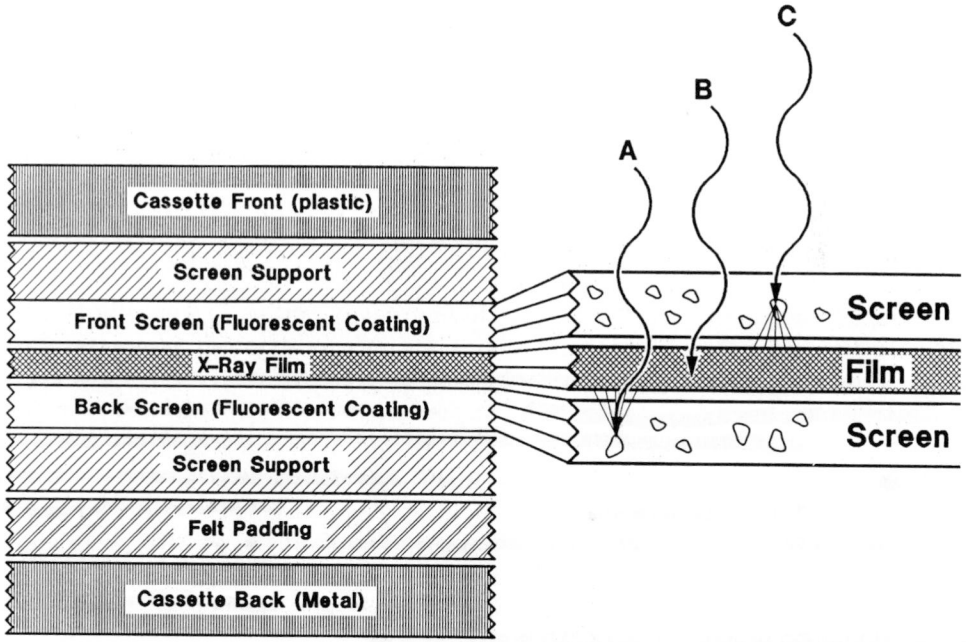

Figure 8–5. Cross section of cassette and diagram showing the effect of x-ray and fluorescent light on the film. X-ray **A** strikes a crystal in the screen behind the film, producing light, which then forms latent images in the silver bromide crystal of the film. X-ray **B** strikes a silver bromide crystal in the film, forming a latent image. X-ray **C** strikes a crystal in the screen in front of the film, producing light, which then forms latent images in the silver bromide crystals of the film.

this case, calcium tungstate, barium strontium sulfate, or rare-earth phosphors—will fluoresce and emit energy in the form of blue, ultraviolet, or green light when they absorb x-rays. Each of these fluorescent crystals, also called **phosphors,** gives off blue, ultraviolet, or green radiations that vary in intensity according to the x-rays in that part of the image. As already observed, screen film is more sensitive to this type of light than to radiation. When the film is sandwiched tightly between two intensifying screens, the x-rays cause the crystals on the screens to fluoresce and return the emitted light to the emulsion to intensify the radiographic image (Fig. 8–5).

The difference in the sensitivity of intensifying screens depends on the size of the crystals, the type of phosphor used, and the thickness of the emulsion. The conventional calcium tungstate screens give off a blue to violet fluorescent light, whereas the new rare-earth phosphor screens give off a green light when energized by x-rays. Several speeds of screens are available. One must be extremely careful to combine the correct film and screen. Some films are sensitive to blue light, whereas others produce best results when exposed to green fluorescent light.

DUPLICATING FILM

Duplicating film, used to reproduce radiographs, is a type of photographic film that appears similar to x-ray film but is exposed by the action of infrared and ultraviolet light rather than x-rays. Only one side of the film is coated with emulsion. During the printing process, the duplicating film is superimposed with its emulsion side toward the radiograph that is to be copied. This process is explained in Chapter 9.

FILM PROTECTION AND STORAGE

As all dental films are extremely sensitive to high temperatures, chemical fumes, and stray radiation, precautions for safeguarding films must be followed. Ideally, all unexposed film should be stored at 50 to 70 degrees Fahrenheit (10 to 21 degrees Celsius) and 30 to 50 percent relative humidity, in an area that is properly shielded, preferably with lead. All intraoral film should be placed on edge so that the expiration date can be seen. The oldest film should be used first. The extraoral films are packaged with or without interleaving paper folders, hermetically sealed, and enclosed in an outer cardboard box that is dated and shows the type of film and speed. Because there are so many types of extraoral films, this information should be considered before selecting a film and removing it from its box. Unlike intraoral films, the extraoral ones can only be removed from their boxes under safelight conditions.

Normally only a small amount of film is kept near the x-ray machine. A lead-lined dispenser or film safe can be placed near the operator. The only time that the film does not need to be protected from radiation is when it is being exposed.

Film dispensers and storage boxes vary in size and complexity. The simplest storage box is a lead-lined container with a removable lead-lined lid. Slightly more complex is a wall-mounted radiation-resistant container. Films are loaded from the top and stacked vertically into a film chute that holds about 150 single or double film packets. A dispensing mechanism delivers one film out of the slot at the bottom of the dispenser each time a plunger is pressed and released. This type of dispenser is available with chutes to fit the most commonly used films. A more complex dispenser is designed to handle #0, #1, and #2 films simultaneously. It contains an additional storage area for bitewing and occlusal film.

A small lead-lined safe or receptacle may be used to protect exposed film from additional exposure while other radiographs are being made on the same patient. Such receptacles usually hold a maximum of 24 to 30 films. Infection control procedures should be followed to prevent contamination when using these safes.

FILM REQUIREMENTS

There is no hard and fast rule for the number of films required to make a full-mouth set of radiographs. One rule is to use the largest films that can be placed effectively and tolerated by the patient. This will enable the operator to complete the survey with a minimum of exposures. However, the operator should remember that because of the curvature of the mouth, normally only two or three teeth—and occasionally only one tooth—can be viewed on any single film without distortion. Normally, one places the films in the mouth so that each overlaps the next, to show some of the same structures.

A minimum of 14 periapical films are required—more if the narrow #1 films are used in the anterior regions—for a full-mouth survey of adults with all their teeth. Such a survey includes a minimum of two bitewing films. The ideal full-mouth series consists of 18 to 21 films.

For children, the type of film varies with their age, size, and emotional stability. Generally such examinations include two bitewing films and at least ten #0 periapical films.

Conditions may require more or less film for any examination. For example, development of x-rays may reveal unusual or unexpected conditions that make more exposures necessary. The dentist, the operator, or both determine the number and type of films to be used and the duration of the exposures. To save time and embarrassment, the operator should always check the film safe to verify that a sufficient quantity of film of the required size or sizes is available before bringing the patient into the x-ray room.

CHAPTER SUMMARY

There are several methods of classifying dental x-ray films: (1) by method of exposure, whether directly by x-rays or indirectly by both x-rays and fluorescent light; (2) by the method used to position the film, intraorally or extraorally; (3) by the function that the film is to perform inside the mouth, namely periapical, bitewing, or occlusal; (4) by the function that the film is to perform outside the mouth, that is, cephalometric, panoramic, and so forth; and (5) by size and film speed grouping.

All x-ray films have a polyester base that is coated with a gelatin emulsion containing silver bromide (halide) crystals that absorb the energy of the x-rays during the exposure to form the latent image. The grain size is an important factor in determining the sensitivity (speed) of the film. The larger the grains used, the faster the film speed. However, a greater degree of definition (sharpness) of the image results when smaller grains are used in the emulsion. Radiation safety is achieved by shortening the patient's exposure time through the use of faster films; however, the penalty may be a small loss of diagnostic detail. The amount and type of information required by the dentist in each individual case determines the type of film to be selected. ASA film speeds range from A for the slowest through F for the fastest. Currently only D- and E-speed films are available in the United States.

Intraoral films vary in size to suit the needs of children, adolescents, and adults. Three types are used: periapical, to examine the entire tooth and surrounding tissues; bitewing, to disclose proximal tooth surfaces; and occlusal, to survey larger areas.

Extraoral films are much larger and, with the exception of Ready-Pack, are not enclosed in protective wrapping. These films are used for panoramic, cephalometric, and lateral jaw exposures, and so forth, and, with the exception of Ready-Pack film, must be placed in cassettes. Most cassettes contain two intensifying screens that are coated with an emulsion containing phosphors that glow when energized by x-rays and produce a blue, violet, or green fluorescent light that acts on the film that is sandwiched between intensifying screens in the panels of the cassette. The recently developed rare-earth phosphor screens (sensitive to green light) are more efficient in using the x-rays than are calcium tungstate screens. This interaction between the x-rays and the phosphors increases the light intensity within the cassette and makes shorter exposures possible.

All x-ray films are sensitive to light and radiation, chemical fumes, heat, and handling pressure. Care must be exercised in storing and in handling the film during and after exposure.

KEY WORDS

Bitewing radiograph

Cassette

Duplicating film

Extraoral

Film sensitivity

Film speed

Halide

Intensifying screen

Intraoral

Latent image

Nonscreen film

Occlusal radiograph

Pedodontic film

Periapical radiograph

Phosphors

Screen film

REVIEW QUESTIONS

1. Which of these is contained in the film emulsion used for dental radiographs? (a) barium sulfate, (b) calcium tungstate, (c) silver bromide, (d) silver nitrate.

2. What is the function of the lead foil in the x-ray packet? (a) moisture protection, (b) protection against backscatter, (c) protection against central ray, (d) protection against fluorescence.

3. Which of these films has the greatest sensitivity? (a) B-speed, (b) C-speed, (c) D-speed, (d) E-speed.

4. Which of these film packages is the largest? (a) periapical film, (b) bitewing film, (c) occlusal film, (d) pedodontic film.

5. Which of these films is best suited when the dentist requests a radiograph of a specific tooth and its surrounding structures? (a) panoramic, (b) occlusal, (c) cephalometric, (d) periapical.

6. What term describes the crystals used in the emulsion on intensifying screens? (a) halides, (b) phosphors, (c) sulfates, (d) bromides.

7. Which type of film is used to copy a radiograph? (a) duplicating film, (b) screen film, (c) nonscreen film, (d) x-ray film.

8. What is the ideal storage temperature for x-ray films? (a) under 32°F (0°C), (b) from 32 to 50°F (0 to 10°C), (c) from 50 to 70°F (10 to 21°C), (d) from 70 to 80°F (21 to 26.5°C).

9. Which of these is a screen film? (a) occlusal, (b) bitewing, (c) panoramic, (d) periapical.

10. Which of these films can produce an image with the greatest degree of definition? (a) duplicating film, (b) D-speed film, (c) pedodontic film, (d) E-speed film.

11. The three types of intraoral films are the _periapical_, the _bitewing_, and the _occlusal_.

12. Which of these films use the shortest exposure time? (a) nonscreen film, (b) screen film.

BIBLIOGRAPHY

Manny EF, Carlson KC, McClean PM, et al: *An Overview of Dental Radiology.* Washington, DC: National Center for Health Care Technology (FDA/BRH), 1980

Eastman Kodak: *Exposure and Processing for Dental Radiography.* Rochester, NY: 1993

Dental X-ray Film Processing

INTRODUCTION

The image on a dental x-ray film cannot be seen or evaluated diagnostically by the dentist until the film has been processed. Most processing is accomplished in a darkroom equipped with special lights. A sequence of steps involving developing and fixing chemicals must be rigidly followed. The technique is simple, but even the smallest error can spoil the end result.

At present three methods are used: (1) the traditional manual processing, still followed in many offices; (2) the chair-side, rapid processing, favored by many endodontists and oral surgeons as an adjunct to routine processing techniques; and (3) the newer automatic processing, used in most offices and clinics.

FUNDAMENTALS OF FILM PROCESSING

Radiographic films are extremely sensitive to light and can be processed only in a properly equipped darkroom or in special processing units that are equipped with light-obstructive devices. Processing transforms the **latent image** (*latent* means "hidden"), which is produced when the x-ray photons are absorbed by the **silver halide crystals** in the emulsion, into a visible, stable image by means of chemicals.

The processing of radiographic film is based on five simple facts: (1) compounds of silver and halogens are sensitive to x-radiation; (2) a radiographic film consists of a polyester base covered with emulsion of silver halide crystals suspended in a solution of gelatin; (3) the function of the gelatin is to keep the silver halide crystals evenly suspended over the base; (4) the gelatin will not dissolve in cold water but swells, thus exposing the silver halide crystals to the chemicals in the developing solution; and (5) the gelatin shrinks as it dries, leaving a smooth surface that becomes the radiograph.

During the chemical processing a selective reduction of the exposed silver halide crystals takes place. **Selective reduction** means that the nonmetallic elements, the halides, are removed. Only the exposed silver remains (Fig. 9–1).

The exposed silver halide crystals on the film are reduced to black metallic silver when immersed in the **developer** for five minutes at 68 degrees Fahrenheit (20 degrees Celsius). A predetermined time–temperature cycle is used. The unexposed halide crystals (in film areas opposite metallic or dense structures that absorb and prevent the passage of x-ray photons) are unaffected at this time. After brief rinsing (20 to 30 seconds) to remove any developer remaining on the film, the film is immersed in the fixer

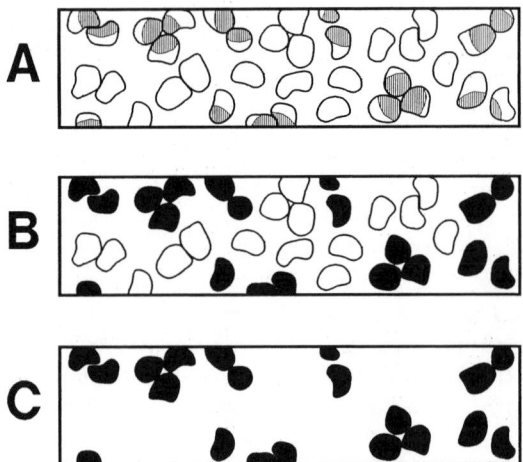

Figure 9–1. Cross section of dental x-ray film emulsion. **(A)** X-rays strike silver bromide crystals forming latent image sites (shown in gray). **(B)** After development, crystals struck by x-rays (latent image sites) reduced to black metallic silver. **(C)** Fixer removes unexposed, undeveloped crystals leaving the black metallic silver.

for 10 minutes. The unexposed halide crystals are removed during this interval, leaving behind only the metallic silver, which is not disturbed by the chemicals of the fixer solution. After the film is completely fixed, it is washed in running water for a minimum of 20 minutes to remove any remaining traces of the chemicals of the fixer and then is allowed to dry.

Thus, the images on the film are made up of microscopic grains of black metallic silver. The amount of silver deposited will vary with the thickness of the tissues penetrated. Where only soft tissues were between the source of the radiation and the emulsion, the film will be black. Where passage of x-rays was blocked by metal fillings or restorations, the film will be white.

As we have already seen in Chapter 4, the amount of light transmitted through the film varies according to the thickness of tissues penetrated by the radiation and accounts for the shades of black, gray, and white. Dark areas are spoken of as **radiolucent** and light areas as **radiopaque.**

DARKROOM AND EQUIPMENT

Until recently, a darkroom was absolutely necessary for processing films. Now one can do "chair-side processing" in normal light with certain rapid-processing units and daylight-loader–equipped automatic processors. However, a darkroom is still required to load and unload the cassettes, to process certain films, and to do manual processing if the automatic processing equipment malfunctions.

In some offices the darkroom is a large, well-equipped room; in others it is just an afterthought. Certainly the size and equipment of the darkroom will contribute little to the production of good radiographs if exposure or processing is poor, but a well-equipped room makes good, standardized processing much easier. As with all things, some darkroom equipment is essential, and some is merely nice to have.

Cleanliness and orderliness are essential. Because the films are handled in almost complete darkness, usually with just a very dim safelight, all needed materials must be within easy reach, and the person doing the processing must know where each item is kept. The workbench must be absolutely free of water, dust, chemicals, or any other substance that can come in contact with unwrapped film. Particular care must be taken not to splash chemical solutions or water on the bench when moving films from one insert of the processing tank to the other. A messy darkroom is not only unpleasant to work in but can stain and damage clothes. More seriously, dirty darkrooms can produce worthless radiographs.

The ideal darkroom is the result of good planning. It is large enough to meet the requirements of the office, is arranged with ample work space, is equipped with the correct types of lighting, is well ventilated, and has adequate storage space for films and radiographic supplies. The darkroom should be an adequate distance from the nearest x-ray machine and should not be used as a general storage area, especially not for materials that produce dust or give off chemical fumes.

The following items are absolutely essential in the darkroom: (1) a normal electric light for use when the films are not being processed, (2) a darkroom safelight, (3) a processing tank, (4) a utility sink, (5) racks for film hangers for holding and drying the radiographs, (6) brushes to clean the tank, (7) paddles to stir the solutions, (8) drip pans to place under wet hangers, (9) storage racks for the film hangers, (10) a timer, (11) two thermometers, and (12) a wastebasket or waste disposal chute. Not essential but nice to have are (1) an electric fan or film dryer, (2) additional safelights—preferably with foot control switches, (3) a built-in view box or illuminator, (4) controls for regulating the temperature of the water entering the processing tank, (5) a safety "in-use" light or lock on the door, and (6) ample storage facilities for films and radiographic supplies.

DARKROOM ILLUMINATION

The control of darkroom illumination is important because any light, whether white or filtered safelight, can blacken the film or cause it to have a fogged appearance, thus diminishing or destroying its diagnostic value. Although many darkrooms are painted black, if they are completely sealed to white light, a lighter-colored paint should be used, as it will reflect more usable safelight than black paint. Felt strips may have to be installed around the door or any other area where a light leak is discovered. Fluorescent overhead lighting should not be used because of its afterglow.

Two forms of illumination are desirable in the darkroom: (1) a white ceiling light that can be used when cleaning tanks, filling them with chemicals, or performing darkroom housekeeping chores; and (2) a safelight that gives off a form of light to which the film is virtually insensitive. The **safelight** provides enough light in the darkroom to perform the minimum essential activities without exposing or damaging the film. Filters function to protect the film from light. A variety of safelights with different types of filters are available. Some are designed to work best with intraoral films, others with extraoral films, and others are universal and can be used for both.

Darkroom users must not only be familiar with the chemical solutions and the type of film and safelight filter used, they must also be aware that the emulsion can be damaged by prolonged exposure even to filtered light. For example, the Kodak GBX-2 can only be used in manual processing, provided that the film handling is limited to 2 1/2 minutes under safelight conditions (Fig. 9–2). The type of safelight required is indicated in the film processing instructions or printed in bold type on the outside of the film package.

Other factors, in addition to the film emulsion, that influence the degree to which a film may become fogged while exposed to a safelight are (1) the wattage of the bulb; (2) the distance between the lamp and the film—the rule is 2 1/4 watts per foot (0.3 m) and a 4-ft (1.2-m) minimum distance; (3) the color of the filter; (4) the condition of the filter—it must be free of scratches; and (5) the length of time that the film is subjected to safelight exposure—any exposure over 2 1/2 minutes is likely to fog the radiograph.

Some darkrooms are equipped with wall-type view boxes or illuminators. These emit considerable light, and care must be taken not to unwrap films or leave the cover of the processing tank off when they are turned on. If the darkroom can be locked, this should be done before processing is started to prevent anyone from entering and inad-

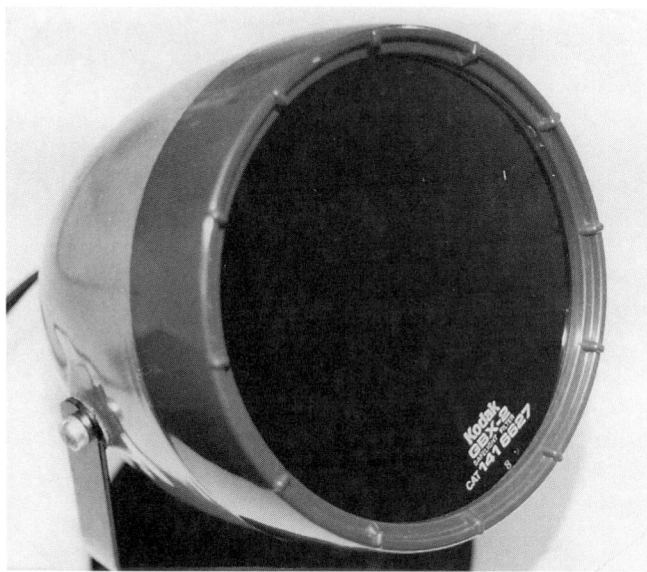

Figure 9–2. This bracket-type lamp can provide either direct or indirect illumination. It can be equipped with either a MORLITE 2 or a GBX-2 Safelight Filter, depending on the types of x-ray film to be handled under this illumination. The safelight lamp should be located at least 4 ft (1.2 m) from the nearest working surface and equipped with a bulb wattage of either 15 or 7 1/2 watts, depending on the type of emulsion to be handled.

vertently spoiling the films through exposure to light; otherwise, the "in-use" light must be turned on.

PROCESSING TANKS

Several types and sizes of processing tanks are available. Most used in dental offices are large enough to accept an 8-by-10 in. (20-by-25 cm) extraoral film. They hold 1 gal (3.8 L) of developer and 1 gal (3.8 L) of fixer in separate compartments, with a large central area in between for rinsing and washing the films (Fig. 9–3).

The processing tank may be made in one piece or with two removable inserts. It may be made entirely of hard rubber, have a hard rubber core with stainless-steel inserts, or be made entirely of stainless steel with welded and polished joints to prevent a reaction with the processing chemicals. Most tanks have removable inserts to facilitate cleaning, and a small hole at the bottom of the insert lets the solution drain into the central compartment when a small rubber plug is pulled out. The central section is connected to the water intake and to the drain. When the tank is in use, fresh water circulates continuously. An overflow pipe keeps the level of the water constant when the tank is full. Some tanks are equipped with a temperature control device, a water-

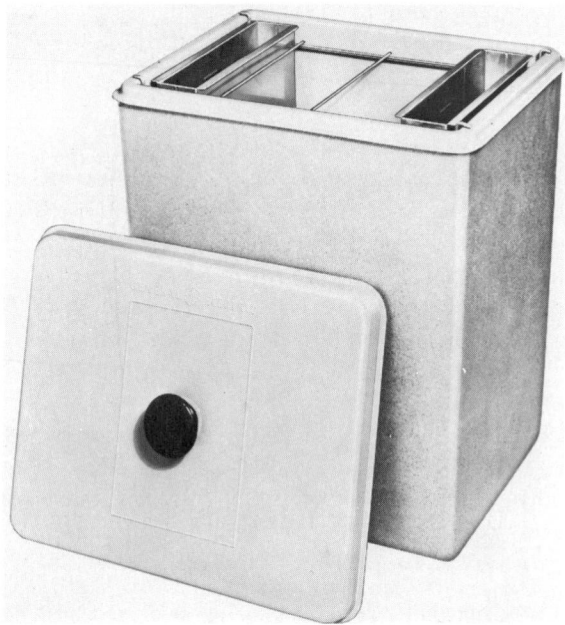

Figure 9–3. Developing tank with removable inserts. The central compartment holds the rinse water. Generally the insert on the left is filled with the developer solution, and the insert on the right is filled with the fixer solution. *(Courtesy of General Electric Company, Medical Systems Division.)*

mixing valve that mixes the hot and cold water in the pipes to any desired temperature. A close-fitting lightproof cover completes the tank assembly.

CARE OF TANKS AND PROCESSING SOLUTIONS

The operator should always wear a protective plastic or rubber apron when cleaning the tank or changing the solutions. The tank and its inserts should be scrubbed each time the solutions are changed. A solution made up of 1.5 oz (45 mL) of commercial hydrochloric acid, 1 qt (0.95 L) of cold water, and 3 qt (2.85 L) of warm water is sufficient to remove the deposits that frequently form on the walls of 1 gal (3.8 L) inserts. To clean the processing tank, first pull the plug and drain the inserts; then thoroughly scrub all portions of the tank, inserts, and cover. Never use cleansing powders, as they will leave a residue that contaminates the processing chemicals. If the inserts appear to be coated, fill them with acid-cleaning solution and let them soak for half an hour; then drain out the cleaning solution and rinse them with plenty of water. All parts of the tank, including the cover, should be wiped clean before the plugs are replaced and the inserts filled.

After the developer and the fixer are poured into the inserts until the level of the solutions reaches a mark on the side of the insert that indicates the full level (about 1 in. from the top), the central compartment must be filled with water. When that is done, the processing tank is ready for use. Most operators drain the central compartment at the end of each working day.

Whenever possible, the processing tank should remain covered to prevent the possibility of oxidation, evaporation, or contamination of the processing solutions. The developer especially is subject to oxidation in the presence of air and loses some of its effectiveness. **Oxidation** is the union of a substance—in this case, the developer—with the oxygen in the air. The cover should be removed only when adding solutions to the proper level, when checking the temperature of the developer or the water, and when inserting, removing, or changing the film hangers from one compartment or insert to another. The cover should be replaced immediately after any of these steps is completed.

Chemical contamination is an ever-present threat in film processing. Stirring paddles and thermometers must be cleaned after each use. Film hangers must be thoroughly rinsed to prevent chemicals from sticking to the handles before they are dried and ready for attaching the film. Care must be taken not to rotate the cover when it is removed, thereby causing a drop or two of condensed developer to fall into the fixer, or vice versa. The operator can minimize this threat by labeling the inserts and the cover and by always refilling the inserts with the same solution that was originally placed in them and making sure that the part of the cover over the developer is always placed there. Never use the same stirring paddle in both the developer and fixer without first cleaning it thoroughly. If the paddles are made of wood, separate ones must be used for each solution to prevent cross-contamination.

X-RAY PROCESSING SOLUTIONS

As already indicated, the chief processing chemicals are in the **developer,** which is slightly alkaline, and in the **fixer**, which is slightly acidic. Both the developer and fixer contain four constituents, each of which makes a specific contribution to the developing or fixing process. The preferred vehicle for mixing these ingredients is distilled water; however, tap water is often used, provided it is known to contain no interfering chemicals, especially when run through filters.

The main purpose of the developer is to convert the exposed silver halide crystals into metallic silver grains. Four constituents are required to accomplish this: (1) a **developing agent** (also called a reducing agent), (2) a **preservative,** (3) an **activator** (also called an alkalizer), and (4) a **restrainer.**

The **developing agent** reduces the exposed silver bromide crystals to metallic silver but has no effect on the unexposed crystals at recommended time–temperatures. It contains two chemicals—hydroquinone and elon. The hydroquinone works slowly but steadily to build up density and contrast in the film, while the elon works fast to bring out the gray shades (contrast) of the image. Although both chemicals are more active at higher rather than lower temperatures, the hydroquinone becomes extremely active when the temperature of the solution is raised and is inactive at lower temperatures.

Therefore, the temperature of the developer is critical. Thus, the higher the temperature, the less time is required to develop the film.

The **preservative,** sodium sulfite, protects the developing agents by slowing down the rapid oxidation rate of the developer.

The **activator,** usually sodium carbonate, provides the necessary alkaline medium required by the developing agents. It also softens and swells the gelatin, letting more of the exposed silver bromide crystals come into contact with the developing agents.

The **restrainer,** potassium bromide, slows down the action of both development agents and inhibits the tendency of the solution to chemically fog the film.

The function of the **fixer** is to (1) stop further development—thereby establishing the image permanently on the film; (2) remove (dissolve) the undeveloped silver halide crystals (those that were not exposed to x-rays); and (3) harden (fix) the emulsion. Four constituents are required to accomplish this: (1) a **fixing agent,** (2) a **preservative,** (3) a **hardening agent,** and (4) an **acidifier.** The result of this process is a negative (radiographs are negatives, whereas photographs are positives) that shows a graduation of light and dark corresponding to the layers of microscopic silver deposited.

The **fixing (clearing) agent,** sodium thiosulfate, also known as "hypo" or hyposulfate of sodium, removes all unexposed and any remaining undeveloped silver bromide crystals from the emulsion.

The **preservative,** sodium sulfite (the same chemical as used in the developer), slows down the rate of oxidation and prevents the deterioration of the hypo and the precipitation of sulfur.

The **hardening agent,** potassium alum, shrinks and hardens the emulsion. This hardening continues until the film is dry, thus protecting it from abrasion.

The **acidifier,** acetic acid, provides the acid medium required to neutralize the alkali of the developer and stop further development.

Two other chemicals are sometimes used in processing radiographs—a wetting agent and a cutting reducer. A **wetting agent** (a form of detergent) reduces the surface tension of the film. A teaspoon of wetting agent added to the developer will hasten film development. Moreover, the fully processed film will dry much faster if, after being properly washed, it is immersed for one minute in a pan of water to which a few drops of wetting agent have been added.

A **cutting reducer** is a combination of potassium ferrocyanide and fixer. It can be used in an emergency to lighten films that have been accidentally overexposed or overdeveloped. The use of a cutting reducer is indicated only when the film is too dark to diagnose and it is impossible or inadvisable to retake the film. Because much of the film density is lost when a reducer is used, this procedure should be attempted only as a last resort. The procedure varies slightly with the brand. Instructions should be carefully checked.

The chemicals used in development and fixation may be obtained in powder form, ready mixed in jugs, or in liquid concentrate form. The concentrate form (Fig. 9–4) is used in most offices. It is easy to store, is fresh, and can be prepared in a few minutes. In many cities, regular tank cleaning and solution-changing services are available.

The processing solutions should be changed every 4 weeks or more often if the

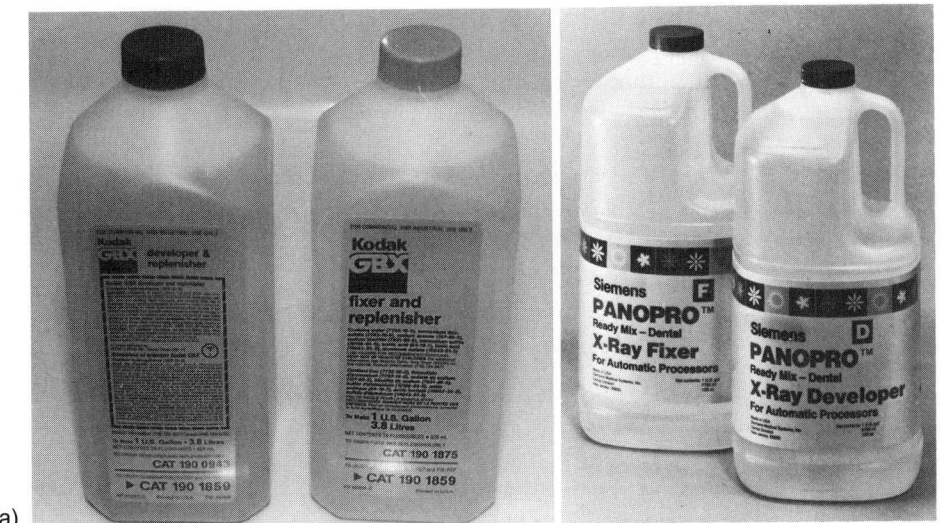

(a)   (b)

Figure 9–4. Processing chemicals. **(a)** Typical concentrate forms of developer and fixer for manual processing. Each bottle is mixed with sufficient water to make 1 gal (3.8 L) of solution, which is the normal capacity of an insert. **(b)** Panopro ready-mix developer and fixer for automatic processors. *(Courtesy of Siemens Medical Systems, Dental Division, Iselin, NJ.)*

workload is extremely heavy. Four things affect the useful life of the solution: (1) the original quality or concentration of the solution, determined by how carefully the proportions are measured and how the solution is stirred; (2) the freshness of the solution; (3) the number of films that are processed in it; and (4) contamination of the chemicals.

A small but significant amount of developer is lost daily through evaporation and by drops of developer adhering to the film surfaces and the film hanger as they are transferred to the rinse compartment. The loss in the fixer is smaller; actually, some dilution takes place by rinse water clinging to the film and hanger when they are transferred to the fixer. Since some fixer is lost when the film hanger is subsequently removed, these factors about balance. The main loss of the fixer is from evaporation; the gradual dilution weakens the solution.

The strength and level of the solutions can be maintained by daily or periodic replenishment, the addition of a superconcentrated solution of developer or fixer (**replenisher**). Depending on whether the chemicals are primarily intended for use in manual, rapid, or automatic processors, special hardeners may have been added to facilitate the transportation of the films through the roller systems of the automatic units. Processing solutions are now available in which the replenisher is already added to the developer and to the fixer. The user must determine which of the many chemicals available is best suited for the type of film and processing technique used.

The first sign of developer exhaustion is a light film with a thin image. Fixer exhaustion can be recognized when the film has not cleared in 2 minutes and still shows a milky coating.

One hazard of permitting the solution levels to drop is that there may not be sufficient developer or fixer to cover all of the films attached to the uppermost clips of the film hanger. This may go unnoticed in the dim light of the darkroom and result in a partial image on the radiograph. This will not happen if the inserts are topped off daily.

Sometimes technicians overexpose or overdevelop the film when the solutions become weak. They should not, because overexposure subjects everyone to more radiation than necessary. Overdevelopment is inaccurate and results in a loss of diagnostic film quality.

MANUAL PROCESSING PROCEDURES

First a word of caution concerning cross-contamination. In many dental offices the x-ray processing procedures have been aseptically neglected. One should assume any patient could be the carrier of an infectious disease. Exposed dental film packets contaminated with saliva should be placed in a plastic bag or cup and carried to the darkroom. Never carry film in uniform pockets. Gloves should be worn as needed during processing procedures to prevent cross-contamination. When opening the film packets, the wrappings should be placed in a plastic bag or cup, or on a paper towel. Upon completion, all waste materials should be disposed of properly (see Chapter 7).

The completion of the radiograph involves preparation for processing, film processing, and final procedures. Each of these involves a number of steps.

The key to processing dental radiographs is adequate preparation. Preparation includes (1) filling the rinse compartment with fresh circulating water, checking the solution levels, and stirring the developer and fixer thoroughly to prevent the heavier chemical from settling to the bottom; (2) determining the temperatures of the water and the developer; (3) checking the workbench for cleanliness, selecting the proper film hangers, determining the optimum development time and setting the timer, laying out the film on the workbench, and identifying the films on the hanger; and (4) closing the darkroom door, turning off all lights except the selected safelight, and unwrapping the film packets and securing the films to the clips on the hanger. Some of these steps require further explanation.

When developing dental x-ray film, always follow a time–temperature development chart. For conventional solutions, the following chart should be used.

TIME–TEMPERATURE CHART

Temperature		Development Time
60° F (15.5° C)		9 min
65° F (18.3° C)		7 min
68° F (20° C)	optimun	5 min
70° F (21.1° C)		4.5 min
75° F (23.9° C)		4 min
80° F (26.7° C)		3 min

The ideal (optimum) temperature for manual processing is 68 degrees Fahrenheit (20 degrees Celsius) with a development time of 5 minutes. Processing for too long a time or at higher temperatures than recommended results in an increase of film fog. Also, the contrast of the radiograph is reduced when films are processed at either higher or lower temperatures and for longer or shorter times than recommended by the manufacturer. The current trend is toward faster-reacting emulsions and processing chemicals. As changes are frequent and without prior warning, the directions should be consulted each time newly purchased chemicals are used. Following the time–temperature chart, one can see how much more time is required if the water and the developer are colder and how much less if they are warmer. Temperature variations from the ideal of 68° F (20° C) are acceptable as long as the developing time is correspondingly adjusted. Lower temperatures make the chemical reaction sluggish, and with higher temperatures the danger of fogging the film increases. A floating thermometer should be kept in both the developer insert and in the water compartment for frequent temperature reading (Fig. 9–5). The temperature of the developer should be read after stirring.

The water should be allowed to circulate in the tank long enough before the films are placed in it for processing to even the temperatures in all three compartments of the tank. Failure to do so may cause **reticulation**—a cracking of the film emulsion, producing a netlike pattern. Reticulation results when the film is removed from a warm solution (where the gelatin softens) and placed in a cold solution (cracking the gelatin).

The selection of the proper film hanger and the identification of the film must also be considered. Decide what type and how many films are to be processed and select the film hanger that will suit the task. Intraoral film hangers hold between 1 and 16

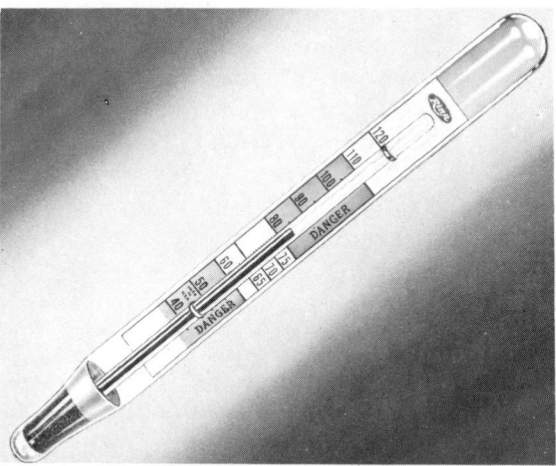

Figure 9–5. Floating thermometer for use in the developer solution or water compartment. When using the time–temperature method, the ideal temperature is 68° F (20° C). *(Courtesy of Rinn Corporation, Elgin, IL.)*

periapical or bitewing films (fewer occlusal films). Most have a white plastic identification tag near the handle on which the patient's name can be entered. This tab can be erased and used again after the film is removed from it and positively identified on a mount or in an envelope. Extraoral films are best identified by fastening an identification plate to one of the lower corners of the face of the cassette. Special lettering sets, made of lead, are available. Minimum identification is the patient's name and the letters *R* (for right) and *L* (for left). These identifications become visible on the processed radiograph.

All radiographs to be processed must be identified in some manner; those that cannot be identified are completely worthless to the dentist. A good procedure is to enter the patient's name and the number of films exposed in a record book kept in the darkroom. This is particularly important in a busy office where the traffic in radiographs is heavy. At the end of the day it is virtually impossible to remember what films were exposed, and unless orderly records are kept, dangerous mix-ups, loss of time, and embarrassment can result. It is not too practical to write or print on the small intraoral films, but offices that specialize or handle a volume of the large extraoral film may use a film identification printer (Fig. 9–6).

Before processing can begin, the films must be removed from their protective wrappers or the cassette and fastened to the selected film hanger (Fig. 9–7). There are four steps in preparing the intraoral film packet for processing: (1) pull up and out on the film tab to tear open the top of the packet; (2) pull on the tab until approximately half of the black paper is out of the packet; (3) hold the black paper away from the film and carefully remove the film from the packet, grasping the film by the edge so as not

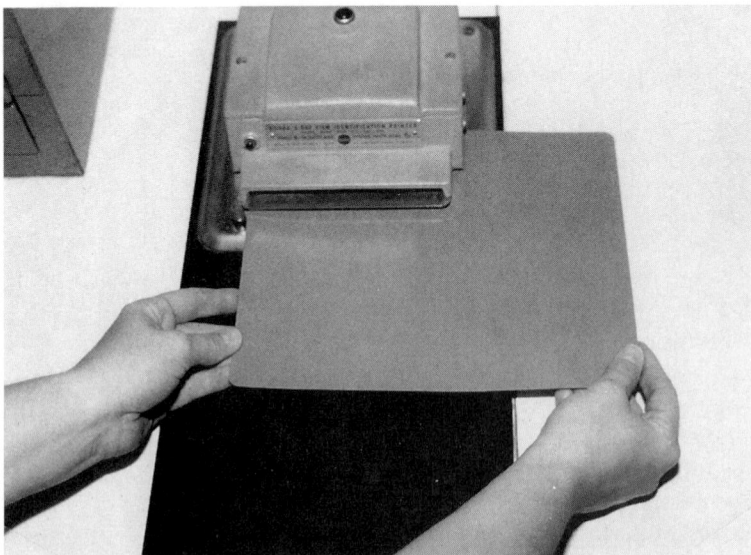

Figure 9–6. Photographic printer for including typed identification information on x-ray sheet film.

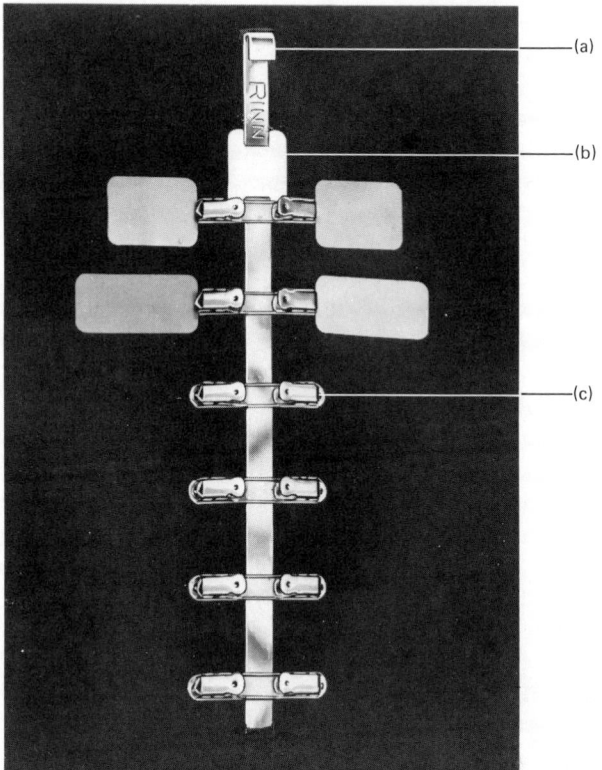

Figure 9–7. Intraoral film hanger with 12 clips. Various hangers ranging in capacity from a single film to 16 films are available. **(a)** Curved portion at the top of the hanger rests on upper rim of tank insert when films are immersed. **(b)** White plastic identification tag on which the patient's name can be written in pencil and later erased. **(c)** Clamps with three-point positive grip hold the film securely in place and parallel to the film base. *(Courtesy of Rinn Corporation, Elgin, IL.)*

to smudge the surface of the film; and (4) clip the film to the hanger, testing each film to check whether it is securely held by the clip—failure to do this may cause the film to be lost at the bottom of the tank. Some film packets contain two films; however, only one film may be attached to each clip. If two films are accidentally fastened to the same clip, only the outside surfaces will be properly developed because the emulsion on the sides of the films that face each other will not come into sufficient contact with the developer and fixer.

Special precautions must be followed with the larger extraoral films. These can only be removed safely from the cassette and processed in minimum light. The operator should be familiar with the light requirement for each type of film used in the office. Extraoral films are placed in special hangers that have channels into which the film fits or are attached to spring clips. To place the film in the hanger, hold the film in the right hand and grasp the hanger with the left. Next, guide the film into the channels until it is all the way into the hanger and the hinged retaining channel over the open end of the hanger can be closed.

Films undergoing processing must hang individually and out of possible contact with other films or with the side of the processing tank. As a rule, when a tank with 1 gal (3.8 L) inserts is used, not more than two hangers loaded with 14 to 16 films should be placed into an insert simultaneously. A slight bending of the bottom of the film hanger toward the wall of the tank will help to prevent films from scraping against the wall.

The steps in the processing of the dental radiograph are (1) development, (2) rinsing, (3) fixation, (4) washing, and (5) drying. Only two of these—development and fixation—generally involve chemicals.

The initial step in the processing sequence is the **development** of the film. This is done by slowly and completely immersing the film in the developer and gently agitating the hanger up and down a few times—taking care not to splash—to eliminate air bubbles from clinging to the film and allow the developer to make contact with all areas of the film. The handle of the film holder should rest on the lip of the insert. This permits the cover to be replaced. Set the activator arm on the timer and leave the film to develop until the timer goes off.

The second step in processing is **rinsing** the film. After the film is removed from the developer, the film hanger is immersed in the circulating water of the middle compartment for at least 20 to 30 seconds and is agitated so that the water can touch all the film. Even the tops of the handles of the hanger should be well rinsed to avoid transfer of developer into the fixer. Before being transferred to the fixer, the hanger should be held above the rinse water and allowed to drain for a few seconds to prevent carrying too much water into the fixer. The purpose of the rinsing is to remove as much of the alkaline developer as possible before placing the film in the fixer, thus preserving the acidity of the fixer and prolonging its useful life.

The third step is the **fixation** of the film. The film is immersed and agitated in the same manner as described for development. The timer is set and started—the common rule is to double the clearing time. A minimum fixation time of 10 minutes is recommended. During the first 2 or 3 minutes in the fixer (the clearing time), the unexposed silver bromide crystals separate from the emulsion, and the film loses its original milky opacity. Several additional minutes are required to diffuse the crystals out of the emulsion and for the gelatin on the film base to harden again. Although the fixing time is not as critical as the developing time, and a film may occasionally remain in the fixer longer than necessary, the recommended time–temperature sequence should be adhered to. When the fixing time is too short, the result can be slow drying, poor hardening of the emulsion, a possible partial loss of detail, and the radiograph will darken; when the time is excessively long, the image will lighten. If the fixer solution is too warm, the gelatin may melt and the image may disappear.

When the radiograph is needed immediately for a quick reading of the x-ray image, the film may be read while it is still wet (wet reading). The film may be removed from the fixer as soon as it clears (usually after 2 or 3 minutes) and should then be rinsed in water for a short interval and taken into the operatory for viewing; however, the film should be returned to the fixer as soon as possible to complete the fixation and permit further shrinking of the emulsion. If this is not done, some of the unexposed silver bromide grains may be left in the film, giving it a fogged and discolored appearance, and the emulsion may not harden completely. Remember to always replace the cover on the tank to retard oxidation of the chemicals and to prevent light from reaching the film.

The fourth step in processing is the **washing** of the film to remove all chemicals left on the radiograph. This is done by placing the films in the circulating water of the rinse compartment for a minimum of 20 minutes. Longer washing is permissible, but the film should always be removed not later than the end of the working day. If the temperature in the darkroom rises on a hot weekend or after the air conditioning is shut off, the water may become warm enough to melt the emulsion, leaving a film without an image. One should also be careful to ascertain that the rinse water is not much colder than the developer. This can cause **reticulation,** the formation of a network of cracks or wrinkles. The emulsion often cracks when subjected to variations in temperature from warm to cold.

The final step is the **drying** of the film. There are several ways to dry film: (1) gently shake the water from the hanger and film, and suspend the hanger from a rod or drying rack, taking care that the film does not contact other films on adjacent racks or brush up against the wall; (2) follow the same procedure but use a fan or blower to expedite the drying; or (3) place the film in a heated drying cabinet, after shaking off the excess water. Films left in the cabinet too long, however, may become brittle. Always use a drip pan when moving the film hangers from the processing tank to the drying area and leave the pan under the film hanger until the film is dry.

The steps in the final procedures include (1) checking to see that none of the films have loosened from the clip and dropped on the floor or the bottom of the tank; (2) cleaning up the work area—wipe up any moisture caused by dripping or accidental splashing of the water or solutions; (3) removing the dry films from the hangers and placing them in properly identified protective envelopes or on film mounts with identifying data (film mounting techniques are discussed in Chapter 11); and (4) removing or erasing identification markings from the hangers and replacing hangers, the timer, or any equipment used, in the proper place. At the end of the working day, turn off the water to the tank, drain the water compartment, and turn off all lights in the darkroom.

RAPID PROCESSING PROCEDURES

As already mentioned, one technique for obtaining a diagnostic radiograph in minimal time during an emergency situation is to remove it from the fixer as soon as it is cleared enough to wet-read the film. A newer technique, made possible by faster-acting chemicals and the introduction of the compact "chair-side darkroom" (Fig. 9–8), makes it possible to process the small intraoral films in normal light within 30 seconds.

Rapid processing is most valuable in endodontic and oral surgery practices. A significant amount of chair time can be saved when it is necessary to expose a series of

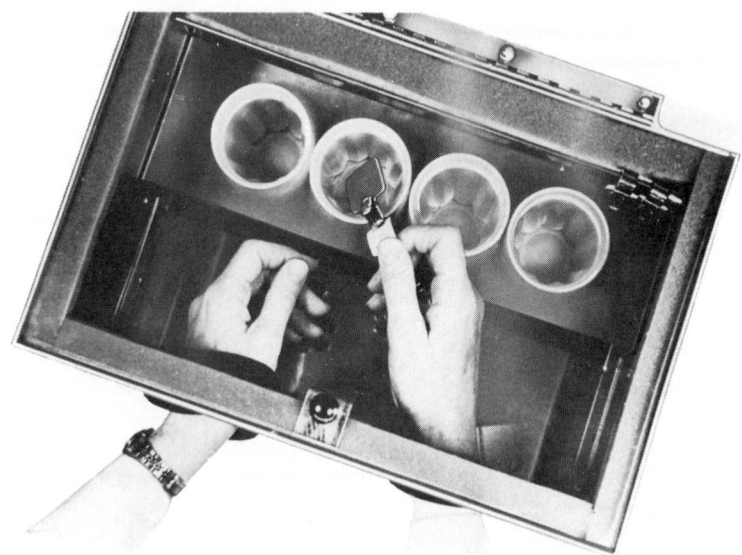

Figure 9–8. Chair-side darkroom unit shown with view through plastic filtered top. The first cup is filled with developer concentrate mixed 1:1 with water, the second with rinse water, the third with fixer concentrate mixed 1:1 with water, and the fourth with wash water. A heater with a thermostat keeps the solutions at optimum temperature for rapid processing. *(Courtesy of Rinn Corporation, Elgin, IL.)*

single films to check the progress in reaming out a root canal during endodontic treatment. Rapid processing enables the oral surgeon to instantly determine the extent or location of a fractured root. The general practitioner occasionally requires rapid confirmation of the success or failure of an operation performed. However, rapid processing has definite limitations and is never intended to replace conventional processing.

Since fast-acting temperatures as high as 92° F (33.3° C) are used, the developing time must be kept short (as brief as 5 seconds). Short developing and fixing times, combined with minimal washing, result in a substandard radiograph. It must be recognized that while rapid processing fulfills the dentist's need to receive rapid information, it is at the expense of image quality. Such films are frequently fogged, have poor image density and contrast, eventually discolor, and are seldom suitable for filing with the patient's permanent record.

The "chair-side darkroom" has two lighttight openings through which the hands can enter the working compartment when the lid is closed. The transparent plastic filtered top permits the operator to see while unwrapping the film packet and transferring it through the four cups filled with developer, rinse water, fixer, and wash water. For best results the solutions are heated to 85° F (29.4° C) by a calibrated heater in the unit. If normal radiographic density is desired, develop for 15 seconds and fix for 30 seconds. In the event that the film is to be retained with the permanent record, it should be refixed for 4 minutes and washed for 20 minutes at normal conventional darkroom temperatures and conditions.

Three precautions are urged: (1) change the water and solutions daily, (2) clean drips or spills after each use to avoid contamination, and (3) close the light filtering top securely before processing the film.

AUTOMATIC PROCESSING

Since the mid-1960s a number of automatic film processing units have appeared on the market. These vary in size and complexity. Some have a limited capacity and process only intraoral or certain types of extraoral films; others can handle any dental film regardless of size. Most are intended for use in the darkroom under safelight conditions; however, those equipped with daylight loaders (Fig. 9–9) have a lighttight baffle for inserting the hands while unwrapping the film and can be used right in the operatory.

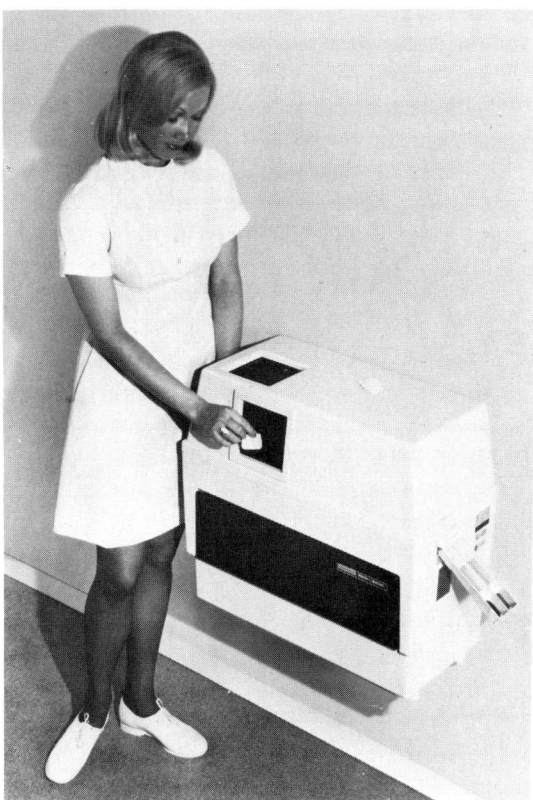

Figure 9–9. This automatic intraoral film processor is equipped with lighttight baffles and does not require special plumbing or a darkroom. *(Courtesy of General Electric Company, Medical Systems Division.)*

Although a large number of dentists have switched to automated processors, many continue to use conventional manual processing. Because automated equipment can, and does, break down occasionally, and because the processor may only handle one or two types of film, the dental office continues to need a conventionally equipped darkroom.

Automated processing has advantages and disadvantages. The advantages are (1) less time required in the darkroom, and (2) a dry film can be viewed in approximately 5 minutes. The disadvantages are (1) artifacts occasionally occur on the radiographs (usually caused by excessive pressure of the rollers on the emulsion), (2) film may become stuck between the rollers and jam up the passage, (3) problems with failure to identify the film, and (4) some processors are difficult to clean and maintain.

Most automated processing systems have a set of rollers or a mechanical rack-type conveyer that transports the film through the processing cycle (Fig. 9–10).

All automatic processors require water. Some can be connected to the plumbing system, whereas in others the water is self-contained. A heating unit warms the processing chemicals to the required temperature. As a rule, a 20-minute warming-up period is required before the unit is operational. On most units the processing cycle is set at approximately 5 minutes for intraoral film. On some units it can be regulated according to the type of film used.

The chemical solutions in automatic processors are heated to temperatures much higher than those used in manual processing—as high as 125° F (52° C) in some units. These chemical solutions differ from those used in manual procedures by being super-saturated and having more hardener in the developer. Fortunately, advanced film technology has produced emulsions that can withstand these temperatures for the short times required in automated processing without excessive softening or melting.

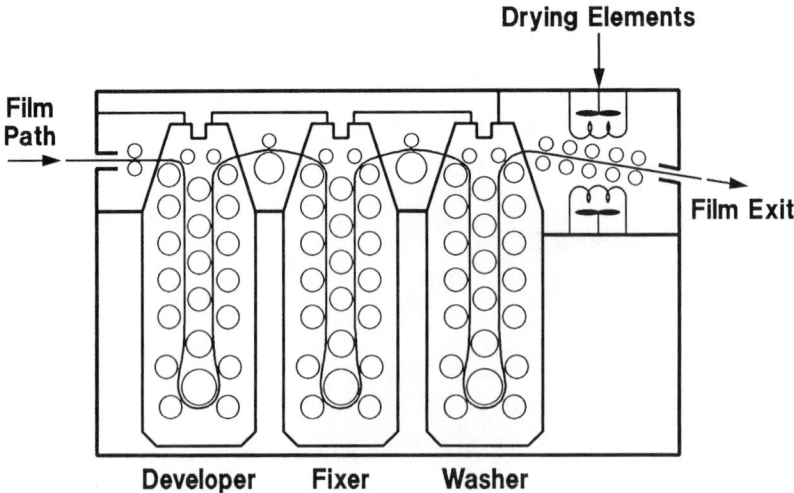

Figure 9–10. Schematic illustration of automatic film processor. Film is transported by roller assemblies.

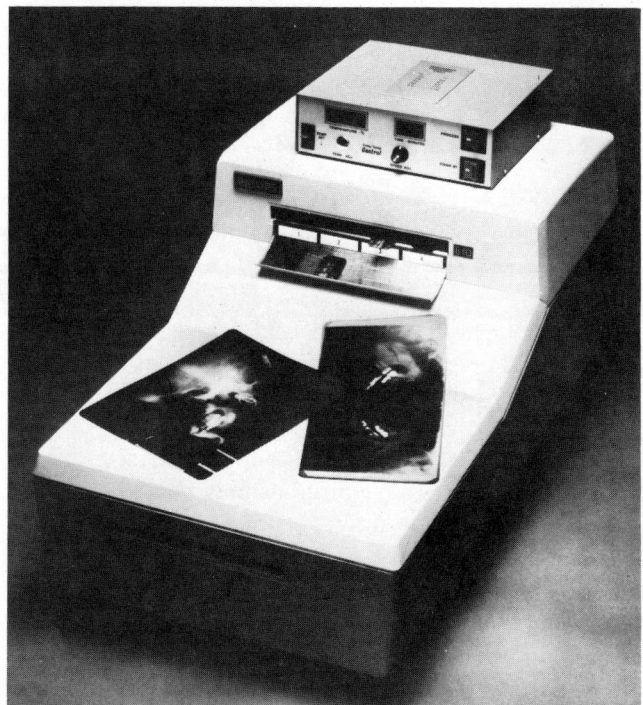

Figure 9–11. This automatic processor, equipped with solid-state time and temperature control, accommodates all films up to 8 in. by 10 in. (20 cm by 25 cm). It is capable of providing damp films for wet reading in just 50 seconds and films of archival quality in 4 1/2 minutes. *(Courtesy of Philips Dental Systems.)*

A recirculation system keeps the solutions agitated and distributed evenly. Some units automatically replenish the solutions; others depend on the operator to keep them at the correct level.

Basic to all units is some form of temperature and time control to produce standardized results that eliminate the human errors of under- and overdevelopment, fixation, improper washing, and drying (Fig. 9–11).

The present trend is toward units to which accessories such as a daylight loader, film loading trays, or a water recirculation system can be added.

Automatic processors can do an excellent job but only if the instructions for maintenance are scrupulously followed. Few pieces of equipment in the dental office require such diligent and regular care. Care must be exercised when filling or emptying the developer and fixer compartments to avoid contamination. If the rollers are not kept clean, the radiographs emerge streaked. For best results a time should be set aside for regular maintenance that includes (1) a check for the proper solution temperature, (2) maintenance of proper solution levels, (3) maintenance of activity of solutions, (4) routine preventive maintenance, and (5) keeping all working parts clean. As these units are becoming more trouble-free, they are finding their way into more and more offices because they save considerable darkroom time.

DISPOSAL OF RADIOGRAPHIC WASTES

Today's dental office team should make every effort to recycle or properly dispose of wastes that may be harmful to the environment. Radiographic wastes include x-ray processing chemicals, intraoral film packets, and discarded radiographs.

The Federal Resource Conservation and Recovery Act (RCRA) of 1976 was enacted to "promote the protection of human health and the environment and to conserve valuable material and energy resources." In the past, the management of radiographic wastes was to discard them with the trash or pour them down the drain. This is no longer appropriate for materials listed by RCRA as hazardous.

In areas that have a municipal sewer system with a secondary biological wastewater treatment plant, x-ray processing solutions may be disposed into the system and considered to be effectively treated. However, the disposal of x-ray processing solutions into a septic tank system could require state regulatory approval. One must be aware that some state and local waste management regulations are more stringent than the federal regulation. Be sure to check with your state Hazardous Waste Management Agency for regulations that exist in your area.

It may be convenient to have processing chemicals removed by a commercial waste disposal company. Contact your state Hazardous Waste Management Agency for a list of licensed companies in your area.

Silver, a metal regulated by most control agencies, is present in the fixing solution and in wash water. The amount of silver will depend upon the number of films processed. Some control agencies may require the removal of silver from the fixing solution before disposal. Silver recovery methods, such as the Kodak Chemical Recovery Cartridge, are available (see bibliography).

Scrap film or discarded radiographs also contain silver and should be collected and recycled. Check with your local health department for a list of silver refiners and buyers.

Intraoral film packets contain plastic and lead foil that should be separated and properly disposed. The plastic components should be recycled. Lead is considered a hazardous waste under RCRA regulations. Dental film manufacturers and local scrap metal dealers are possible sources for recycling lead foil.

Every dental office should dispose of wastes properly, for today's actions will surely affect the quality of tomorrow's environment.

FILM DUPLICATING PROCEDURES

There are increasing requirements for duplicating radiographs on the part of insurance companies and governmental agencies because of third-party payment plans. Also, changes of patients' residence and an increase in malpractice suits require the making of more duplicate radiographs.

New legislation, first enacted in California in 1982, concerning the "patient right of access to dental records," has since been enacted in other states. Consequently, many dentists choose to duplicate films to protect themselves as well as to comply with the law.

The necessity for film duplication has long been recognized. Many dentists solved the problem by using two-film packets, but that did not eliminate the possibility that a radiograph mailed to another dentist at the patient's request might be lost or damaged in transport. Advantages of film duplication are (1) a film can be duplicated as often as necessary without reexposing the patient, and (2) the density of the radiograph can be varied for improved diagnostic quality by changing the time it is exposed to light in the duplicator.

The process of film duplication is simple and rapidly learned. All duplication must be done in the darkroom under a safelight. The minimum equipment is a printing frame and a light source that is about 2 ft (61 cm) from the film. Duplicating film is available in sheet form in a variety of sizes. The film is emulsion-coated on one side only. Under a safelight, the emulsion side looks dull, while the noncoated side looks shiny. Depending on the printing frame and the size film sheet used, it is possible to duplicate either a single radiograph or a full-mouth series at a single printing.

The original radiograph to be duplicated is placed with viewing side up on the glass area of the printing frame. Then, under safelight conditions, the duplicating film is positioned on the original with the emulsion side away from the operator and in contact with the top of the original radiograph. The cover is then closed to keep both radiograph and duplicating film in tight contact during the exposure. The light source is 2 ft (61 cm) from the printing frame and faces the glass on which the original is posi-

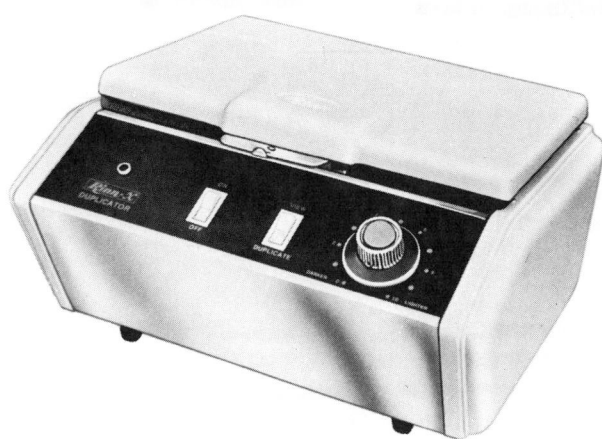

Figure 9–12. Contact printer type of x-ray duplicating unit containing a built-in fluorescent light source and a timer that turns on the lamp for a preset time to permit variations in contrast. This x-ray duplicator provides a convenient means for exposing duplicating film with dental radiographs. *(Courtesy of Rinn Corporation, Elgin, IL.)*

tioned. When turned on, the exposure is made through the original onto the emulsion side of the duplicating film. With such a setup, the exposure is made in 4 to 5 seconds. The time required varies with the type of duplicator used. Ranges as short as 3 and as long as 25 seconds are not uncommon.

Another factor affecting the time is the density of the radiograph that is to be duplicated. A shorter exposure will increase the density (darkness) of the duplicate; a longer exposure will decrease (lighten) the duplicate. This fact can be taken advantage of to lighten an overexposed film or to darken one that was underexposed. After the exposure is complete, the film is removed from the frame and processed in the same manner as a radiograph—manually or automatically. Consult the film instructions for optimum time–temperature cycles.

Better control of film density and standardization of technique can be achieved if a contact printer type of duplicating unit is used (Fig. 9–12) instead of a printing frame and outside light source. A built-in light and a timer control the duration of the exposure.

REMOVAL OF PROCESSING STAINS FROM UNIFORM

Despite all precautions, uniforms will occasionally become soiled with developer or fixer stains. Of the two, the developer is more difficult to remove. Never launder a uniform before trying to remove the spot. The best procedure is to rub a saturated soap solution into the spot as soon as possible, before it becomes permanently set into the fabric. Uniform shops and dental supply houses carry a number of very effective commercial spot removers, such as Fix Off. If such a remover is not available, the spot may be soaked for 5 to 10 minutes in a solution of 1/2 oz (15 mL) of household bleach and 1/2 oz (15 mL) of vinegar to 1 gal (3.8 L) of warm water and then rinsed in plain water. Stubborn stains may require longer soaking. After the spot is removed, the uniform should be laundered as soon as possible.

CHAPTER SUMMARY

Certain preparatory steps are necessary before processing begins. These include cleaning the work area using infection control procedures, stirring the solutions, checking the temperature of the solutions, and selecting the proper safelight for the film to be used. When this is done, the film is removed from its protective wrapping or from a cassette. The sequence followed in all processing is developing, rinsing, fixing, washing, and drying.

An invisible latent image forms when the silver halide (bromide) crystals in the film emulsion are energized by x-rays. The metallic silver, which turns black while the film is in the developer, remains on the film surface. Later, when the film is in the fixer, the unexposed crystals are cleared from the film. The latent image becomes visible during processing. When the processing is finished, the image becomes permanent.

Two processing chemicals are used—an alkaline developer and a slightly acid fixer. The latent image, although quite cloudy in the early stages, starts to become visible while the film is in the developer. The film is rinsed thoroughly to remove the developer before the film is inserted in the fixer. It is here that further development is stopped and the image becomes visible permanently.

With the exception of automatic processors equipped with lighttight baffles, all processing must be done in the darkroom under safelight conditions. Using the proper safelight is important because radiographic films vary in their sensitivity to light. If several different types of film are used in an office, the operator must remember to use the correct safelight to prevent irreversible film damage.

Three techniques are commonly used to make the latent image visible: (1) conventional manual processing, based on full development of the film by the time-temperature method; (2) rapid processing, a method of producing an image rapidly at the expense of quality; and (3) automatic processing, a method that delivers a fully processed and dry film in a matter of minutes.

The chemicals in rapid and automatic procedures are more concentrated and contain more hardener; higher temperatures and shorter processing time are used.

Accurate record keeping and film identification are important during and after processing. The original radiographs are a part of the patient's record and should be kept with it always. A radiograph can be copied on duplicating film whenever it is necessary to send one out of the office to another dentist, insurance company, law firm, and so forth. A special duplicating film is placed in contact with the radiograph to be duplicated and is briefly exposed to light in a frame or duplicator. It is then processed in the same manner as a radiograph—either manually or automatically.

KEY WORDS

Acidifier

Activator

Cutting reducer

Developer

Fixer

Halide

Hardening agent

Latent image

Oxidation

Preservative

Radiolucent

Radiopaque

Reduction

Replenisher

Restrainer

Reticulation

Safelight

Selective reduction

Wetting agent

REVIEW QUESTIONS

1. Which term best describes the process by which the latent image becomes visible? (a) reticulation, (b) reduction, (c) sensitivity, (d) preservation.

2. What happens to the radiograph when a film is exposed to a safelight too long? (a) radiograph appears white, (b) radiograph becomes fogged, (c) radiograph becomes reticulated, (d) radiograph becomes attenuated.

3. How far above the work area in the darkroom should the safelight be located? (a) 6 to 8 in. (15 to 20 cm), (b) 1 1/2 ft (46 cm), (c) 2 1/2 ft (76 cm), (d) 4 ft (1.2 m).

4. Which of these is the correct processing sequence? (a) rinse, fix, wash, develop, dry; (b) fix, rinse, develop, wash, dry; (c) develop, rinse, fix, wash, dry; (d) rinse, develop, wash, fix, dry.

5. Which of the following reduces the exposed silver bromide crystals? (a) the developer, (b) the wetting agent, (c) the fixer, (d) the cutting reducer.

6. Which developing chemical becomes extremely active when the temperature is raised? (a) sodium sulfite, (b) potassium bromide, (c) elon, (d) hydroquinone.

7. Which ingredient of the developer is alkaline and causes the emulsion to soften and swell? (a) the developing agent, (b) the preservative, (c) the activator, (d) the restrainer.

8. What is the ideal temperature when film is processed manually? (a) 60° F (15.5° C), (b) 68° F (20° C), (c) 75° F (23.9° C), (d) 83° F (28.3° C).

9. Chemically, what is the major difference between solutions used for manual processing and those used for rapid and automatic processing? (a) there is more acid in rapid processing solutions, (b) manual processing solutions contain more preservative, (c) rapid and automatic processing solutions contain more hardener, (d) manual processing solutions are more alkaline.

10. Which term describes a fully processed radiograph that shows a network of cracks or wrinkles on its surface? (a) fogged, (b) reticulated, (c) restrained, (d) proliferated.

11. Which items of darkroom equipment are essential for manual processing? (a) safelight, view box, and water-mixing valve; (b) film hanger, film drier, and illuminator; (c) timer, water-mixing valve, and "in-use" light; (d) paddles, thermometers, and timer.

12. What is the major problem encountered with automatic processors? (a) overdevelopment of films, (b) underdevelopment of films, (c) amount of maintenance required, (d) films getting stuck between the rollers.

13. What is the appearance of duplicating film when viewed under safelight conditions? (a) the nonemulsion side appears dull, (b) the nonemulsion side appears pebbly, (c) the emulsion side appears shiny, (d) the emulsion side appears dull.

14. Gloves should be worn during processing procedures to prevent _cross contaminatⁿ_

15. Radiographic wastes include _x-ray proc. chem_ , _x-ray film packets_, and _discarded Radiographs_.

BIBLIOGRAPHY

Eastman Kodak: *Exposure and Processing for Dental Radiography*. Rochester, NY: 1993

Eastman Kodak: *Management of Photographic Wastes in the Dental Office*. Rochester, NY: 1991

Eastman Kodak: *X-rays in Dentistry*. Rochester, NY: 1985

CHAPTER 10

Quality Assurance in Dental Radiography

OBJECTIVES

By the end of this chapter the student should be able to

1. Differentiate between quality assurance and quality control.
2. Describe who is responsible for carrying out quality assurance programs.
3. Name four requirements for an acceptable radiograph.
4. Describe who benefits from quality assurance programs.
5. Name at least three equipment failures.
6. Name at least five causes of processing errors.
7. Describe how to test for light leaks in the darkroom.
8. Make a checklist useful in quality assurance.
9. List at least four chair-side operator errors.
10. Make a step wedge with cardboard and lead foil and demonstrate how to use it.

QUALITY ASSURANCE AND CONTROL

In dental radiography the terms quality assurance and quality control are often used interchangeably. The difference is slight. **Quality Assurance** is defined as the planning and carrying out of procedures to assure high-quality radiographs with maximum diagnostic information (yield) while minimizing the exposure to dental patients and personnel. This takes the conservative view that the minimum of radiation should be used to get the job done. Remember the ALARA concept, where ALARA stands for "as low as reasonably achievable." Quality assurance includes both quality administration procedures and quality control techniques.

Quality control is defined as a series of tests to assure that the radiographic system is functioning properly and that the radiographs produced are of an acceptable level of quality. These tests include the monitoring of x-ray equipment and the x-ray processing system. A log of all tests performed, including dates, results, and corrective actions should be made.

The objectives for these tests are to:

1. Identify any problems in the radiographic system before image quality is compromised.
2. Maintain a high standard of image quality within the dental office.
3. Keep patient and occupational exposures to a minimum.
4. Reduce the x-ray retake rate.

ADVENT OF QUALITY ASSURANCE PROGRAMS

The concept of quality assurance has developed slowly. At first the only ones who presented ideas on how good and safe radiographs could be produced were educators and progressive professionals—the dentists and auxiliary personnel who attended continuing education workshops and seminars. Now, however, quality assurance programs are being set up in many dental offices and clinics.

It is the responsibility of the dentist and the auxiliaries to consistently practice quality assurance. This is a legal as well as a moral obligation. The entire office personnel should be aware of the causes of failure and of corrective measures that may have to be taken. The goal is to achieve maximum diagnostic yield so that the patient gains the benefit of a correct diagnosis.

It should be a matter of pride in each office that the radiographs be of at least standard quality and that the exposure levels to radiation be held to the absolute minimum. This goal can be achieved if all concerned are adequately trained and dedicated to implementing quality control measures. The quality assurance program must have the support of the dentist and auxiliary personnel in order to be successful. The duties of each individual must be clearly defined.

Because the dentist usually delegates most radiographic procedures to the dental assistant and/or dental hygienist, these tasks become a shared responsibility—even if the final responsibility legally rests with the dentist.

REQUIREMENTS FOR AN ACCEPTABLE DENTAL RADIOGRAPH

Occasionally the dentist will accept a substandard film rather than submit the patient to more radiation from additional exposures; this is particularly so when the film was exposed in order to determine the location of an embedded tooth or the absence of a deciduous tooth.

An acceptable radiograph should: (1) show the entire area to be studied with minimal distortion; (2) have proper film blackening, or density; (3) exhibit sufficient definition, sharpness; and (4) have sufficient contrast between adjacent areas.

Unfortunately, many dental radiographs are substandard. The failure to achieve desired goals may be due to problems with the equipment, the processing, the personnel, or even the patient. Most problems can be easily corrected.

NECESSITY FOR TRAINED PERSONNEL

It is said that the technique for producing an acceptable radiograph is unforgiving, that each of the numerous steps is of equal importance. An error anywhere along the way will result in some degree of failure. Even a trained and dedicated worker may have an occasional failure. Therefore personnel must be trained to recognize problems, their causes, and how to correct them. Such training generally works out best if done on a one-on-one basis in the dental office. A novice should seek assistance and be shown what was done wrong. Retakes should not be made without knowing why. Ideally, each film exposed is recorded in a log and this log should be periodically reviewed and the cause of problems detected and corrected.

Office personnel should be familiar with the following quality assurance guidelines.

1. Radiographic quality should be continuously monitored against a standard reference film.
2. Processing chemicals should be evaluated daily.
3. A daily log of all retake radiographs should be maintained.
4. On a monthly basis, the darkroom (including the safelight), all viewboxes, cassettes, and screens should be checked.
5. There should be comprehensive testing of the x-ray machine on a yearly basis or as state regulations require.

A number of tests have been developed by which auxiliaries can detect problems that are about to happen. Obviously, there are problems that can only be solved by an expert repairman or a qualified radiation monitor.

The dentist, with the assistance of his or her staff, should develop a list of things that must be checked at the start of each day to promote quality assurance. Depending on the amount of radiographic traffic in the office, such a list could be checked in approximately 15 or 20 minutes. Some tests, such as determining the potency of the processing solutions, should be carried out at the start of each work day; other tests, such as determining the output of the x-ray machine, may be made annually.

CAUSES OF SUBSTANDARD RADIOGRAPHS AND PREVENTIVE MEASURES

Some substandard radiographs can be traced to malfunction of the x-ray machine. Such failure is usually gradual and may remain undetected because the operator gets used to substandard results and accepts them as normal. There may be defects in the tube or the transformer, such as loose or worn wires. The tube head may shake or drift. Minor malfunctions include slight variations in the **output** of the x-ray machine. (Output is the amount of radiation calculated in coulombs per kilograms per second [roentgens per second], measured at the open end of the position indicating device [PID]). There may be timing errors or the dials may register inaccurate mA or kVp readings. All of these require the services of expert repair technician or qualified health physicist.

Periodic comprehensive testing of the x-ray machine is essential to a quality assurance program. These tests should include beam alignment, collimation, filtration (beam quality), output, timer accuracy, and tube head stability. State and local health departments may provide x-ray equipment testing as part of their registration or licensing programs. If necessary, a health physicist should be hired to perform these tests.

In the past, it was often necessary to make equipment or structural changes to assure radiation safety. With the advent of high-speed film, the timers were not fast enough and had to be replaced. Except in Third World countries, this is no longer a factor because most of these machines have been replaced in recent years.

Radiation monitoring badges should be worn by all persons in the office. These badges may be the first to give a warning that something may be wrong.

Lead aprons and thyroid collars should be inspected and maintained on a regular basis. Make sure they are cleaned and stored properly.

Quality control is extremely important in processing the dental x-ray films because even a single variation from the prescribed procedures can affect the quality of the radiograph. Such a seemingly small thing as a speck of dirt on the workbench, dried chemical residue on a film hanger, insufficient or weakened chemicals, or the failure to maintain proper chemical temperature can, and all too often does, spoil what would otherwise have been an excellent radiograph. Several simple tests can be made to determine whether the conditions for film processing are acceptable. Some should be performed daily, others as the occasion demands.

One of the first things to check is the integrity of the darkroom. This includes determining that it is beyond the reach of stray radiation, adequately ventilated, free from chemical fumes, within the prescribed temperature range, and lighttight. Also, check to see that the safelight and filter are not defective or giving off too much light.

Whether the darkroom is lighttight can be determined by closing the door and turning off all lights, including the safelight. Light leaks, if present, become visible after about five minutes when the eyes become accustomed to the dark.

To find out if the safelight is really safe, turn off all lights, unwrap an unexposed dental film, and place a coin on the film emulsion surface. Turn on the safelight for approximately the time you take to unwrap a full-mouth series of film (about 4 minutes); then process the film. If the outline of the coin appears, the safelight is not safe for use with that type of film. The filter may be scratched, the wattage of the bulb may be too great, the light may be too close to the work area, or the film may not be designed for use with that particular light and filter combination.

Another area to check is the processing equipment. If manual processing is used, determine whether the thermometer and timer are accurate, whether wet or dry chemicals are adhering to the mixing paddles and film holders, and whether the work area is clean and free of dust. In addition, determine if the water is circulating and is at the desired temperature.

If automatic processing equipment is used, check to see if the water circulating system is working properly and that correct solution levels, replenishment, and temperatures are maintained. Follow the manufacturer's procedure and maintenance directions. When cleaning, be careful to keep oil and grease off the rollers.

Regardless of what processing method is used, check the solutions as needed, maintain the solution levels by replenishment, and above all, avoid cross-contamination of the chemicals.

Not to be overlooked is the viewing equipment (viewbox or viewer). If functioning properly it should give off a uniform, subdued light. Some viewers have fluorescent light tubes that will glow after the light is turned off. Film emulsions are sensitive to this afterglow and can be damaged.

Still another thing to check daily is the degree of density and contrast shown on freshly developed radiographic films. Visual perception varies from person to person, and some dentists prefer radiographs that are slightly lighter or darker. However, there is a medium density range that is acceptable to most. Unfortunately, many radiographs exhibit poor density and are either too light or too dark. This makes it difficult to see the contrast between adjacent areas and to diagnose the radiograph properly. There are three common causes for light or dark radiographs: (1) failure of the x-ray operator to evaluate correctly the density of the patient's bone structure; (2) improper setting of exposure factors: milliamperage, kilovoltage, exposure time, and target–film distance; and (3) processing errors caused by weakened chemicals or failure to follow the correct time–temperature cycle.

If the radiographs appear to be too dark though the solutions are fresh, it indicates that the film was overexposed. Properly exposed films will show the correct density, unless the film used was old (outdated) and appears light after processing or unless the film was fogged by light or stray radiation and then appears excessively dark.

QUALITY ASSURANCE TESTING METHODS

A test to measure the output of the x-ray unit and to monitor film processing is to expose a film daily using a calibrated **sensitometer** (a steplike instrument used to measure the film's sensitivity to radiation) and develop the film immediately. The developed film can then be read with a **densitometer**, an instrument used for measuring the degree of darkening of processed x-ray film, which uses a photocell to measure the light transmitted through a given area of the film. A **step wedge** device (Fig. 10–1) can be very useful for quality control in manual processing. Such a step wedge can be obtained commercially or be made in the dental office by: (1) dividing a piece of cardboard the size of a #2 x-ray film into thirds, (2) leaving the first third uncovered and covering the remaining two thirds with two pieces of lead backing from a discarded film packet, and (3) covering the final third with three additional pieces of lead backing and taping them down. This results in a device that can be used to check the qual-

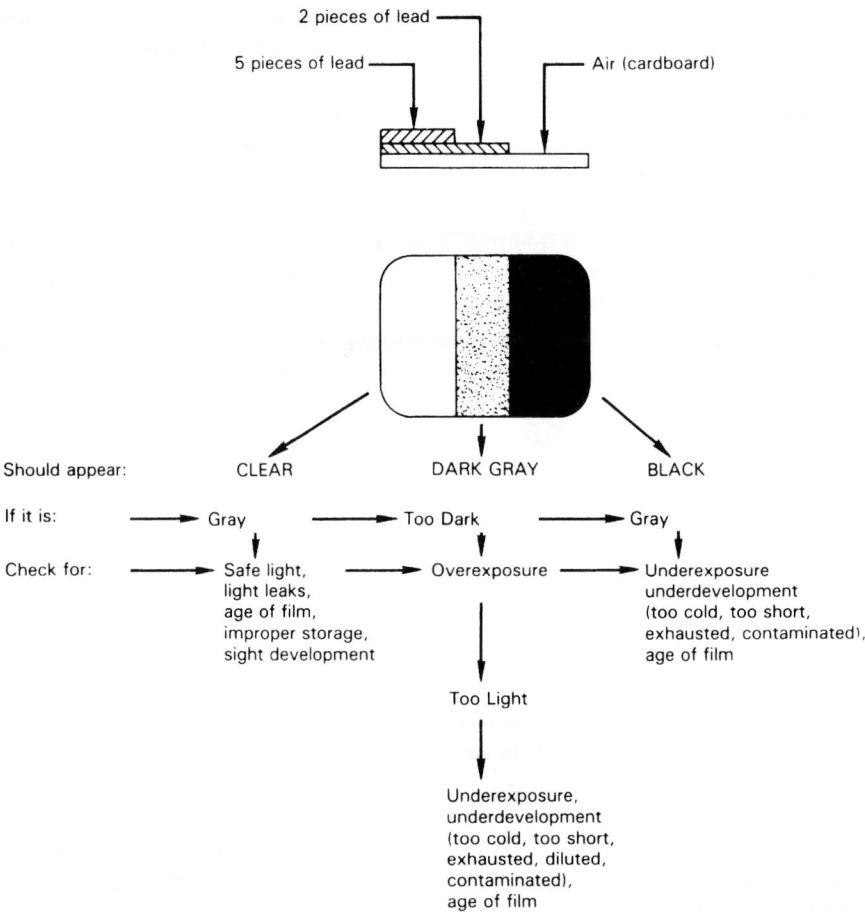

Figure 10–1. Sketch of a step wedge useful in making visual comparisons for quality control. (Courtesy of Dr. A. Peter Fortier, Louisiana State University School of Dentistry, and Department of Dental Diagnostic Science, School of Dentistry, University of Texas at San Antonio.)

ity of the developing solutions. It can also be used to measure the consistency of the x-ray machine.

In order to determine whether the fault lies with the x-ray machine or with the processing chemicals, place the step wedge on top of the x-ray packet and expose it by using the same exposure factors used for a molar view of an adult patient. Repeat this procedure six or eight times to create a supply of films for future testing. These become the control films to monitor inconsistencies in image quality. Develop only one of these films; then develop the others later as needed, whenever the quality of the processed films appears to be substandard. One of the film packets saved can now be developed in the same solutions in which the film with questionable density was developed. If it is of poor quality the processing solutions are bad; otherwise the x-ray machine should be tested.

Two daily tests are helpful when using automatic processors. Begin by processing an unexposed film. The film should come out of the return chute clear and dry. If it does not, check the solutions, the safelight, or look for possible light leaks. If the film is still moist, check the dryer temperature. Then process a film that has been exposed to light. This film should be black and dry after processing. If not, check both the solutions and the temperature of the dryer. A convenient checklist of problems with density is shown in Table 10–1, and another checklist of problems with marks on the film surface is presented in Table 10–2. Table 10–3 is a checklist for film drying problems.

Rough film handling can cause severe problems, particularly when automatic processing is used. Many operators slightly bend a corner of the film to make it easier to place and conform with the contour of the palate. Such bending, while undesirable, is acceptable when manual processing is used. The film may show a pressure mark but generally not in an area of diagnostic interest. Much greater care must be used when feeding films into automatic processors. Bent films tend to become stuck and jam up in the rollers. It is best to feed the films in slowly and make sure that they go in straight

TABLE 10–1. A GUIDE TO FILM DENSITY PROBLEMS

Problem	Cause	Correction
1. Light films.	a. Developer nearing exhaustion.	a. Drain developer solution, clean tank, and fill with new developer solution.
	b. Developer contaminated.	b. Same as above.
	c. Developer temperature too low.	c. Be sure standby switch on. Be sure heater pad plugged in. Check thermostat—adjust or replace. Check heating pad and replace if defective.
	d. Processing speed too fast.	d. Increase total processing time.
	e. Exposure time too short.	e. Increase exposure time in 20% steps.
2. Dark films.	a. Exposure time too long.	a. Decrease exposure time in 20% steps.
	b. Fixer in developer.	b. Change developer.
	c. Thermostat failure, causing solutions to overheat.	c. Replace thermostat.
3. Fogged film.	a. Incorrect safelight filter or bulb.	a. Use a 6B filter with 15-watt bulb.
	b. Excessive light.	b. Check that safelight bulb is of proper wattage. Be sure no light leaks in darkroom.
	c. Developer temperature too high.	c. Check thermostat—adjust or replace.
	d. Light leak between processor and daylight loader.	d. Block light leak with black tape.
4. Gray films.	a. No water in wash section.	a. Add water.

Courtesy of Dr. A. Peter Fortier, Louisiana University School of Dentistry, and Department of Dental Science, School of Dentistry, University of Texas at San Antonio.

TABLE 10–2. A GUIDE TO PROBLEMS WITH FILM SURFACE MARKS

Problem	Cause	Correction
1. Pressure marks.	a. Foreign material on roller. b. Rough handling of film before processing.	a. Clean rollers. b. Due to sensitivity of film emulsions, gentle handling should be practiced.
2. Film with greenish-yellow hue.	a. Depleted fixer. b. Improper film. c. Wrong fixer. d. Processor speed too fast.	a. Replace fixer. b. Use film made for automatic processing. c. Use rapid-process fixer. d. Reduce processor speed.
3. Emulsion peeling.	a. Deposits on developer roller. b. Solution temperature too high. c. Wash water temperature too high. d. Improper film.	a. Clean roller. b. Turn off standby switch. Check thermostat. c. Reduce wash water temperature. d. Use film made for automatic processing.
4. Film scratches.	a. Rough handling of film before processing. b. Sticking roller. c. Foreign material on roller. d. Burr on input slot.	a. Gentle handling of films should be practiced. b. Check racks, gears, and gear mesh. c. Clean rollers. d. Remove burr.
5. White chalky film.	a. Lack of wash water. b. Fixer precipitated.	a. Check water supply. b. Replace fixer.

Courtesy of Dr. A. Peter Fortier, Louisiana State University, and Department of Dental Diagnostic Science, School of Dentistry, University of Texas at San Antonio.

TABLE 10–3. A GUIDE TO FILM DRYING PROBLEMS

Problem	Cause	Correction
1. Films damp or wet.	a. Processor speed too fast. b. Defective dryer fan heater. c. Improper film. d. Wrong developer and/or fixer.	a. Increase processing time. b. Replace defective fan heater. c. Use film made for automatic processing. d. Use only rapid-processing developer and fixer.

Courtesy of Dr. A. Peter Fortier, Louisiana State University School of Dentistry, and Department of Dental Diagnostic Science, School of Dentistry, University of Texas at San Antonio.

and in the right direction. Failure to insert the films into automatic units in the right sequence or order can result in serious problems in identification.

PROBLEMS CAUSED BY OPERATOR ERRORS

Quality assurance begins at chair-side, for it is here that the initial steps are taken that determine whether the final product is of excellent, medium, or poor quality. No amount of excellent processing is going to salvage a film that was positioned backwards. Assuming that the film to be used is fresh, and all x-ray and processing equipment is functioning properly and used correctly, there remain a number of chair-side operator errors that must be guarded against.

Frequent procedural errors include: (1) selecting the wrong film for the task at hand—too large a film is difficult to position and causes patient discomfort, whereas too small a film fails to cover the area completely and give the required diagnostic yield; (2) failure to correctly center the film packet over the designated area—this can result in failure to include the correct teeth for the area; (3) incorrect vertical or horizontal positioning of the position indicating device (PID), resulting in elongation, foreshortening, "cutting off" apical or occlusal areas, or overlapping of the image; and (4) failure to place the identification dot on the film packet into the incisal or occlusal area.

Not to be overlooked is the necessity for patient cooperation. Failure to inform the patient about what is to be done is a frequent cause of retakes. This is especially true with young patients. The operator should take the time to explain the necessity of what is to be done, tell the patient how long the procedure lasts, and caution the patient against movement—turning of the head or releasing pressure on the biteblocks. Be gentle when positioning the film and make the exposure promptly to avoid the danger of gagging. On rotational panoramic units, check to determine that the rotating tubehead does not engage the lead apron or thyroid collar. Keep your eye on the patient during the exposure and watch from an area of safety.

Less frequent procedural errors include (1) accidental exposure to radiation through failure to protect the film by using a film safe; (2) using the wrong exposure factors where several x-ray units of different manufacturers are used and controls differ; (3) contamination of the film by moisture through failure to blot saliva from the packet after exposure; (4) positioning the film backwards; (5) failure to turn on the "in-use light" or locking the darkroom door when processing film.

BENEFIT OF QUALITY ASSURANCE PROGRAMS

Quality assurance programs are undergoing changes that are suggested by various study groups. Such programs at present are voluntary; however, it would not be surprising if some portions of them became mandatory.

Programs must be flexible and allow for change as new techniques come into being. There is a necessity for the dentist and the entire staff—assistants, hygienists, and clerical personnel—to meet on a regular basis to discuss the effectiveness of the programs and to evaluate them. The records or log of all unsatisfactory radiographs and the reason for the retakes should be examined. If such examination shows any pattern of one particular error being made repeatedly—or by the same person—corrective measures are in order. Films should be indexed and properly filed so that they can be rapidly located. Everyone concerned benefits from a well organized program. Once the office personnel is trained properly, such programs take as little as 15 to 20 minutes per day. Quality assurance programs are cost-effective once initial expenditures have been made. The resulting improved image quality helps the dentist to see what otherwise might be missed or misinterpreted. Retakes can often be reduced as well as the radiation dose to the patient and operator, a further important benefit.

CHAPTER SUMMARY

The interest in quality assurance programs is getting more attention as its benefits are realized. Several specific measures or tests can be employed by the operator to determine that the radiograph becomes a satisfactory diagnostic tool for the dentist and at the same time minimizes the number of unproductive exposures to dental x-rays.

It is the responsibility of the dentist and the auxiliaries to continuously practice quality assurance and control. Substandard or unacceptable films are often the result of errors that can be attributed to the equipment, darkroom errors, chair-side errors, and uncooperative patients. Although a few errors are traceable to mishaps, most can be avoided if proper measures are followed. A few simple tests can be made daily, or as required, to check the processing and the accuracy and function of the equipment.

The price of obtaining a superior radiograph is meticulous attention to detail. Quality assurance, if practiced faithfully, ensures standard results and images of the highest quality.

The majority of errors made at chair-side during exposure can be avoided if the operator is well trained, skillful, and dedicated. The production of radiographs of high quality with high diagnostic yield should always be the goal of each operator. This can be implemented whenever quality assurance measures are used. It is then a win situation with benefits for all.

KEY WORDS

Densitometer
Output
Quality assurance
Quality control
Sensitometer
Step wedge

REVIEW QUESTIONS

1. T F   The entire office staff should be dedicated to the concept of quality assurance.

2. T F   The goal of quality assurance is to achieve maximum diagnostic yield from each radiograph.

3. T F   Any radiograph that is less than perfect should be retaken immediately.

4. T F   The output of the x-ray machine should be tested weekly.

5. T F   The drifting of the tube head should be corrected by a trained repair person.

6. T F   Automatic processors require little or no servicing.

7. T F   A step wedge is a valuable tool to use in quality control tests.

8. In radiography, film blackening is called _density_.

9. A steplike instrument used to measure the film's sensitivity to radiation is called a _Sensitometer_

10. Exposed intraoral film packets are often contaminated by _saliva_, blood, or chemicals on the workbench.

11. Which testing device is used in quality control to compare the density of the radiographic image? (a) a safelight, (b) a step wedge, (c) a viewer, (d) a photoreceptor plate.

12. Which device, used in quality assurance programs, measures the degree of darkening in a processed film? (a) monitoring badge, (b) densitometer, (c) dosimeter, (d) collimator.

BIBLIOGRAPHY

American Academy of Dental Radiology Quality Assurance Committee: Recommendations for quality assurance in dental radiography. *Oral Surg* **55:**421–426, 1983

Farman AG, Hines VG: Radiation safety and quality assurance in North American dental schools. *J Dent Educ* **50:**304–308, 1986

Quality Assurance for Diagnostic Imaging Equipment: Recommendations of the National Council on Radiation Protection and Measurements, Bethesda, MD: NCRP Publications, 1988. NCRP Report no. 99

Eastman Kodak: *Quality Assurance in Dental Radiography.* Rochester, NY: 1991

CHAPTER 11

Identification of Anatomical Landmarks for Mounting Radiographs

OBJECTIVES

By the end of this chapter the student should be able to

1. Describe why it is important to recognize and identify normal anatomical landmarks of the face and head.
2. Recognize and identify the facial and cranial bones.
3. Name all of the anatomical landmarks of the maxilla and mandible.
4. Differentiate between the terms radiopaque and radiolucent.
5. Differentiate between cortical and cancellous bone.
6. Recognize and describe the radiographic appearance of all structures of the teeth and the alveolus.
7. Name and identify all landmarks or structures normally seen on radiographs of the maxillary and mandibular tooth areas.
8. Determine whether a periapical radiograph is of the right or left side.
9. Identify any given periapical radiograph according to its exact location in the maxilla or mandible and describe how to position it on a film mount.
10. Describe how to block out excess light during film viewing.

IMPORTANCE OF IDENTIFICATION OF ANATOMICAL LANDMARKS

The dental auxiliary should be able to recognize and identify normal anatomical landmarks that may be seen on radiographs of the teeth, the jaw structures, or the skull areas.

There are two major reasons for this: (1) to ensure that the film was positioned and exposed in such a manner that all the desired areas and anatomical structures are clearly visible so that the radiograph thus produced is of diagnostic value and (2) to assist in determining into which frame of the x-ray mount each radiograph is to be mounted.

Before the dental radiographs can be arranged in meaningful sequence and secured to their proper frames in the film mounts, the auxiliary must identify each separate tooth area portrayed. The general configuration of the dentition, the size or shape of the crowns and the root, and certain landmarks typical of a given area help to provide the clues needed for mounting. It is assumed that most students using this text will be studying dental and cranial anatomy and have access to a skull and an anatomy text. The student should periodically review the major landmarks of the face and the structures surrounding the teeth until he or she is completely familiar with them and able to identify them positively on a skull, radiograph, or patient.

In any text on anatomy, the illustrations show numerous protuberances, ridges, depressions, sutures, grooves, canals, and other landmarks. Only a portion of these are commonly used in mounting dental radiographs. Indeed, many of them are not visible on the average radiograph.

Only commonly used landmarks are labeled in illustrations in this chapter. Auxiliaries planning to work for certain specialists or in dental offices where highly sophisticated radiographic techniques are employed will require additional training to recognize less common structures. Numerous excellent texts are available for advanced training.

SIGNIFICANT NORMAL ANATOMICAL LANDMARKS

Anatomical landmarks in this chapter are separated into the following groups: (1) landmarks of the face, (2) landmarks of dental interest on the skull, (3) specific landmarks of the maxillae, and (4) specific landmarks of the mandible.

Facial Landmarks

The surface landmarks of the face cannot be distinguished on a radiograph, but they help the radiographer to rapidly locate a number of important planes and structures. Such landmarks (Fig. 11–1) as the tip of the nose, the ala (wing) of the nose, the inner canthus of the eye, the outer canthus of the eye, the tragus of the ear, and the symphysis of the chin are often used in certain techniques of placing the film and directing the position indicating device (PID).

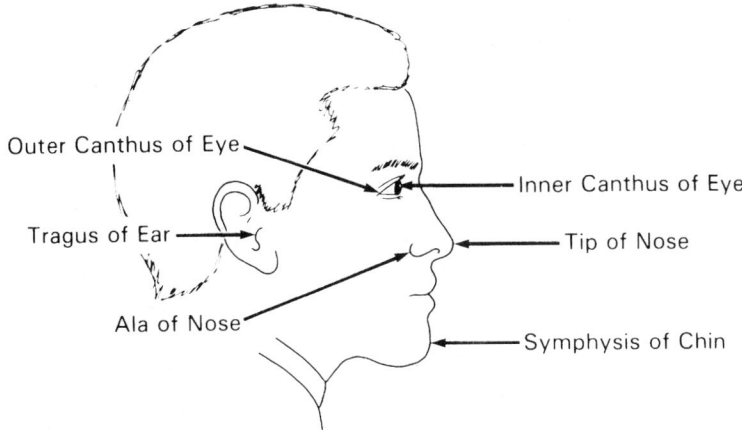

Figure 11–1. Landmarks of the face.

The positioning of the patient's head during intraoral radiographic procedures is often determined by aligning the midsagittal plane perpendicularly and the ala–tragus line parallel to the floor. Plane alignments and film positioning are explained in Chapters 14 and 15.

Bones and Anatomical Structures of the Cranium and Face

Although most anatomical landmarks that can be used to interpret or mount intraoral radiographs are located on the maxillae or the mandible, the auxiliary should also be able to recognize and identify the major bones and anatomical structures of the cranium and face. Such knowledge is useful when making cephalometric, temporomandibular joint, or panoramic exposures.

With some practice, skill in recognizing the names of the bones and anatomical structures can be achieved by comparing the labeling on the illustrations that follow with their appearance on a dry skull. To make it easier to locate these bones or structures, turn the skull so that it is oriented in the same direction as the illustration at which you are looking. Many structures can be seen readily; others may only be seen from one specific direction. You should be aware that not all of these can be identified on dental radiographs. For an in-depth study, an anatomy text is suggested.

One of the first steps is to become familiar with the names and locations of the cranial and facial bones that may be seen on dental radiographs. Using Figure 11–2 (frontal view of the skull), attempt to locate the following bones on the skull: the frontal bone, the right and left parietal bones, the right and left zygomas (zygomatic bone, also called malar bone or cheekbone), the sphenoid bone, the right and left nasal bones, the right and left maxillae, and the mandible.

Use Figure 11–3 (lateral view of the skull), to locate the following bones and structures: the frontal bone, the parietal bone, the temporal bone, the occipital bone, the

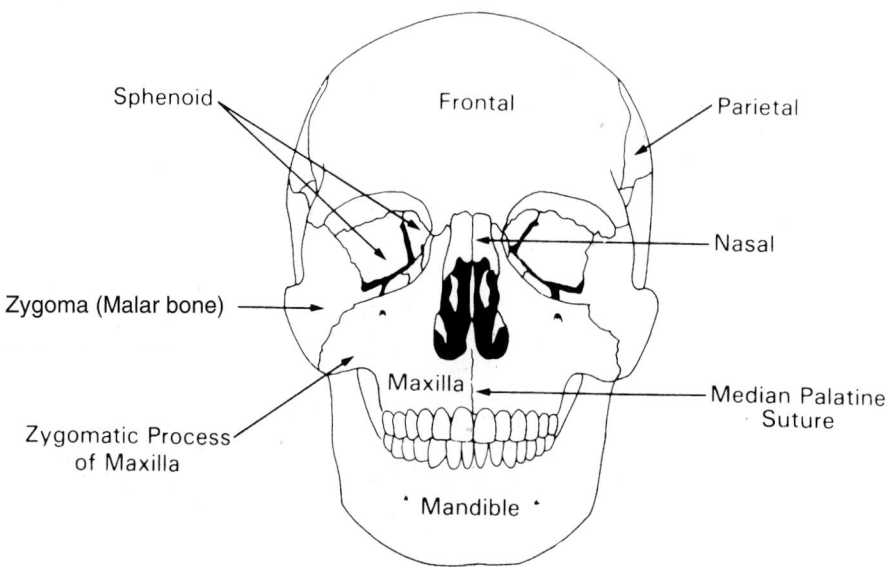

Figure 11–2. Frontal view of the skull.

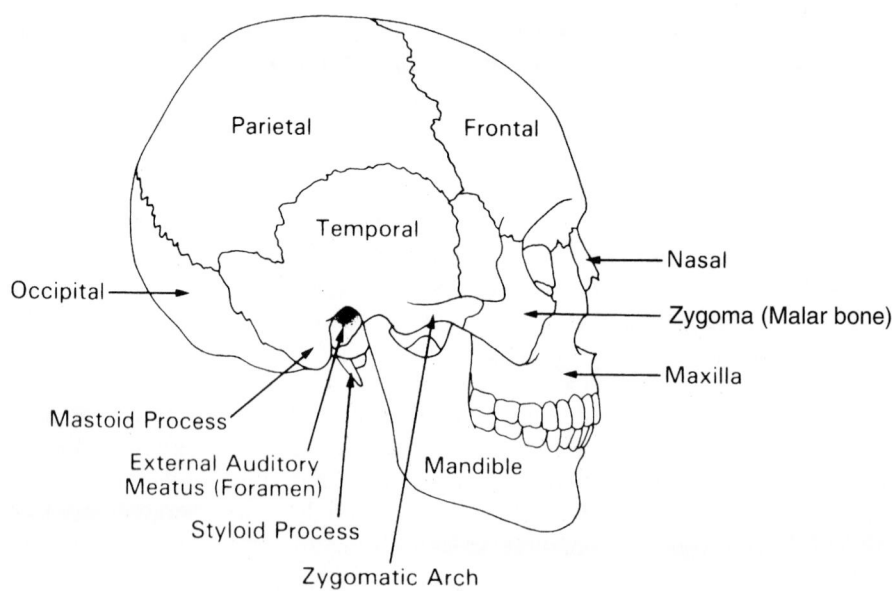

Figure 11–3. Lateral view of the skull.

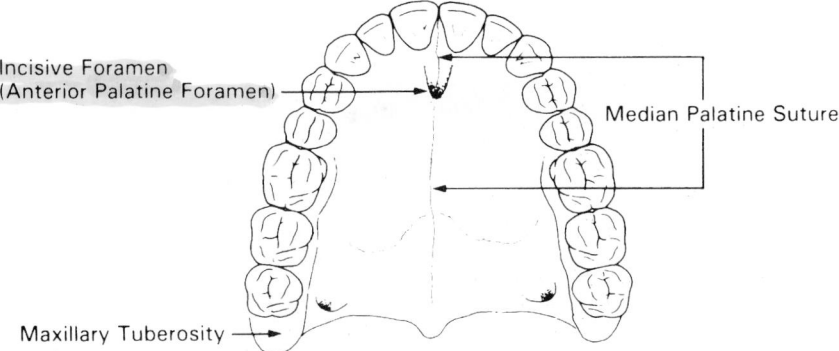

Figure 11–4. Palatal view of maxilla.

nasal bone, the zygoma (zygomatic bone, malar bone, or cheekbone), the maxilla, the mandible, the zygomatic arch, which is made up of the temporal process of the zygoma and the zygomatic process of the temporal bone, the external auditory meatus (foramen), and the styloid and the mastoid processes of the temporal bone.

Landmarks of the Maxillae and Mandible

The teeth are located within the alveolar processes of the maxillae and the mandible; thus most dental radiographs include portions of these bones. The maxillae are two bones, a right and left maxilla, whereas the mandible is a single bone. Generally, but not always, the same structures appear on both sides.

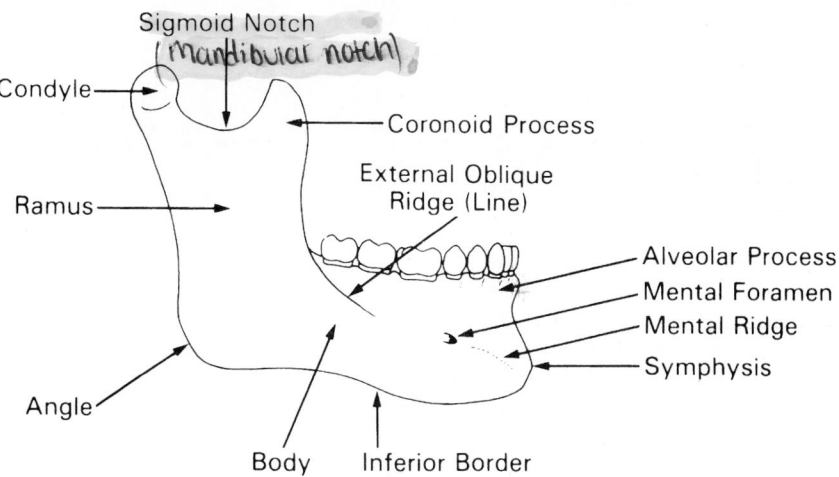

Figure 11–5. Lateral view of detached mandible.

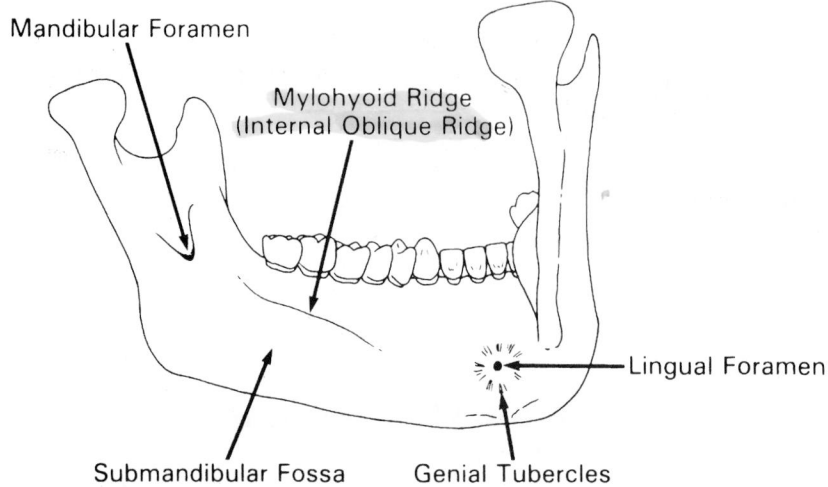

Figure 11–6. Lingual view of detached mandible.

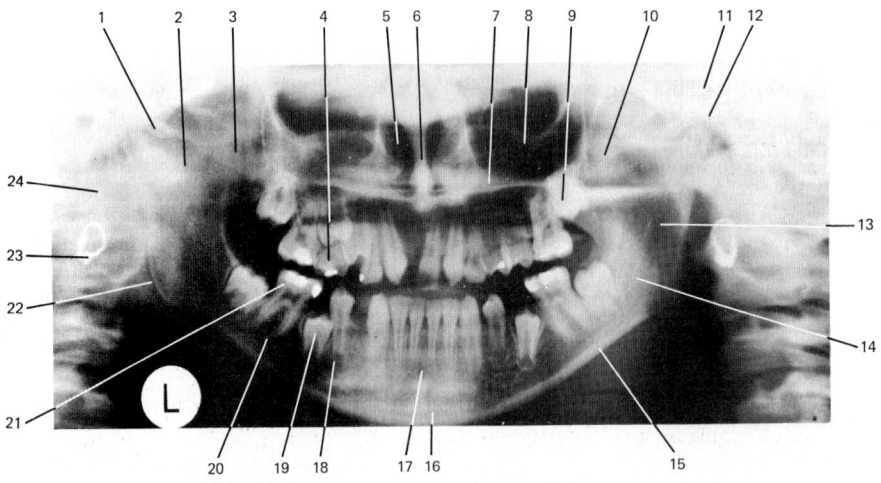

Figure 11–7. Panoramic-type radiograph produced with Orthopantomograph. Landmarks indicated by numbers: **1** zygomatic arch, **2** sigmoid notch, **3** maxillary tuberosity, **4** deciduous second molar, **5** nasal fossa, **6** septum, **7** hard palate, **8** maxillary sinus, **9** unerupted permanent second molar, **10** coronoid process, **11** glenoid fossa, **12** mandibular condyle, **13** mandibular foramen, **14** mandibular canal, **15** inferior border of mandible, **16** mental symphysis, **17** lingual foramen, **18** mental foramen, **19** unerupted second premolar, **20** submandibular fossa, **21** metal restoration, **22** angle of mandible, **23** earring, **24** cervical vertebra. *(Courtesy of Siemens Medical Systems, Inc., Dental Division, Iselin, NJ.)*

Compare the labeling on Figure 11–4 and locate the following structures on the maxilla: the median palatine suture, the maxillary tuberosity area, and the incisive (anterior palatine) foramen. The maxillary sinus is an empty space within the maxilla.

Next compare the labeling on Figures 11–5 and 11–6 and attempt to locate the following areas and structures on a mandible: the body, the ramus, the inferior border, the alveolar process, the angle of the mandible, the condyle, the coronoid process, the sigmoid (mandibular) notch, the mandibular foramen (the mandibular canal is located within the mandible between the mandibular foramen and the mental foramen), the mental foramen, the mental ridge, the symphysis, the lingual foramen, the genial tubercles, the external oblique ridge (line), the mylohyoid ridge (internal oblique ridge or line), and the submandibular fossa.

The location of these structures of the maxillae and mandible should be memorized, and identification should be practiced frequently. Some of the landmarks listed are visible only in the larger occlusal and extraoral radiographs. The number shown on any radiograph depends on the size of the film and the area exposed. Typical maxillary and mandibular structures, as well as some teeth and restorations, are identified in the panoramic-type film shown in Figure 11–7.

RADIOGRAPHIC APPEARANCE OF THE ALVEOLAR BONE AND TOOTH AREA

As explained in Chapter 4, the terms radiolucent and radiopaque are used to describe the appearance of all areas exposed to any radiograph. **Radiolucent** is defined as that portion of the processed radiograph that is **dark** because the exposed structures lack density; it refers to a substance that permits the passage of x-rays with little or no resistance. The opposite term is **radiopaque,** which is defined as that portion of the processed radiograph that appears **light** because the structures in the path of the x-rays are dense and absorb or resist the passage of the x-ray beam. Obviously, the majority of structures in the path of the x-rays are not of equal density; therefore most structures will appear as some shade of gray rather than just black or white.

Before considering the specific bones and structures visible in a full-mouth series of radiographs, it is important to recognize and identify the normal appearance of alveolar bone and the structures of the teeth. Compare the drawing of this area (Fig. 11–8) with a radiograph of the same area (Fig. 11–9).

Although bones appear solid, they are solid only on the outside and are honeycombed within. Bone is classified as **cortical bone,** a compact or dense form of bone, such as that which lines the outside layers of the maxillae and the mandible, and **cancellous** or spongy bone, which forms the bulk of the inner bone. Small, interconnected **trabeculae** (bars or plates of bone) form a multitude of various-sized compartments that account for the honeycomb appearance. These trabecular spaces are usually filled with fat, blood, or bone cells, which accounts for the difference in the radiographic appearance of bone. All bone tissues appear radiopaque. The compact or cortical outside layer appears extremely radiopaque (white), whereas the cancellous bone varies in radiopacity (shades of gray) according to the size and number of the trabecular spaces.

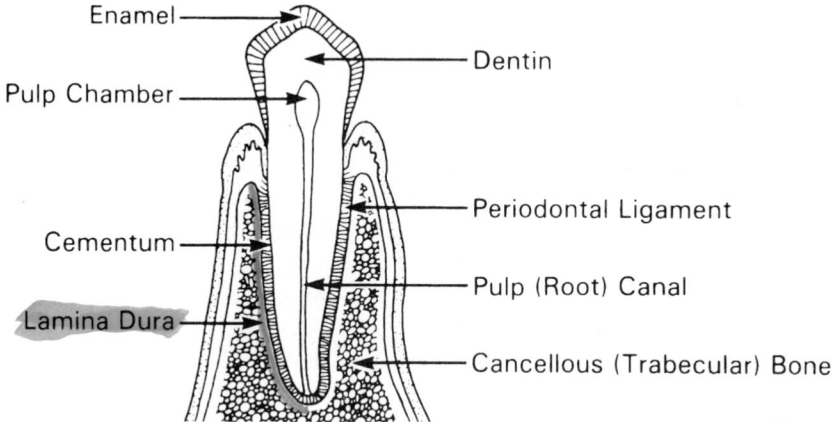

Figure 11–8. Drawing of mandibular premolar tooth and alveolar bone.

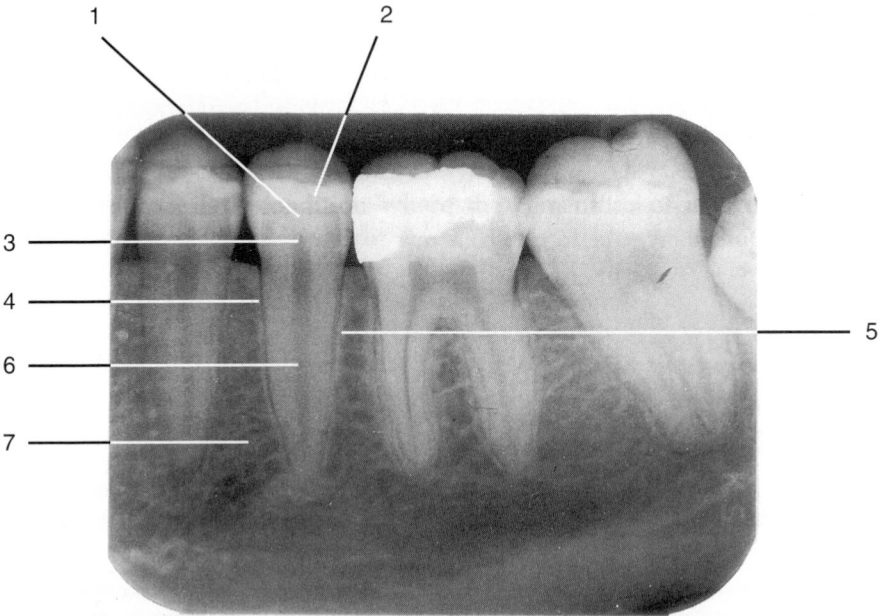

Figure 11–9. Radiograph of mandibular premolar (bicuspid) area shows **1** dentin, **2** enamel, **3** pulp chamber, **4** periodontal ligament, **5** lamina dura, **6** pulp (root) canal, and **7** cancellous (trabecular) bone. Note: Because only a very thin layer of cementum covers the root, it is indistinguishable from the underlying dentin.

The area may even appear almost radiolucent (black) if these spaces are very large or if the bone is thin, as is the case in the submandibular fossa.

By definition, the **alveolar process** is that portion of the maxilla or mandible that surrounds and supports the teeth. It is composed of the **lamina dura** and the **supporting bone.** The lamina dura is the hard, **cortical** bone that lines the **alveolus** (the tooth socket). On radiographs the **lamina dura** appears as a thin radiopaque (white) border that outlines the shape of the alveolus (the root of the tooth). The supporting bone is **cancellous** and varies in density in the different parts of the alveolar process.

The teeth are attached to the lamina dura by the fibers of the **periodontal ligament,** which is so thin that sometimes it is not radiographically visible. When visible, it has the appearance of a thin radiolucent (dark) border between the lamina dura and the roots of the teeth.

The tooth structures are enamel, dentin, cementum, and pulp. **Enamel,** the hardest body structure, covers the crown and is very radiopaque. The underlying **dentin** is not as dense and appears less radiopaque. The **cementum** that covers the roots is even less dense. Because only a thin layer of cementum covers the root, it is generally indistinguishable from the underlying dentin. Although all three highly calcified tooth structures vary in radiopacity in direct proportion to the thickness of each structure in

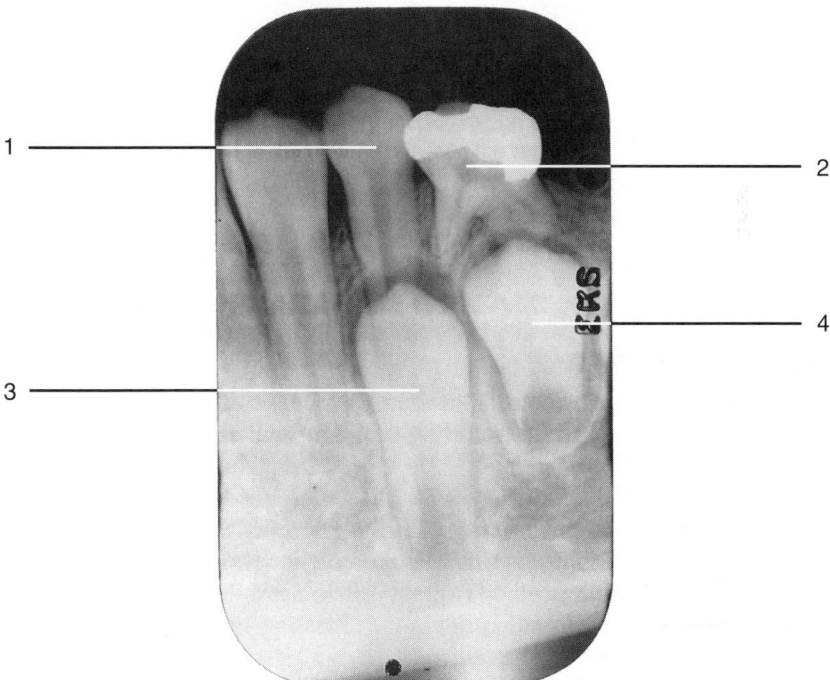

Figure 11–10. Radiograph of mixed dentition in mandibular canine (cuspid) area shows **1** deciduous canine (cuspid), **2** deciduous first molar with partially resorbed roots, **3** permanent canine (cuspid), and **4** permanent first premolar (bicuspid) with incomplete root formation.

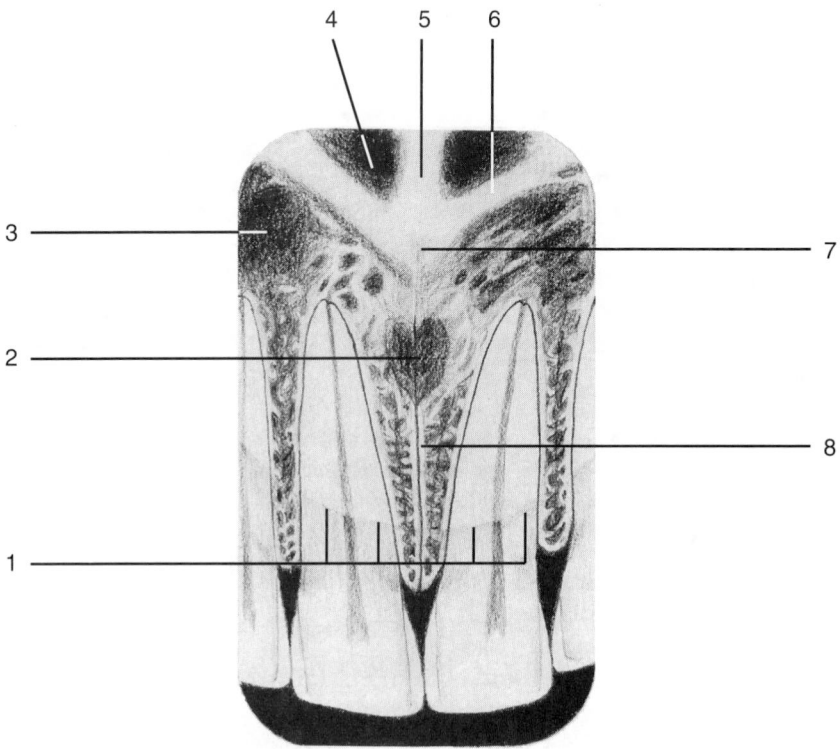

Figure 11–11. Drawing of maxillary midline area. **1** outline of nose, **2** incisive foraman (anterior palatine foramen), **3** lateral fossa, **4** nasal fossa, **5** nasal septum, **6** border of nasal fossa, **7** nasal spine, and **8** median palatine suture.

the path of the x-ray beam, for descriptive purposes enamel, dentin, and cementum are considered radiopaque.

The **tooth pulp** that occupies the pulp chamber and the root canals is the only noncalcified tooth tissue. As this soft tissue offers only minimal resistance to the passage of x-rays, it appears radiolucent. The end of the root canal is called the **apical foramen.** This foramen permits the passage of nerves and blood vessels that nourish the tooth structures.

Nutrient canals are thin radiolucent lines of fairly uniform width that sometimes exhibit radiopaque borders. They contain blood vessels and nerves that supply the teeth, bone, and gingivae. Nutrient canals are most often visualized in the anterior of the mandible and in edentulous areas.

To correctly identify and interpret the radiographs, one needs to understand the dentition. Young children have 20 deciduous (baby or primary) teeth that are gradually lost as they grow older. During the transition years they have a mixed dentition—that is, both deciduous and permanent teeth. A radiograph may show several deciduous teeth with partially resorbed roots, which are in a process of **exfoliation,** as well as permanent teeth, whose roots are not yet fully formed, which are in the process of eruption. This is a normal phenomenon and is to be expected in radiographs of chil-

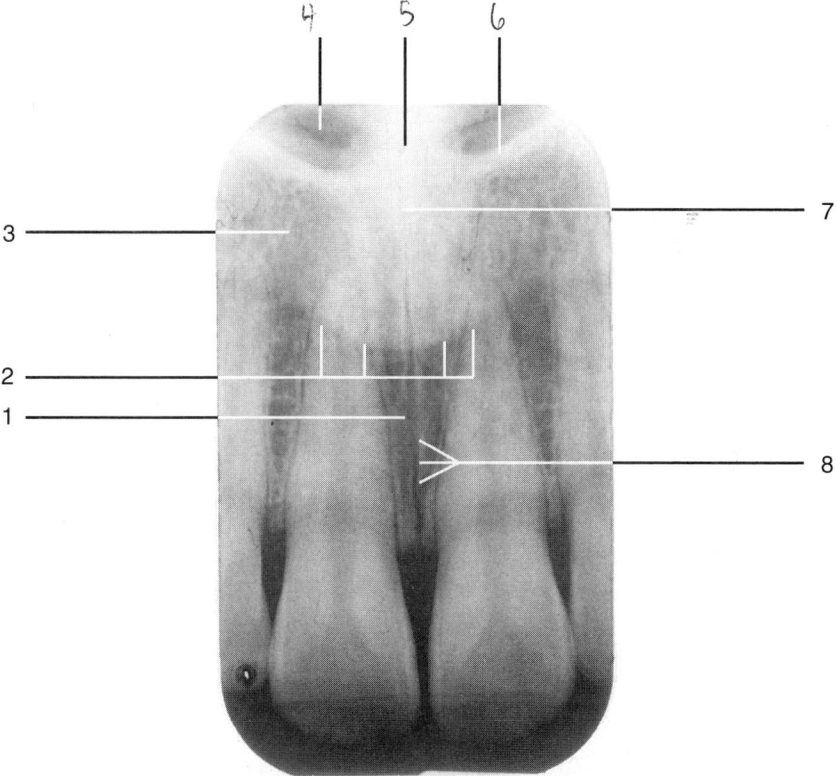

Figure 11–12. Radiograph of maxillary incisor area shows **1** incisive (anterior palatine) foramen, indicated by an irregularly-shaped, rounded radiolucent area, **2** outline of the nose, **3** lateral fossa, **4** nasal fossa (radiolucent), **5** nasal septum (radiopaque), **6** border of nasal fossa, **7** nasal spine, and **8** median palatine suture.

dren 10 to 12 years old and younger (Fig. 11–10). Such radiographs are often very difficult to identify and require a sound knowledge of dental anatomy. There are 32 permanent (secondary or succedaneous) teeth, provided that all four of the third molars (wisdom teeth) are formed. These are frequently missing or malpositioned.

Occasionally, teeth form but are unable to erupt: these are described as **impacted** teeth. Some people have one or more extra teeth; these are called **supernumerary** teeth. Another deviation is the congenital absence of certain teeth, described as **anodontia.** These conditions occur so frequently that, although not desirable, they are not considered pathological (see Chapter 12).

RADIOGRAPHIC APPEARANCE OF MAXILLARY LANDMARKS

The normal landmarks visible in radiographs of the maxilla vary in radiopacity or radiolucency in direct proportion to the densities of the exposed tissues. Individual difference, the manner in which the film was positioned, and the angle at which the expo-

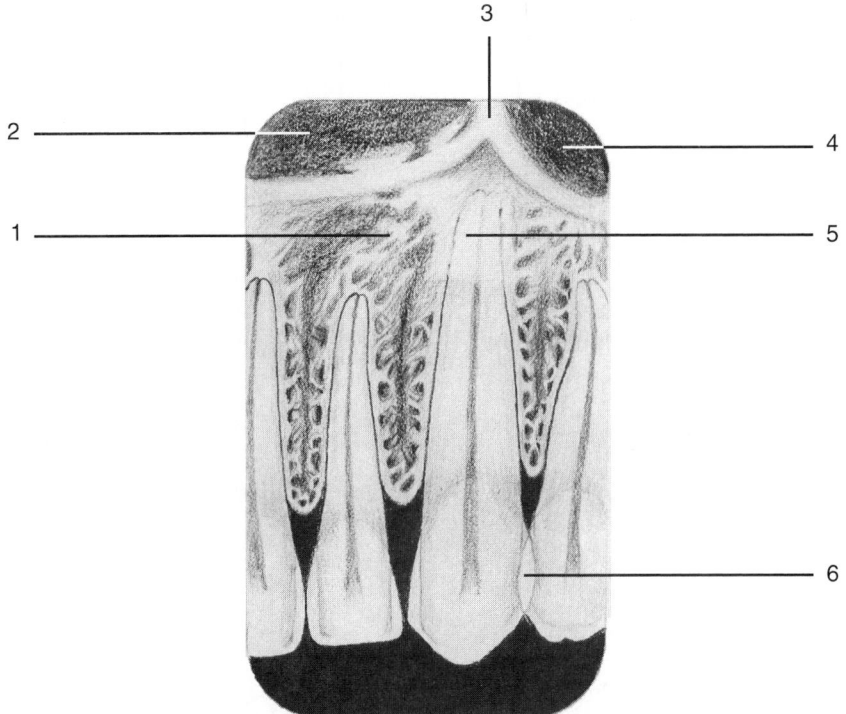

Figure 11–13. Drawing of maxillary canine (cuspid) area. **1** lateral fossa, **2** nasal fossa, **3** inverted Y (border of nasal fossa and maxillary sinus), **4** maxillary sinus, **5** canine (cuspid) eminence, and **6** dense radiopaque area caused by overlapping of the mesial surface of the first premolar over the distal surface of the canine (cuspid).

sure was made determine which landmarks may be visible on a radiograph of any given film placement area. Indeed, the expected landmark may not be visible at all, or perhaps on only a radiograph of the right or the left side.

Each normal structure is identified at least once on the drawings shown in Figures 11–11, 11–13, 11–15, and 11–17. Study the radiographs following each drawing to become proficient at recognizing and identifying normal maxillary anatomical landmarks (Figs. 11–12, 11–14, 11–16, 11–18, and 11–19).

Beginning with a radiograph of the incisor area and progressing posteriorly toward the molar area, it is generally possible to observe several or all of the following maxillary radiopaque structures: (1) the **nasal septum,** a dense cartilage structure that separates the right nasal fossa from the left; (2) the **anterior nasal spine,** a V-shaped projection from the floor of the nasal fossa in the midline; (3) the **inverted Y,** an important landmark seen in the canine-premolar area, made up of the lateral wall of the nasal fossa and the anterior-medial wall of the maxillary sinus; (4) the thin, dense bone forming the **floor** or **inferior border** of the sinuses; (5) sometimes a **septum** (wall or partition) may be seen separating the maxillary sinus into two or more compartments; (6) the **zygomatic process** of the maxilla, appearing as a broad U-shaped band often seen above the roots of the first and second molars; (7) the **zygoma** (malar bone or

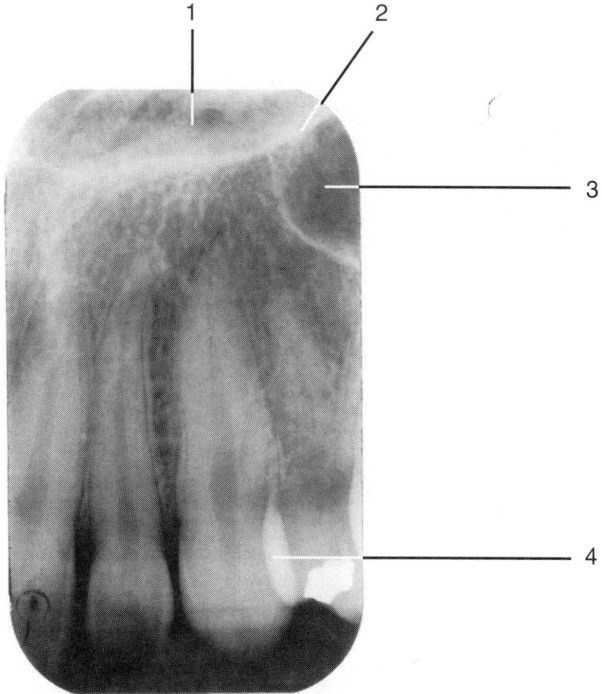

Figure 11–14. Radiograph of maxillary canine (cuspid) area shows **1** nasal fossa, **2** inverted Y (border of the nasal fossa and maxillary sinus), **3** maxillary sinus, and **4** dense radiopaque area caused by overlapping of the mesial surface of the first premolar over the distal surface of the canine (cuspid).

cheekbone), which extends laterally and distally from the zygomatic process of the maxilla; (8) the **zygomatic arch,** which is continuous with the zygoma and extends distally; (9) the **maxillary tuberosity,** the extension of the alveolar bone behind the molars that is covered by the oral mucosa and marks the posterior limits of the maxillary arch; (10) the **pterygoid plates** of the sphenoid, of which the **hamulus** (or hamular process, which is a downward projection of the medial pterygoid plate) appears as a hooklike structure that serves as a muscle attachment; and (11) sometimes the **coronoid process** of the mandible can be seen overlapping the maxillary tuberosity.

The following structures appear **radiolucent** on radiographs of the maxillary areas: (1) the **median palatine suture,** a thin line that delineates the midline of the palate and the junction of the right and left maxilla, frequently seen between the central incisors; (2) the **incisive foramen** (anterior palatine foramen), a round or pear-shaped opening that varies greatly in size, serves for the passage of nerves and blood vessels, and is often visible near or between the apices of the central incisors (this foramen can easily be mistaken for an abscess, cyst, or granuloma); (3) the **nasal fossa,** a large air space divided by the nasal septum, often visible above the roots of the incisors; and (4) the **maxillary sinus,** a large air chamber inside the maxilla, visible in the areas from the canines to the molars.

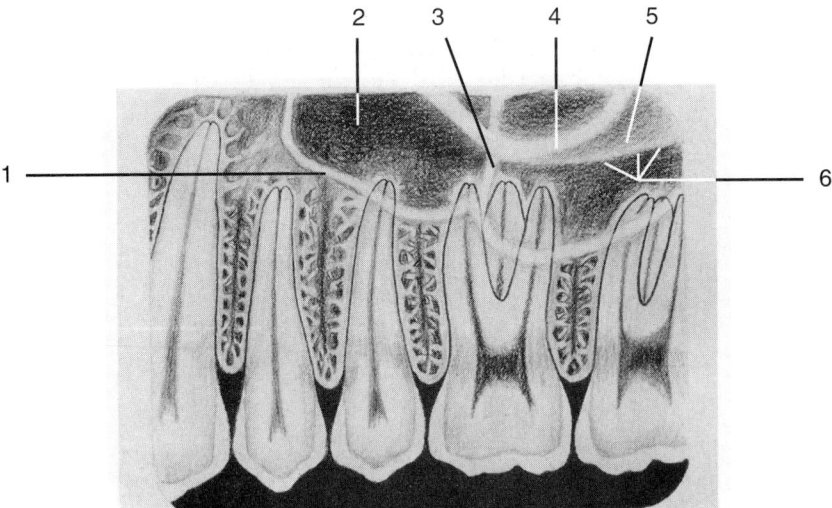

Figure 11–15. Drawing of maxillary premolar (biscuspid) area. **1** border (floor) of maxillary sinus, **2** maxillary sinus, **3** septum in maxillary sinus dividing the sinus into two compartments, **4** zygomatic process of maxilla, **5** zygoma, and **6** lower border of zygomatic arch.

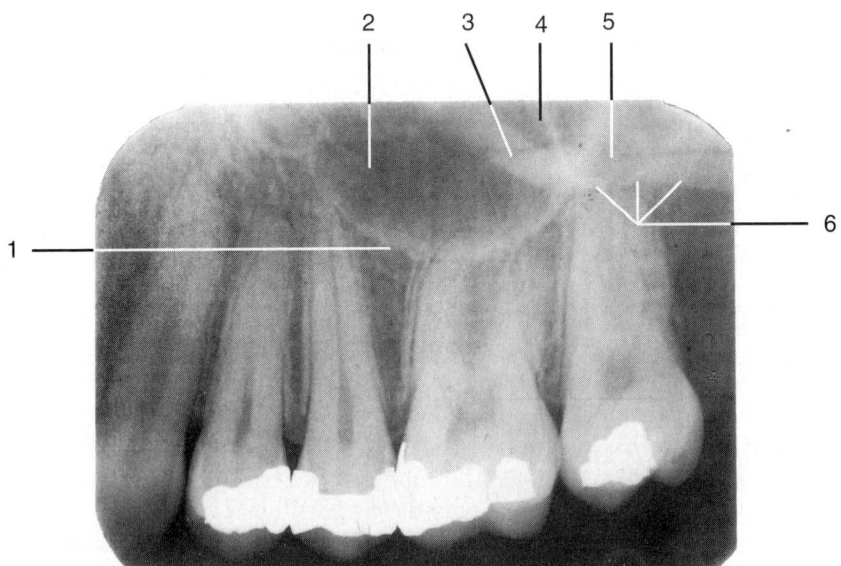

Figure 11–16. Radiograph of maxillary premolar (bicuspid) area shows **1** border (floor) of maxillary sinus, **2** maxillary sinus, **3** zygomatic process of maxilla, **4** septum in maxillary sinus dividing the sinus into two compartments, **5** zygoma, and **6** lower border of zygomatic arch.

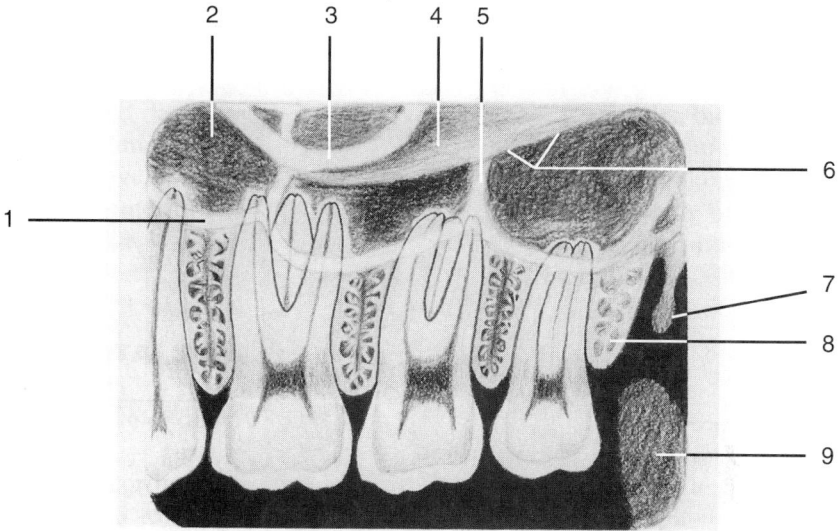

Figure 11–17. Drawing of maxillary molar area. **1** border (floor) of maxillary sinus, **2** maxillary sinus, **3** zygomatic process of maxilla, **4** zygoma, **5** septum in maxillary sinus, **6** lower border of zygomatic arch, **7** hamulus (hamular process), **8** maxillary tuberosity, and **9** coronoid process (mandible).

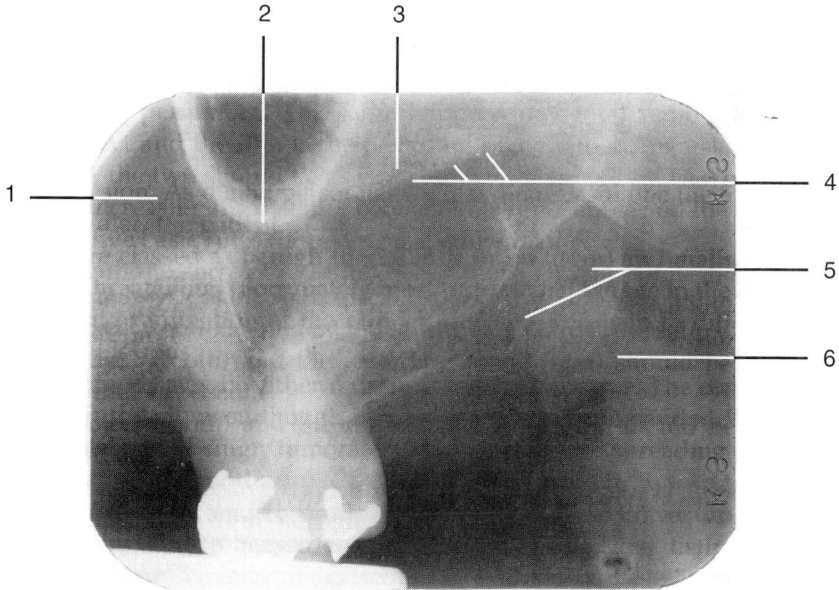

Figure 11–18. Radiograph of maxillary molar area shows **1** maxillary sinus, **2** zygomatic process of maxilla, **3** zygoma, **4** lower border of zygomatic arch, **5** maxillary tuberosity, and **6** coronoid process of the mandible.

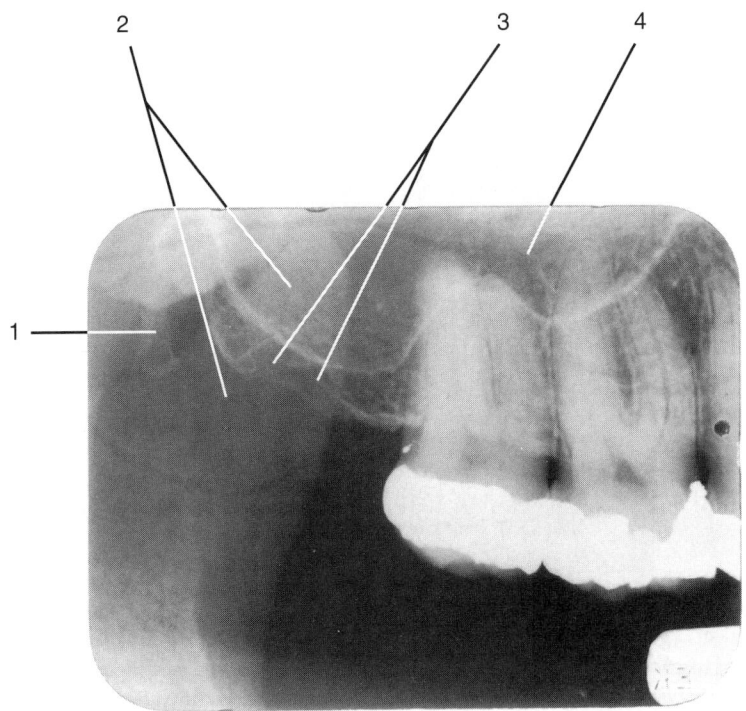

Figure 11–19. Radiograph of maxillary molar area shows **1** hamulus (hamular process), which is a downward projection of the medial pterygoid plate, **2** coronoid process of the mandible, **3** maxillary tuberosity, and **4** maxillary sinus.

RADIOGRAPHIC APPEARANCE OF MANDIBULAR LANDMARKS

Each mandibular landmark is identified at least once on the drawings shown in Figures 11–20, 11–22, 11–24, and 11–27. Study the radiographs following each drawing to become proficient at recognizing and identifying normal mandibular anatomical landmarks (Figs. 11–21, 11–23, 11–25, 11–26, 11–28, and 11–29).

Continuing the method used to identify and mount the maxillary radiographs, it is generally possible to observe several or all of the radiopaque structures on radiographs of the mandibular tooth areas: (1) **genial tubercles,** four small bony crests on the lingual surface that serve for muscle attachments, generally visible as a round radiopaque "doughnut" at the midline below the apices of the central incisors; (2) the **mental ridge** on the lateral surface, which appears as a radiopaque line extending from the premolar region to the symphysis; (3) the **external oblique ridge,** a continua-

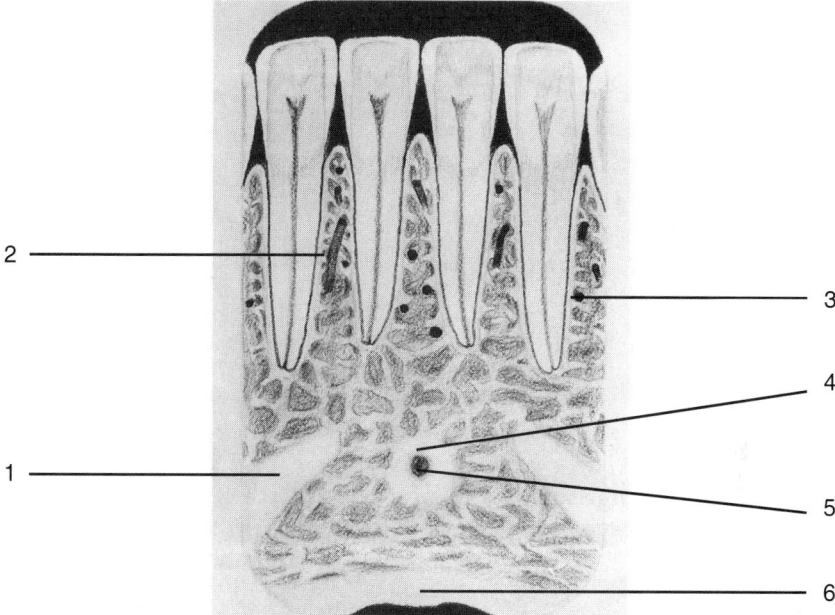

Figure 11–20. Drawing of mandibular midline area. **1** mental ridge, **2** nutrient canal, **3** nutrient foramen, **4** genial tubercles, **5** lingual foramen, and **6** inferior (lower) border of mandible.

tion of the anterior border of the ramus that extends downward and forward on the lateral surface of the mandible and appears as a radiopaque line of varied width across the molar region; (4) the **mylohyoid ridge** or **internal oblique ridge,** an irregular crest of bone for muscle attachments on the lingual surface of the mandible in the molar re-gion, which appears as a radiopaque line parallel and always below the external oblique ridge; and (5) the **inferior border** of the mandible, a heavy layer of cortical bone, visible only if the radiograph is deeply depressed in the floor of the mouth.

The following structures appear radiolucent on radiographs of the mandibular ar-eas: (1) the **lingual foramen,** a very small circular area surrounded by the genial tuber-cles, occasionally seen in the central incisor area but often so small that it goes unno-ticed; (2) the **mental foramen,** a small opening on the lateral side of the body of the mandible, often seen near the apices of the premolars; (3) the **submandibular fossa,** a large irregularly shaped area below the mylohyoid ridge and the roots of the mandibular molars, in which the bone is quite thin and can easily be mistaken for a le-sion; and (4) the **mandibular canal,** a canal for the passage of the mandibular nerve and blood vessels, outlined by very thin layers of cortical bone, which can often be seen in the premolar-molar areas below the apices of the teeth.

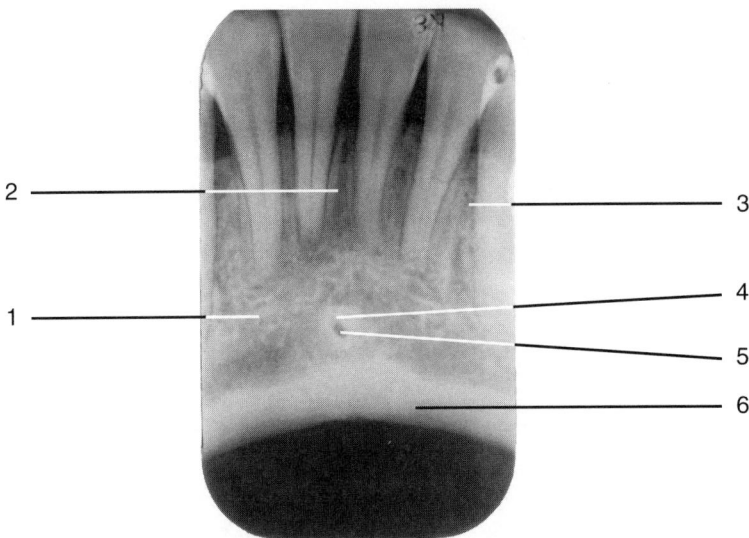

Figure 11–21. Radiograph of the mandibular incisor area shows **1** mental ridge, **2** nutrient canal, **3** nutrient foramen, **4** genial tubercles surrounding the lingual foramen, **5** lingual foramen, and **6** inferior (lower) border of the mandible (radiopaque band of dense cortical bone).

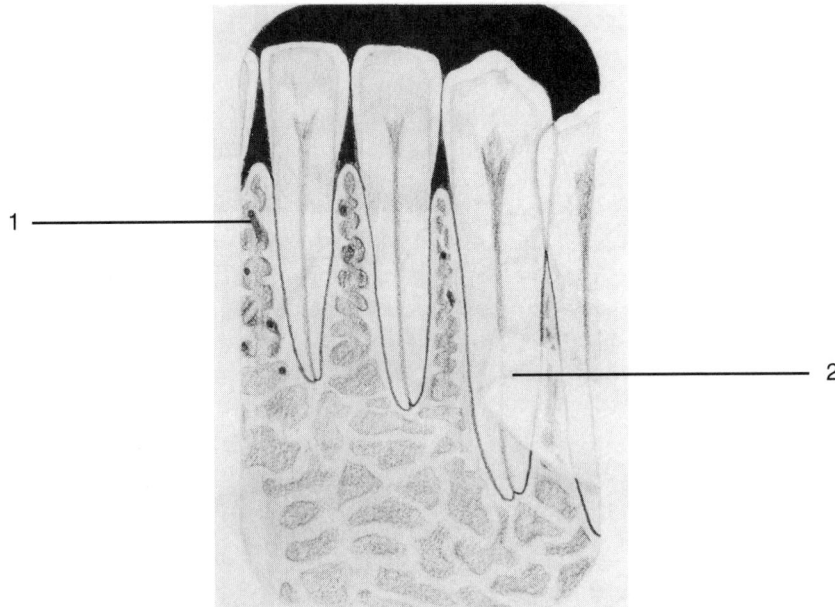

Figure 11–22. Drawing of mandibular canine (cuspid) area. **1** nutrient canal, and **2** torus mandibularis (lingual torus).

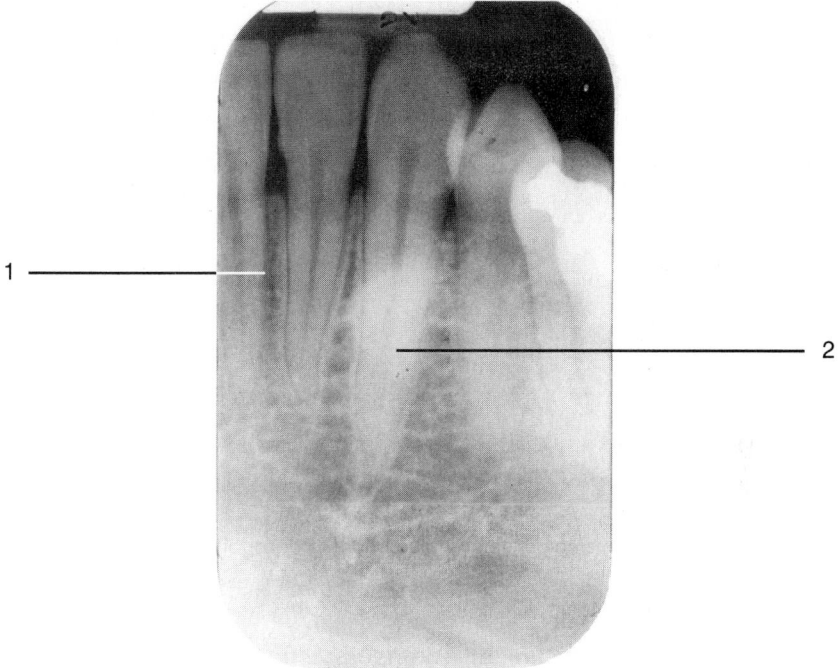

Figure 11–23. Radiograph of mandibular canine (cuspid) area shows **1** nutrient canal, and **2** torus mandibularis (lingual torus).

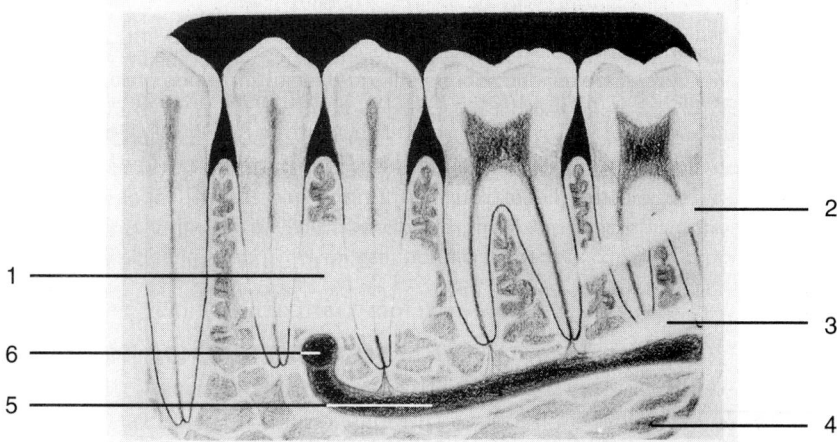

Figure 11–24. Drawing of mandibular premolar (bicuspid) area. **1** torus mandibularis, **2** external oblique ridge, **3** mylohyoid ridge (internal oblique ridge), **4** submandibular fossa, an area where the bone of the mandible is extremely thin and offers little resistance to the passage of radiation and therefore appears radiolucent instead of radiopaque as denser bone does, **5** mandibular canal, and **6** mental foramen.

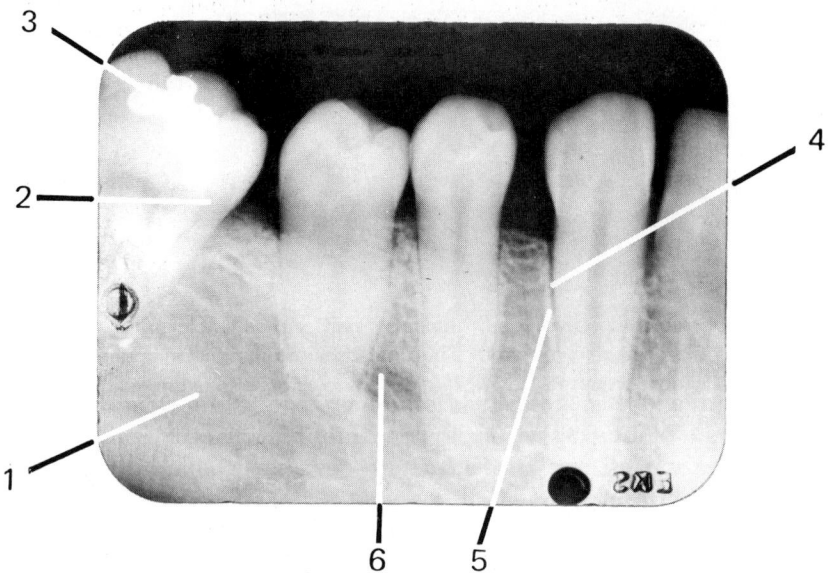

Figure 11–25. Radiograph of mandibular premolar (bicuspid) area shows **1** submandibular fossa, an area where the bone of the mandible is extremely thin and offers little resistance to the passage of radiation and therefore appears radiolucent instead of radiopaque as denser bone does, **2** cervical burnout at cemento-enamel junction (radiolucent), **3** metal restoration, **4** thin radiolucent line indicating periodontal ligament space, **5** thin radiopaque line as the lamina dura, and **6** small radiolucent circle as the mental foramen.

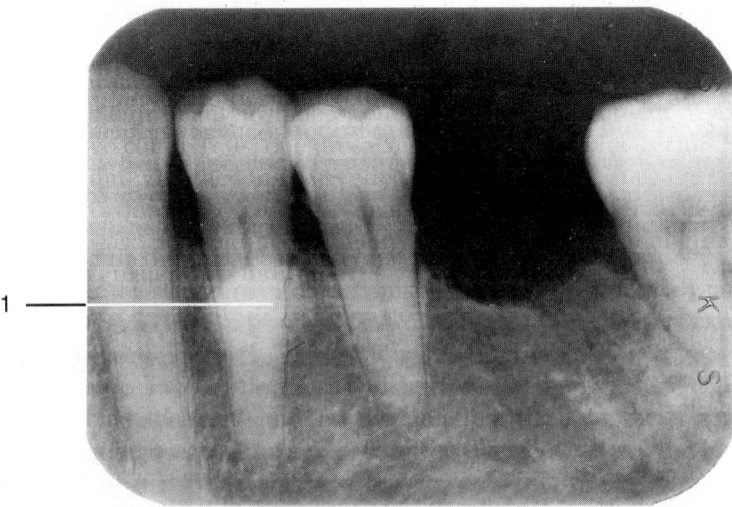

Figure 11–26. Radiograph of mandibular premolar (bicuspid) area shows **1** torus mandibularis (lingual torus).

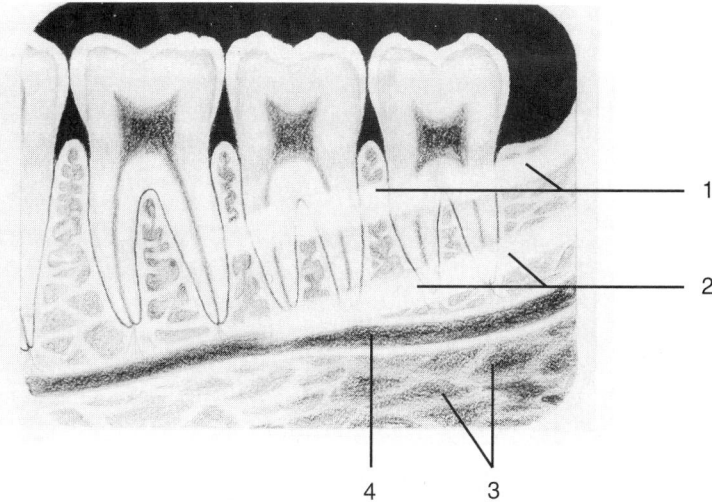

Figure 11–27. Drawing of mandibular molar area. **1** external oblique ridge, **2** mylohyoid ridge (internal oblique ridge), **3** submandibular fossa, an area where the bone of the mandible is extremely thin and offers little resistance to the passage of radiation and therefore appears radiolucent instead of radiopaque as denser bone does, and **4** mandibular canal, a wide diagonal radiolucent area outlined above and below by a thin radiopaque line.

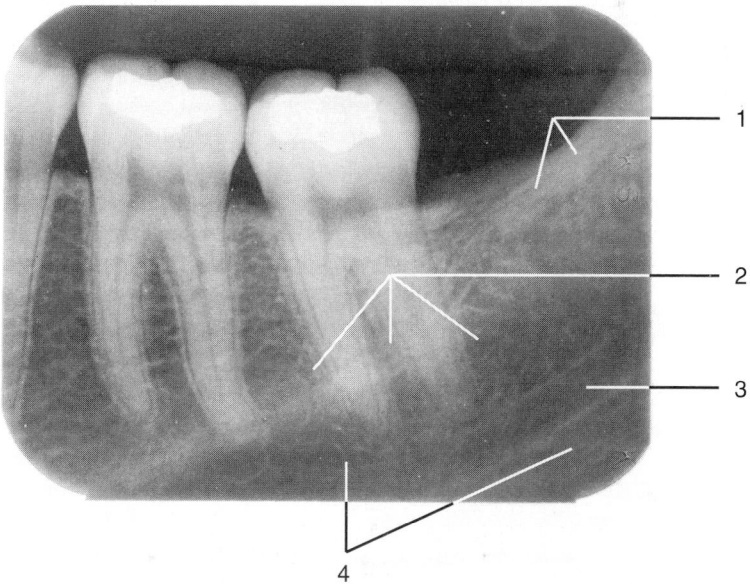

Figure 11–28. Radiograph of mandibular molar area shows **1** external oblique ridge, **2** internal oblique ridge, **3** mandibular canal, and **4** submandibular fossa, an area where the bone of the mandible is extremely thin and therefore appears somewhat radiolucent.

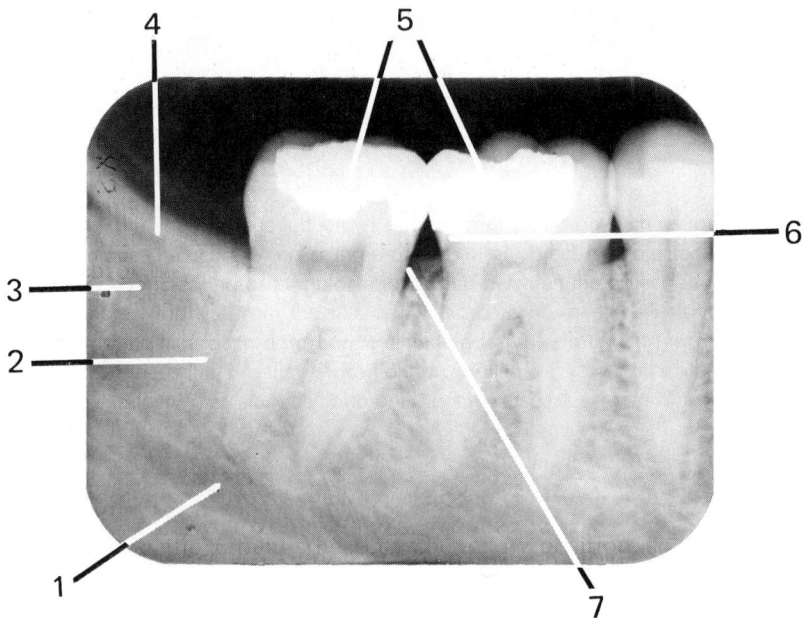

Figure 11–29. Radiograph of mandibular molar area shows **1** mandibular canal, a wide diagonal radiolucent area outlined above and below by a very thin radiopaque line, **2** mylohyoid ridge, diagonal radiopaque thickening of the mandibular bone, **3** cone-shaped, slightly radiolucent area denoting the site where a third molar was removed and the bone has not completely regenerated, **4** external oblique ridge, indicated by diagonal radiopaque band of bone, **5** metallic restorations (appearing radiopaque), **6** small radiolucent area beneath metal restoration denoting either cervical burnout or recurrent caries—differentiation can be made by digital inspection with explorer, the radiographic appearance on another film exposed at a slightly different angle, or both, and **7** radiolucent area between root of second molar and alveolar crest indicating a slight degree of vertical bone resorption.

MOUNTING THE RADIOGRAPHS

Mounting is extremely important so that each of a series of radiographs can be arranged in proper anatomical relationship to all other radiographs exposed on a patient at a given time. Correct mounting helps to eliminate embarrassing errors caused by confusing radiographs of the patient's right and left sides. When mounted, radiographs are easier to view and interpret.

Film mounts are celluloid, cardboard, or plastic holders with frames or windows for the radiographs. Attaching the radiographs to the film mounts is called **mounting**. Film mounts are available in many sizes and with numerous combinations of windows or frames to fit films of different sizes. Most mounts are large enough to accommodate a full-mouth series of radiographs, although some hold only a few or even a single radiograph. Standard ready-made mounts are used in most dental offices; however, several firms will make custom mounts to suit special needs. Black mounts are often preferred because they can block out extraneous light from the viewbox.

The task of mounting the radiographs is not difficult once the novice becomes familiar with the appearance of the anatomical structures and masters a few simple procedures. First, one must be able to distinguish which films are of the patient's right and which are of the left side. A little identification dot near the edge of the film appears convex or concave depending on the side from which the film is viewed. When the film is mounted with the convex dot toward you, the patient's left side is on your right (Fig. 11–30).

In the past, two systems of film mounting were commonly used. The first method, now obsolete, had the radiographs mounted so that they gave the effect of viewing the patient from behind. In this arrangement, the concave side of the dot faces the viewer. The second method, now taught by all dental colleges, mounts the radiographs so that they are viewed from the front of the patient. The convex side of the dot faces the viewer. All national organizations, including the American Dental Association, recommend the latter method.

Mounting generally refers only to intraoral films. The large extraoral films are already identified through the use of metal lettering and are usually placed in a protec-

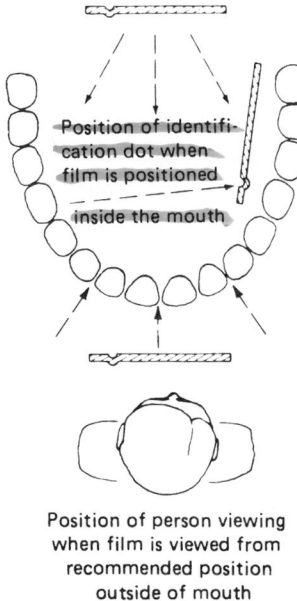

Position of person viewing
when film is viewed from
recommended position
outside of mouth

Figure 11–30. Regardless of the tooth area involved, whenever an x-ray film is positioned in the mouth, the raised portion of the identification dot (the convexity) must face the x-ray tube and the source of radiation. Therefore, when the film is viewed from outside the mouth or from in front of the patient, the convex side of the dot faces the person viewing the film.

tive envelope. The patient's name and the date of the exposure are always written on the outside of these envelopes. Occasionally, single intraoral radiographs are not mounted but are slipped into a coin envelope and attached to the record card. However, it is better to mount even a single or a small group of radiographs; a full-mouth series should always be mounted for easier and faster viewing. Obviously, each film mount must be identified with at least the patient's name, case number if applicable, and the date. Few things are as useless in a dental office as unidentifiable radiographs.

The auxiliary generally follows a routine when mounting a set of radiographs. First, wash hands to prevent smudging the films and lay a clean towel over the workbench in front of an illuminator. To avoid confusing radiographs, remove only one patient's films from the clips of the film hanger at one time (sometimes films of different patients are processed on the same hanger). Then arrange the films so that all the identification dots face in the same direction, with the convex side toward the viewer.

The radiographs must be arranged just as the teeth in the mouth are; the anterior teeth must be mounted in the middle frames and the posterior teeth in the frames on either side of the mouth. The maxillary teeth must be positioned so that the incisal edges or occlusal surfaces point downward and the roots upward. The mandibular teeth are mounted the opposite way, with the incisal or occlusal surfaces pointing up and the roots pointing to the bottom of the mount.

Several distinctive tooth characteristics and bone structures make mounting easier: (1) the roots and crowns of the maxillary anterior teeth are larger than those of the mandibular teeth; (2) the maxillary molars generally have three roots and the mandibular molars only two; (3) most roots curve toward the distal; (4) the large radiolucent areas denoting the nasal fossa or the maxillary sinus indicate that the radiograph is of a maxillary area; (5) the radiolucent mental foramen indicates that the film belongs in the mandibular premolar (bicuspid) area; and (6) the body of the mandible has a distinct upward curve toward the ramus in the molar area.

With these characteristics firmly in mind, the auxiliary holds the radiographs up to the illuminator and separates them into three groups: (1) the anterior films, (2) the posterior films, and (3) the bitewing films. The radiographs of each of these groups are then identified as right or left, maxillary or mandibular. They are put into proper order and placed on the mount one by one. Some auxilaries like to mount the bitewings first, so there is a base of reference for mounting periapicals by comparing restorations or carious lesions. The auxiliary should handle films by their edges to avoid smudging them. After the last radiograph has been mounted, the entire film mount should be carefully checked to ensure that no films were reversed accidentally or mounted upside down and that the name and date are on the mount.

The method just described is particularly recommended for beginners. As their skills increase, many auxiliaries develop simpler and faster techniques.

VIEWING THE RADIOGRAPHS

The importance of using a good illuminated viewbox for mounting and interpreting the radiographs cannot be overemphasized. Many types of viewboxes are available, both built-ins and portables. The preferred type for the dental office use has a dark,

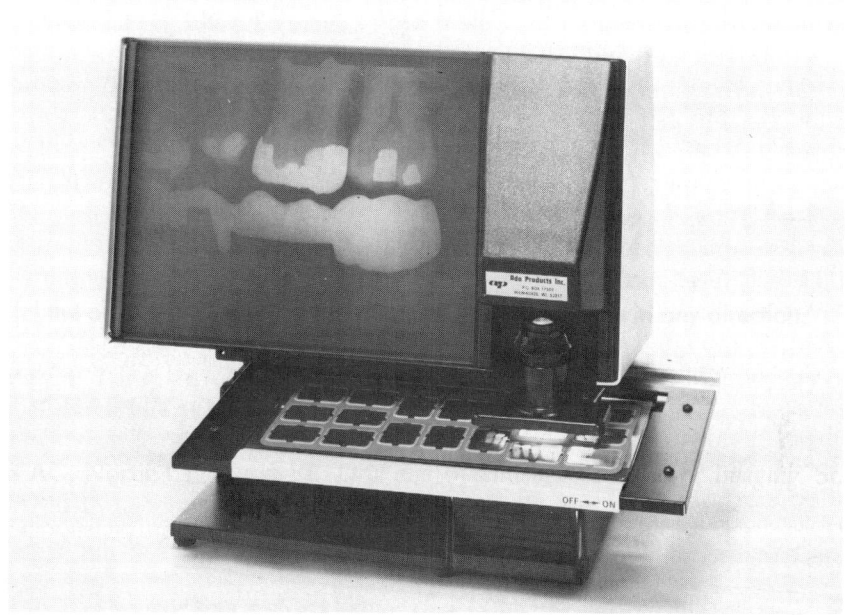

Figure 11–31. Viewer-enlarger-projector. Used as a viewer, the radiographs can be observed on a 9-by-12-in. (32-by-38-cm) screen. High-low light control gives the image the brightness needed for diagnosis. Used as an enlarger, the size of the radiograph is increased eight times. By removing the viewing screen, the unit can be converted into a projector. *(Courtesy of Ada Products, Inc.)*

nonreflective frame, a frosted glass panel, and a rheostat to vary the intensity of the light. Blocking out excess light reduces glare and facilitates viewing. The use of black cardboard or frosted film mounts also helps to reduce glare and enhances the detail of the images. Some viewers are also equipped with a magnifying device (Fig. 11–31).

Mounted radiographs show the relations between major tooth areas and reveal each in its entirety, clearly and with a minimum of distortion. If circumstances permit, substandard radiographs should be retaken before being submitted to the dentist. Depending on the auxiliary's status and responsibility in the dental office, the individual may now proceed to make a preliminary interpretation and discuss it with the dentist. After this, the film mount should be placed in a properly identified protective envelope and filed until needed at the patient's next visit.

FILING AND STORAGE OF DENTAL RADIOGRAPHS

After the radiographs are mounted, they should be placed in a protective envelope and given to the dentist to examine before they are discussed with the patient. The radiographs should be in the operation room along with other records each time the patient visits the office.

After the appointment, the radiographs should be filed until needed again. They may be stored along with the record folder or in a separate x-ray filing cabinet. The radiographs may be filed by either name or case number, as long as they can be located rapidly when needed. The need for an orderly filing system cannot be overstressed; missing radiographs can be a source of much annoyance. Some dentists store current radiographs in one file and older ones in another. When new radiographs are exposed, the old ones are often removed from the mounts and placed into smaller envelopes, identified and dated, to conserve space.

All radiographs should be handled with care to prevent smudging or scratching and should be protected from heat damage by storage in cool, well-ventilated areas. Although radiographs are seldom used after more than 6 months or 1 year because oral conditions change constantly in most patients, they are valuable for comparing present with previous conditions. Sometimes they are needed in a court of law. Therefore, dentists should preserve them until they are certain that the statute of limitations for their state has expired.

CHAPTER SUMMARY

A knowledge of the anatomical landmarks of the face and skull is needed to properly position the film packet and direct the radiation through the proper point of entry. This can be acquired through practice and study by using a skull and a textbook and followed by clinical exercises. With this training and experience, dental auxiliaries can learn to identify most landmarks and structures of the maxillae and mandible. This is essential for mounting the processed films.

Dental anatomical landmarks are separated into the following groups: (1) face, (2) skull, (3) maxillae, and (4) mandible. Although facial landmarks cannot be distinguised on a radiograph, they help the radiographer locate important planes and structures when placing the film and directing the PID. Knowledge of skull landmarks is useful when making cephalometric, temporomandibular joint, or panoramic exposures. One must be familiar with all radiopaque and radiolucent landmarks of the maxillae and mandible in order to interpret or mount intraoral radiographs.

It is customary to arrange the radiographs of a full-mouth series in anatomical order on some form of film mount. These mounts vary in size and number of frames, but all have space for identifying information: patient's name and date of exposure. Each film has an identification dot in one of the corners by which it is possible to determine on which side of the face it was exposed. When the radiograph is mounted with the convex side of the dot toward the viewer, the radiographs of the patient's left side are on the right side of the mount as seen by the viewer. As experience is gained, the auxiliary should be able to differentiate between normal and abnormal structures of the jaws, teeth, and periodontium and recognize most restorative materials. Recognition is facilitated if a viewbox with magnification and a variable light intensity control is used.

KEY WORDS

Ala

Alveolar bone

Alveolar process

Alveolus

Angle of mandible

Apical foramen

Cancellous bone

Cementum

Condyle

Cortical bone

Dentin

Enamel

External auditory meatus (foramen)

External oblique ridge

Film mount

Foramen

Fossa

Genial tubercles

Glenoid fossa

Hamulus

Identification dot

Incisive foramen (anterior palatine foramen)

Inferior border of mandible

Lamina dura

Lingual foramen

Mandibular canal

Median palatine suture

Mental foramen

Mylohyoid ridge (internal oblique ridge)

Periodontal ligament

Process

Radiolucent

Radiopaque

Ramus

Septum

Sinus (maxillary)

Submandibular fossa

Symphysis

Trabecular bone

Tragus

Tubercle

Tuberosity (maxillary)

REVIEW QUESTIONS

1. Which of these terms describes the ability to read a radiograph? (a) case presentation, (b) prognosis, (c) dissertation, (d) interpretation.

2. Which of these is a facial landmark? (a) coronoid process, (b) glenoid fossa, (c) tragus, (d) mylohyoid ridge.

3. Which of these is not a mandibular landmark? (a) incisive foramen, (b) lingual foramen, (c) coronoid process, (d) mental foramen.

4. Which of these structures appears radiolucent? (a) enamel, (b) dental pulp, (c) dentin, (d) alveolar bone.

5. Which of these structures appears radiopaque? (a) maxillary sinus, (b) nasal fossa, (c) maxillary tuberosity, (d) mental foramen.

6. Which of these appears most radiopaque? (a) trabecular bone, (b) cementum, (c) dentin, (d) enamel.

7. A bony projection that extends downward and slightly posterior in many maxillary molar radiographs is the (a) mastoid process, (b) styloid process, (c) condylar process, (d) hamular process.

8. In a radiograph of the maxillary molars, the following structure may obscure the roots of the teeth. (a) zygomatic process of the maxilla, (b) maxillary tuberosity, (c) mastoid process, (d) mylohyoid ridge.

9. All dental schools now teach that for viewing, radiographs should be mounted as though (a) you are seated on the tongue looking out, (b) you are facing the patient, (c) you are viewing the patient from behind, (d) you are viewing the patient from the side.

10. Which of these helps to determine whether the radiograph is of the patient's right or left side? (a) the lamina dura, (b) the film emulsion, (c) the location of the septum, (d) the identification dot.

BIBLIOGRAPHY

Farman AG, Nortje CJ, Wood RE: *Oral and Maxillofacial Diagnostic Imaging.* St. Louis, MO: CV Mosby, 1993

Goaz PW, White SC: *Oral Radiology: Principles and Interpretation,* 3rd ed. St. Louis, MO: CV Mosby, 1994

Kasle, MJ: *An Atlas of Dental Radiographic Anatomy,* 2nd ed. Philadelphia, PA: WB Saunders, 1983

CHAPTER 12

Preliminary Interpretation of the Radiographs

By the end of this chapter the student should be able to

1. Differentiate between preliminary interpretation and diagnosis of the radiograph.
2. Identify all radiopaque- and radiolucent-appearing restorative materials.
3. Identify the radiographic appearance of dental caries.
4. Identify at least four types of cysts.
5. Describe the appearance of at least eight anomalies.
6. Differentiate between normal and pathological resorption of bone structures and teeth.
7. Differentiate between calcifications and ossifications.
8. Describe the radiographic appearance of odontogenic tumors.
9. Describe the radiographic appearance of dental injuries.
10. Identify two methods used to localize objects in the jaws by applying the buccal-object rule.

PRELIMINARY INTERPRETATION BY AUXILIARY PERSONNEL

Just a few years ago, and even still in many dental offices, all that was expected of a competent auxiliary was to recognize sufficient anatomical landmarks or structures to be able to mount the radiographs correctly. Although radiographic interpretation is legally forbidden, many dentists today expect their auxiliaries to have a sound knowledge of the normal and also the abnormal or pathological conditions that may occasionally be visible on dental radiographs.

Chapter 11 dealt with the radiographic appearance of normal anatomical structures and landmarks. In this chapter the emphasis is on the recognition of the radiographic appearance of restorative dental materials, dental caries, cysts, anomalies, the more common diseases of the periodontium, bone pathology, and dental injuries.

The complete interpretation of dental radiographs is the task of dentists, whose years of training and study have prepared them to render a diagnosis. However, according to the recent concept of expanded duties, in some states a preliminary interpretation can be made by the trained dental auxiliary. Final responsibility for the diagnosis remains with the dentist.

The terms **interpretation** and **diagnosis** are often used interchangeably. This book, however, defines interpretation only as the ability to read the radiographs; diagnosis means the correlation of the patient's case history, clinical findings, test results, and radiographs. The dentist makes the diagnosis only after considering all the evidence pertaining to the patient's condition.

Because dental auxiliaries lack the in-depth training of the dentist and therefore may overlook important factors or err in the interpretation, they must never express interpretive or diagnostic opinions to the patient. However, the dentist should encourage the auxiliary to make a private preliminary interpretation of the radiograph.

To produce consistently good radiographs, the student or auxiliary must not only be familiar with dental anatomy and exposure techniques but must know how to tell whether or not all the desired information appears on the radiograph. One must know how to recognize anatomical landmarks and structures as well as dental caries, restorative dentistry, periodontal disease, and uncomplicated periapical disease arising from tooth involvement.

This text can discuss only common conditions. The study of complete interpretation of dental radiographs is far too complex to be feasible within the scope of this text for dental auxiliary personnel.

Recognizing complex or uncommon pathological conditions is not the responsibility of the auxiliary. Several textbooks listed in the bibliography are excellent sources for reference and additional study. Although primarily written for dental students and dentists, these books are liberally illustrated with helpful radiographs showing normal and abnormal structures and conditions of the jaws, the teeth, and the periodontium. With practice in identifying oral landmarks and structures, many auxiliaries learn to recognize all the common, and occasionally the less common, abnormalities. It is satisfying to have one's own analysis corroborated by the dentist.

Before you attempt to interpret any radiograph, it is highly desirable to have a viewbox with a light source of variable intensity. Furthermore, the light in the room should be reduced so that the eyes will adapt to the light level of the radiograph. A magnifying glass may also be helpful in examining the radiograph.

RADIOGRAPHIC APPEARANCE OF DENTAL RESTORATIVE MATERIALS

The radiographic appearance of normal tooth structures was discussed in Chapter 11. These are readily identified by most auxiliaries. The differentiation between the various restorative materials is a little more difficult and requires additional experience.

Some restorative materials are easy to identify; others can be differentiated only by the size and contour of the restoration, its probable location on the tooth, and the relative degree of radiopacity or radiolucency.

For example, the image outlines of all metallic restorations of approximately equal density appear extremely radiopaque. Thus it is impossible to determine whether the material used was gold, silver, or a base metal alloy. Only by looking at the size and contour of the restoration is it possible to make an educated guess based on what materials are generally used in such circumstances. Furthermore, it is not always possible to determine on which tooth surface the restoration is located. A filling looks the same whether it is on the facial (buccal) or lingual side of the tooth because radiographs are merely shadow pictures. Methods of localization are presented at the end of this chapter.

The image of a restoration on one surface may be superimposed on the image of another large restoration on the same tooth, thus giving the appearance of only one

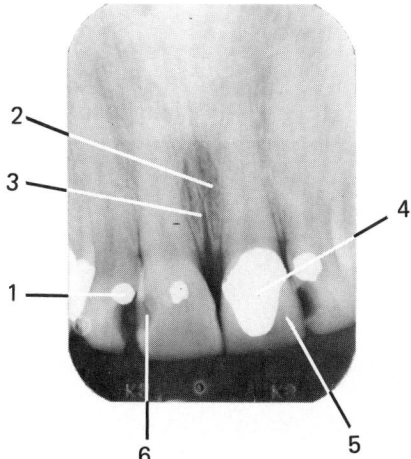

Figure 12–1. Radiograph of maxillary incisor region shows: **1** small radiopaque metallic restoration, which could be gold foil or amalgam; these materials cannot be differentiated on a radiograph and must be determined by a visual inspection; **2** incisive (anterior palatine) foramen; **3** thin dark line as median palatine suture; **4** metal core of porcelain jacket crown; **5** fused porcelain of crown, the most dense of the esthetic (natural appearing) dental restorative materials and described as being slightly radiolucent; and **6** a silicate restoration (radiolucent). Observe that the silicate in the adjacent tooth has partially disintegrated. A visual inspection is required to verify any preliminary interpretation of the radiographs.

restoration instead of two, or even more. Some materials, such as the cements used in dentistry, can be differentiated only by the location on the tooth and the degree of radiopacity, while esthetic materials, such as fused porcelain, silicate, the acrylic resins (plastics), some of the composites, and the sealants may be barely visible or appear quite similar and exhibit only slight differences in radiolucency. Of these, fused porcelain is the most dense and least radiolucent, whereas the acrylic resins are least dense and most radiolucent. The identification of composite resin restorations is difficult because some manufacturers add radiopaque particles to their product so that the

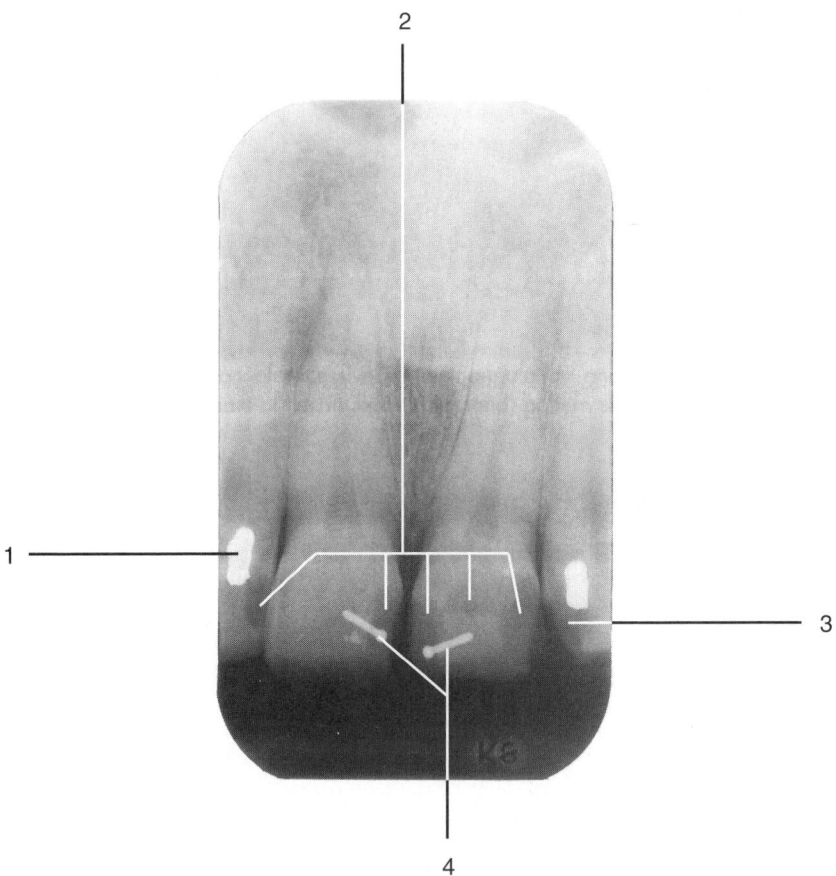

Figure 12–2. Radiograph of maxillary incisor region shows: **1** small radiopaque metallic restoration, probably amalgam on the lingual surface; **2** radiolucent areas, possibly restorative materials (composites, acrylic resins, or silicates) or caries—a visual inspection is required to verify any preliminary interpretation of the radiographs; **3** fractured mesial incisal angle; and **4** radiopaque metallic pins holding the radiolucent composite restorations.

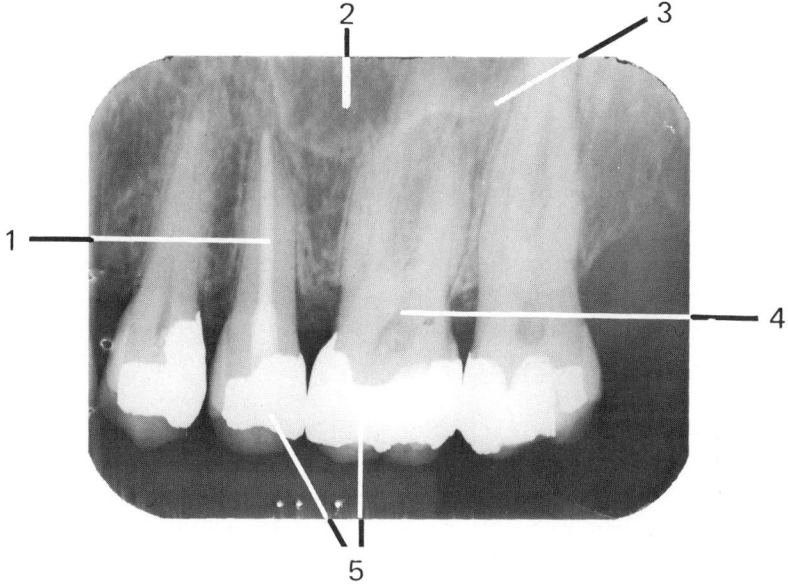

Figure 12–3. Radiograph of maxillary premolar (bicuspid) region shows **1** gutta-percha–filled root canal (radiopaque), **2** maxillary sinus, **3** dense bone lining the inferior border of the maxillary sinus, **4** small radiopaque pulp stone in the center of the pulp chamber, and **5** metallic restorations.

viewer will not mistake it for dental caries. Thus, it should be obvious that a visual and digital examination is required to verify the conditions shown on a radiograph.

All metals used in dentistry—whether in the form of fillings, crowns, bridges, or orthodontic wires, the gutta-percha points used in root canals, the zinc phosphate cements used in bases and for cementation, the zinc oxide–eugenol pastes used as protective bases, or those composite filling materials and calcium hydroxide pastes used in pulp capping that have opaque materials added to them—exhibit some degree of radiopacity and are described as **radiopaque** (light).

The fused porcelains used for crowns and as facings for bridgework, the silicates used for filling anterior teeth, the acrylic resins used for fillings and crowns, many composite fillings, and most calcium hydroxide pastes exhibit some degree of radiolucency and are described as **radiolucent** (dark). Several of these materials are identified on the radiographs in Figures 12–1 through 12–3.

RADIOGRAPHIC APPEARANCE OF DENTAL CARIES

The radiographic appearance of normal tooth structures is often drastically altered by the development of carious lesions (tooth decay). Because the detection of dental caries is based on substantial loss of tooth minerals, all caries visible on radiographs appear radiolucent.

Dental **caries** are the radiolucent lesions most frequently encountered on radiographs. There are three types: (1) incipient caries, the small breaks in the enamel often visible in the areas between the teeth; (2) recurrent caries, decay that occurs under the restoration or around its margins; and (3) rampant decay, the deep cavities that are easiest to recognize (Fig. 12–4).

Dental caries may develop in the enamel and dentin of any tooth surface and occasionally on the cementum, usually near the cementoenamel junction. Because the dense enamel covering of the crowns blocks the passage of the x-rays to a certain extent, caries on the occlusal pits and fissures—unless the caries are quite advanced and large—are often not visible radiographically and can be detected more easily during clinical examination.

The bitewing (interproximal) radiographs, described in Chapter 16, are generally considered to be most useful for early caries detection. Interproximal surface caries are located between the contact point of the tooth and the gingival margin. The shape of interproximal caries is triangular, with the base toward the outer surface of the tooth and the apex toward the dentin–enamel junction (DEJ). Once the caries progresses into

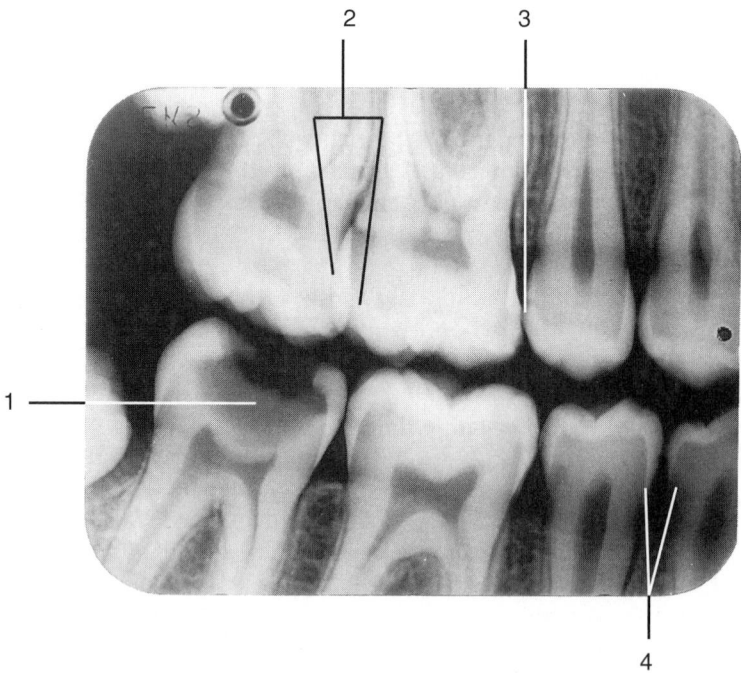

Figure 12–4. Bitewing radiograph shows **1** large occlusal caries; **2** radiolucent lines or mach band effect, an optical illusion caused by overlapped enamel; **3** interproximal caries; and **4** cervical burnout.

the dentin, another triangle is formed. This time the base is toward the DEJ and the apex toward the pulp chamber.

Dental caries are sometimes difficult to diagnose because nonmetallic restorations attenuate the x-ray beam so little that the area in question appears radiolucent, and only a clinical examination can determine what it is. Another factor that complicates caries detection is that large metallic restorations frequently hide decay beneath or behind them.

Two frequently observed radiolucencies that occasionally are mistaken for caries are esthetic restorations in anterior teeth and cervical burnout. Anterior restorations appear radiolucent because they are usually nonmetallic. On radiographs on which **cervical burnout** is noted, an irregularly shaped radiolucent area with a fuzzy outline can be seen on both the mesial and distal surfaces along the cervical line. The cause of cervical burnout is the concavity of the root surfaces, which results in greater penetration by the x-rays (Fig. 12–4).

Another radiolucency that frequently occurs, and may be mistaken for caries, is an optical illusion caused by overlapping teeth. When two interproximal surfaces overlap (caused by natural overlap of misaligned teeth or by improper horizontal angulation of the x-ray beam) there is a dense radiopaque area surrounded by radiolucent lines. These lines are an optical illusion called the **mach band effect** caused by the high contrast between the normal enamel and the dense, overlapped enamel (Fig. 12–4).

RADIOGRAPHIC APPEARANCE OF APICAL DISEASE

Less common than caries or periodontal disease are the radiolucent areas surrounding the apices of the teeth. These radiolucencies indicate pathological changes in the hard (bony) tissues. Their radiographic appearance may be misleading unless carefully correlated with other diagnostic information.

Periapical infections usually result from pulpal inflammation. Bacteria from caries infect the pulp and gain access to the periapical bone by way of the root canals. As a rule, **acute abscesses** (early stages of pulpal or periapical infections) are barely discernible, becoming more radiolucent as they become chronic. In fact, in the very early acute stages there may be no radiographic evidence at all. The earliest sign may be a break in the **lamina dura.** Clinically such teeth are often tender to percussion (Fig. 12–5). **Chronic abscesses** may appear as circular dark areas around the apices and eventually turn into **granulomas,** masses of granulation tissues usually surrounded by a fibrous sac continuous with the periodontal ligament and attached to the root apices. Under certain conditions epithelial elements may proliferate to form a **radicular cyst** (also known as apical cyst, periapical cyst, apical periodontal cyst, or root end cyst)—a cyst around the end of the root. Radiographically all the described lesions assume various configurations, and it is not possible to accurately differentiate between a periapical abscess, a granuloma, or a cyst (Fig. 12–6).

Cysts are epithelium-lined sacs filled with fluid or semisolid material. Because of osmotic imbalance, pressure is exerted in all directions; therefore, cysts tend to be

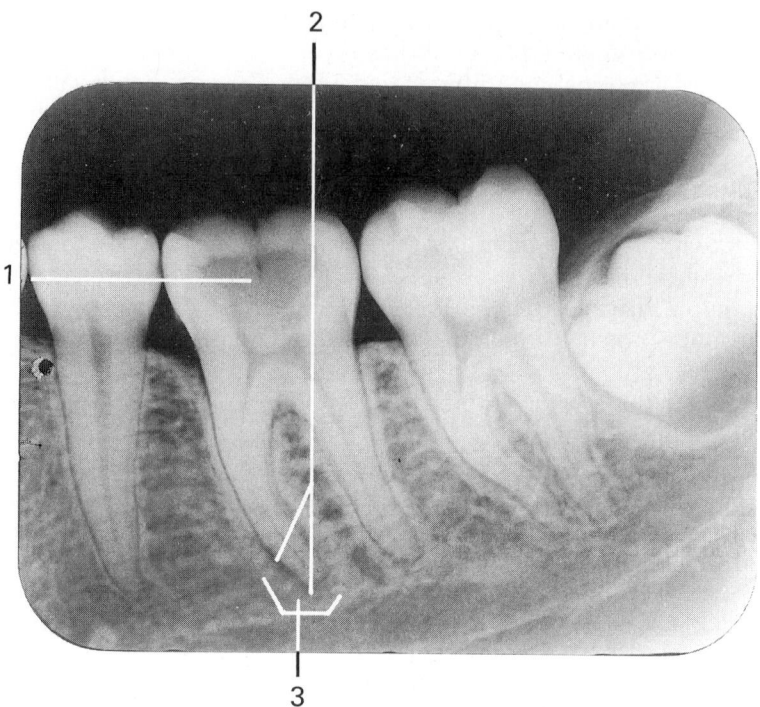

Figure 12–5. Radiograph of mandibular molar region shows **1** deep carious lesion in the first molar resulting in pulpal damage; **2** loss of lamina dura and periapical bone around the mesial root of the first molar, and **3** condensing osteitis—a term used when sclerotic (hardened) bone is formed as a result of infection.

spherical unless unequal resistance is encountered. Cysts follow the path of least resistance. Cysts tend to be slow-growing and push aside adjacent structures. Although usually unilocular (made up of one compartment), cysts may also be multilocular (made up of several compartments). Radiographically cysts may appear as fairly uniform radiolucent cavities within the bone and surrounded by a well-defined radiopaque border that resembles the lamina dura.

There are many types of cysts. The most common are **odontogenic cysts** (of tooth origin); a few of the rarer ones are **nonodontogenic.** A cyst frequently observed on radiographs of young patients is the **dentigerous cyst** (Fig. 12–7). When found, this type of cyst occurs frequently with imbedded teeth—third molars and supernumerary teeth—and is always associated with the crown of a tooth. If the tooth causing the cyst continues to develop and is able to erupt, the cyst is often destroyed by natural means. Hence it is also known as a **follicular cyst** or **eruptive cyst** (Fig. 12–8).

Unless radicular cysts are completely removed at the time of the extraction or surgery, they will remain and are then called **residual cysts.**

Nonodontogenic cysts arise from epithelium other than that associated with tooth

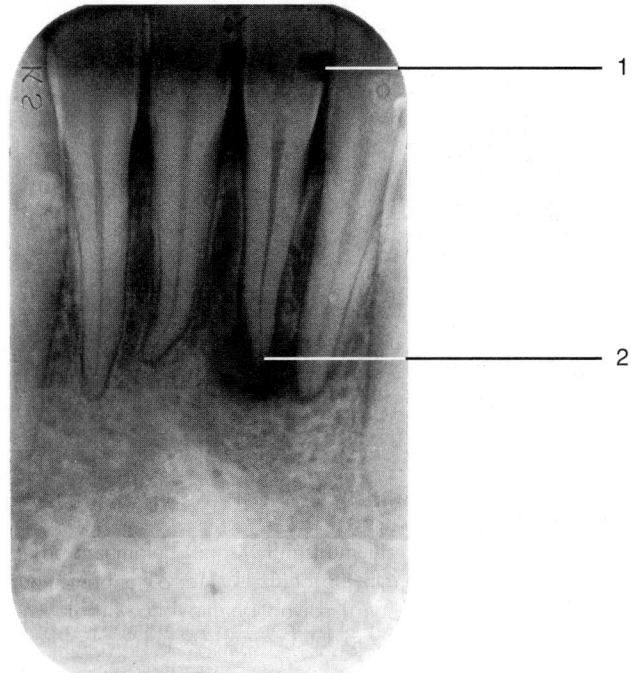

Figure 12–6. Radiograph of mandibular incisor region shows **1** caries on the distal surface of the left central incisor, and **2** a round radiolucent lesion that may be a periapical abcess, a granuloma, or a cyst.

formation. Two types are the **incisive canal** (nasopalatine) **cyst,** located within the incisive canal, and the rare **globulomaxillary cyst,** which arises between the maxillary lateral incisor and the canine (cuspid).

RADIOGRAPHIC APPEARANCE OF ANOMALIES

Anomalies—departures from regular arrangement—are numerous. Such anomalies include **anodontia,** congenitally missing teeth that often include the third molars, the premolars (bicuspids), and the maxillary lateral incisors (Fig. 12–9), **supernumerary teeth** (extra teeth), radiopacities that may or may not resemble normal tooth form, and **mesiodens,** so named because they are located in the maxillary midline, are small extra teeth that are almost always conical in shape (Fig. 12–10).

Complications caused by supernumerary teeth include the possibility of cyst formation and the malposition, noneruption, or both of the normal teeth. Radiographic examination at an early age will reveal the presence of supernumerary teeth so that they may be removed.

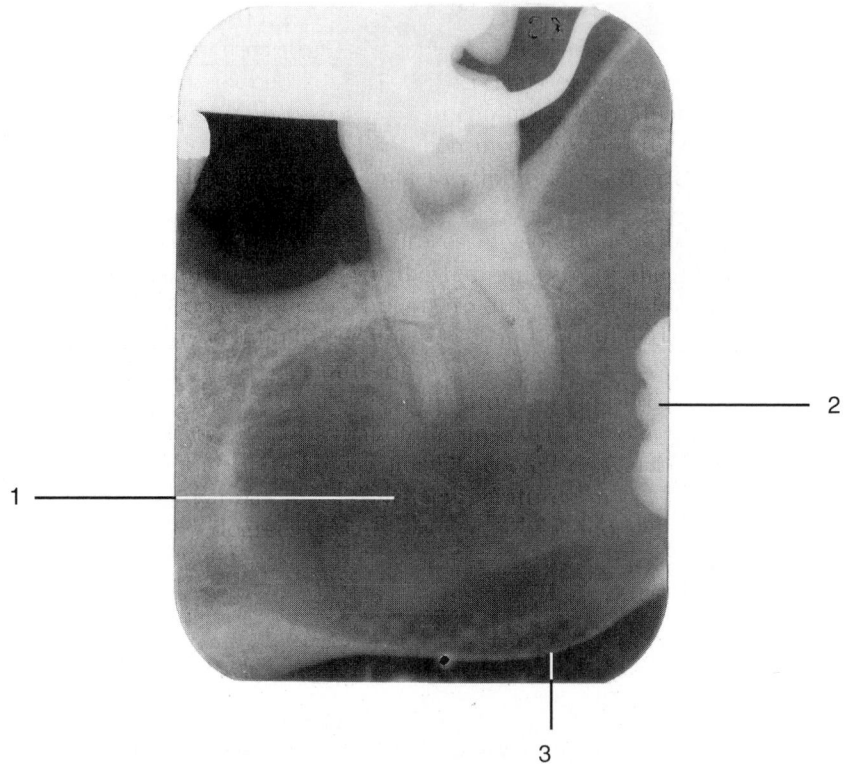

Figure 12–7. Radiograph of mandibular molar region (note film was placed in a vertical position instead of the usual horizontal position) shows **1** dentigerous cyst involving **2** imbedded third molar and **3** expansion and thinning of the cortical bone.

Additional anomalies include the following:

1. **Malposed teeth** are teeth that are often unerupted and not in normal location.
2. **Dens in dente** (dens invaginatus) is, literally, a tooth within a tooth, an invagination of the enamel within the body of the tooth. This anomaly occurs most frequently in the maxillary lateral incisor (Fig. 12–11).
3. **Hypercementosis** usually appears radiopaque and is caused by excessive cementum formation. The excessive cementum on the roots often causes a bulbous enlargement near the apex.
4. **Ankylosis** is a radiopacity produced by the fusion or union of part or all of a tooth to the alveolus. It is caused by mineralization and hardening of the periodontal ligament fibers that normally surround the roots and separate them from the alveolus.
5. **Dilaceration** is a tooth with a sharp bend in the root (see Fig. 12–19). It usually develops as a result of trauma during root formation.

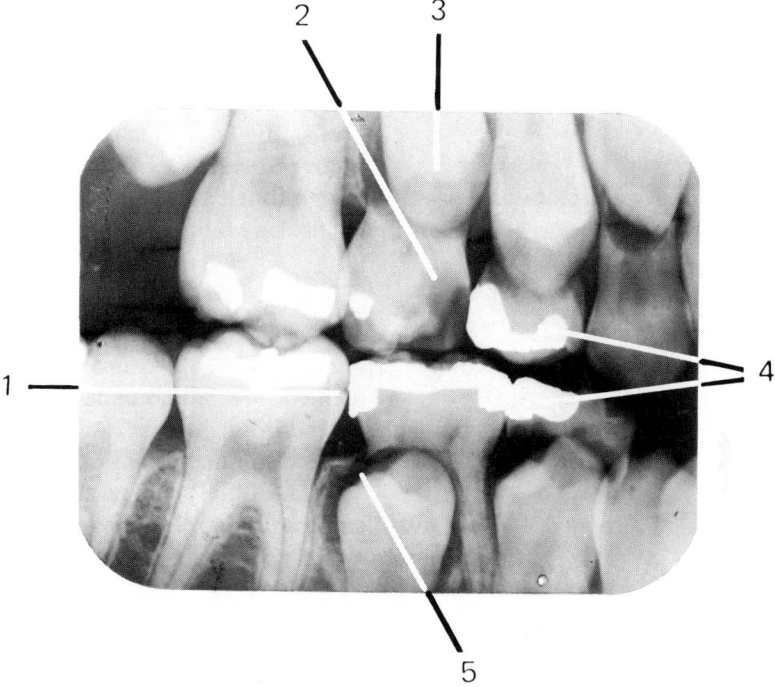

Figure 12–8. Bitewing radiograph of mixed dentition shows **1** incipient caries on permanent molar, **2** deep caries on deciduous second molar, **3** erupting second maxillary premolar, **4** deciduous first molars about to be exfoliated, and **5** follicular (eruptive) cyst around the crown of second mandibular premolar.

Other less frequently encountered anomalies include the following:

1. **Dentinogenesis imperfecta** (hereditary opalescent dentin) is characterized by imperfectly formed dentin that has an opalescent or amber color. Radiographs reveal small, underdeveloped roots and obliterated pulp chambers.
2. **Amelogenesis imperfecta** is characterized by scant or totally missing enamel.
3. **Taurodontia** is characterized by very large pulp chambers and very short roots.
4. **Macrodontia** is characterized by teeth that appear too large for the individual.
5. **Microdontia** is characterized by teeth that appear too small for the individual.
6. **Gemination** (twinning) is a single tooth bud that divides and forms two teeth.

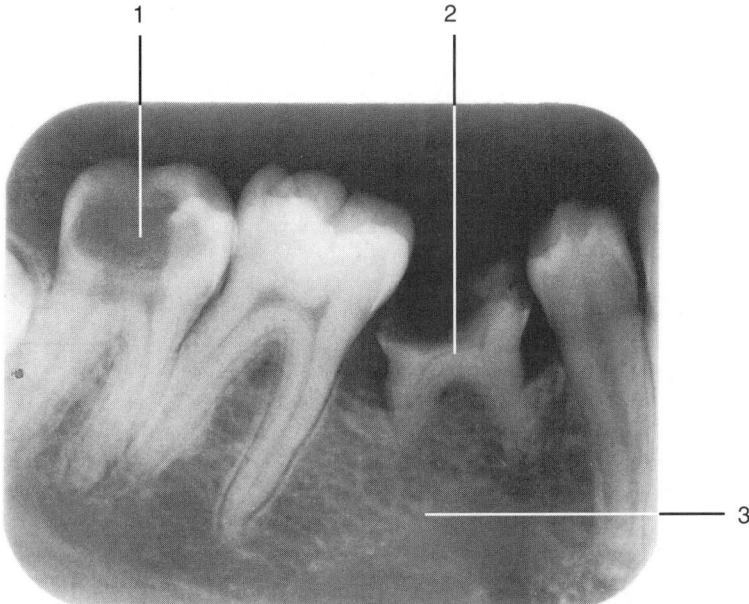

Figure 12–9. Radiograph of mandibular premolar (bicuspid) region shows **1** extensive caries in second molar, **2** second primary molar, and **3** congenitally missing second premolar (bicuspid).

7. **Fusion** is a condition where the dentin and one other dental tissue of adjacent teeth are united.
8. **Concrescence** is a condition where the cementum of adjacent teeth is united.

RADIOGRAPHIC APPEARANCE OF BONE OR TOOTH RESORPTION

Evidence of **resorption** is a common finding in dental radiographs. Resorption, such as the roots of deciduous teeth or the gradual diminution of the alveolar process in the elderly, can be considered normal. Most resorptive processes, however, are the result of infection, trauma, or some unusual condition. An example of such resorption is the gradual destruction of the vertical and horizontal bone loss that is typical of **periodontal disease** (Fig. 12–12).

Other examples include the resorption of the adjacent tooth by pressure from an impacted or erupting tooth, resorption caused by slowly growing tumors, or trauma that causes root-end resorption when teeth are moved too rapidly during orthodontic treatment (Fig. 12–13).

Less common is **idiopathic resorption,** where the cause is unknown (Fig. 12–14).

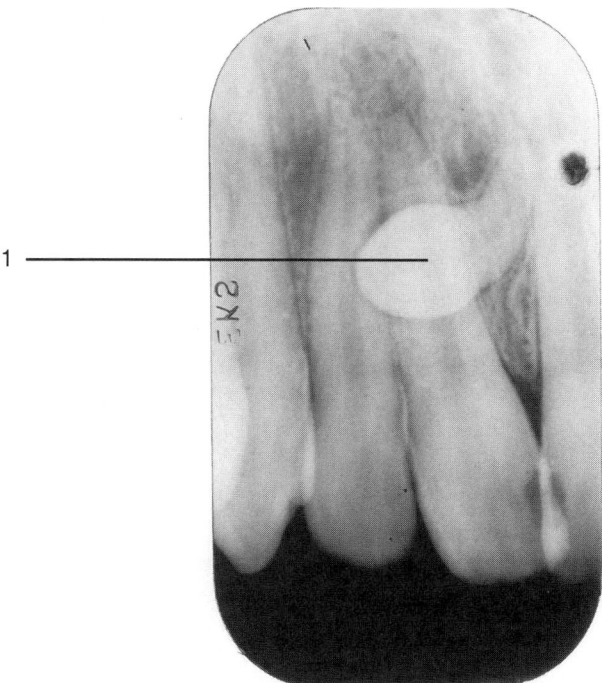

Figure 12–10. Radiograph of maxillary incisor region shows **1** mesiodens, a small, supernumerary tooth located in the midline between the central incisors.

RADIOGRAPHIC APPEARANCE OF CALCIFICATIONS AND OSSIFICATIONS

Calcifications, the deposition of calcium salts from the saliva into the tissues surrounding the teeth, and **ossifications,** the pathological or abnormal conversion of soft tissues into bone, appear radiopaque.

Calculus (Fig. 12–12) is the most frequently observed form of calcification. Calculus, although not classified as a lesion because its formation is a normal process for many persons, is a gradual deposition of calcium and other inorganic salts and organic matter around the gingival areas of the teeth. The accumulation and growth of these calculus deposits contributes to periodontal disturbances. Although there are several forms of supragingival and subgingival calculus, all forms appear radiopaque on the radiographs.

Calcifications in the dental pulp occur in the form of small nodules called **pulp stones** (Fig. 12–3). They appear in the radiograph as radiopaque structures of varied size and may appear singly, but more often are multiple. Pulp stones are very common but of little significance because they never cause inflammation of the pulp. They

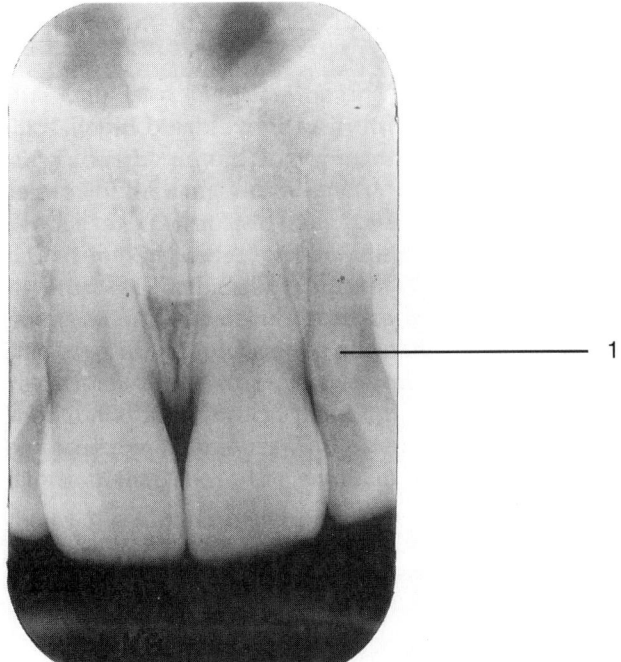

Figure 12–11. Radiograph of maxillary incisor region shows **1** dens in dente, an invagination of the enamel within the body of the lateral incisor.

do present a problem in root canal therapy if they are large and adhere to the pulpal wall.

Other less frequently encountered calcifications are (1) **sialoliths,** depositions of calcium salts in the salivary glands and ducts; (2) **rhinoliths,** stones within the maxillary sinuses; and (3) **phleboliths,** or calcified thrombi, calcified masses that are observed as round or oval bodies in the soft tissues of the cheeks.

Two forms of **ossification** are often radiographically visible: (1) **Condensing osteitis** occurs when **sclerotic** (hardened) bone is formed as a result of infection (see Fig. 12–5). This condition may develop in periapical areas prior to complete pulp degeneration and appear as a widening of the periodontal ligament and surrounded by dense bone. (2) **Osteosclerosis** occurs when regions of abnormally dense bone that are not a direct result of infection form (Fig. 12–15). Although the cause is unknown, it commonly occurs in the interseptal premolar area and may be associated with fragments of retained deciduous roots. This condition tends to remain following extraction of the teeth.

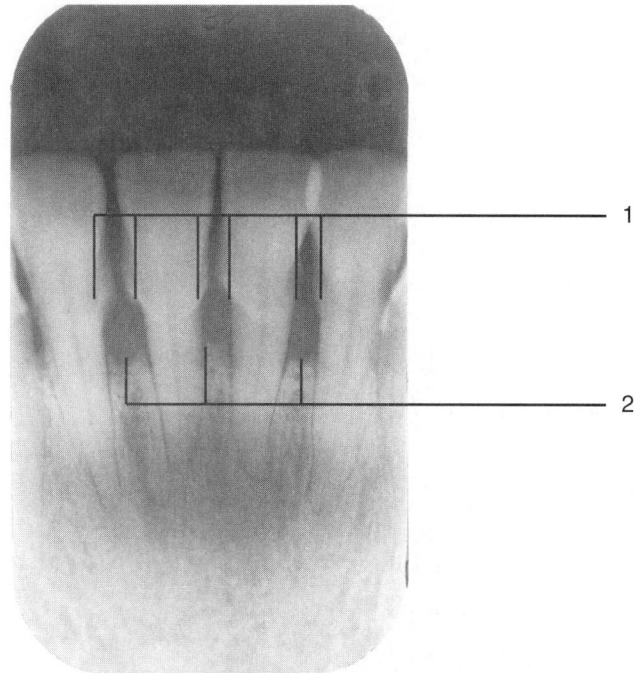

Figure 12–12. Radiograph of mandibular incisor region shows **1** large deposits of calculus around the necks of the teeth, and **2** radiolucent areas indicating vertical and horizontal bone loss that is typical of peridontal disease.

RADIOGRAPHIC APPEARANCE OF ODONTOGENIC TUMORS

Odontogenic tumors result from abnormal proliferation of cells and tissues involved in odontogenesis (the formation of the teeth). The three types occasionally seen on radiographs are (1) ameloblastomas, (2) odontomas, and (3) cementomas. **Ameloblastomas** have the greatest potential for serious implications for the patient. These appear as large radiolucencies of enamel origin. Radiographically, ameloblastomas may be monolocular (one compartment) or multilocular (many compartments). The monolocular form closely resembles dentigerous cyst (Fig. 12–16). The multilocular form has a characteristic "soap bubble" appearance.

  Odontomas are the most common ondontogenic tumors (Fig. 12–17). These are tumors of small misshapen teeth whose number in each odontoma varies widely. These toothlike structures appear radiopaque and are located within a radiolucent fibrous capsule that often resembles a cyst.

  Cementomas, also called cementifying fibromas, are derived from the periodontal ligaments of fully developed and erupted teeth. Early cementomas are radiolucent and

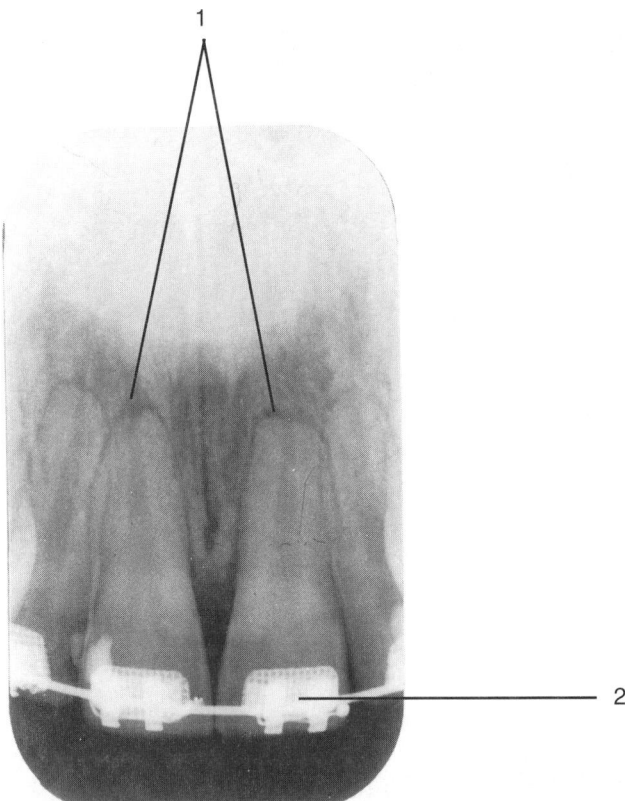

Figure 12–13. Radiograph of maxillary incisor region shows **1** root-end resorption caused by trauma of orthodontic treatment and **2** orthodontic appliance.

appear identical to radicular cysts. In the later stages of development cementomas appear as radiopaque masses surrounded by a radiolucent line (Fig. 12–18). Cementomas occur most frequently in the mandibular incisor region of women. The teeth are vital and the cementomas need no treatment.

RADIOGRAPHIC APPEARANCE OF NONODONTOGENIC TUMORS

The tumors described here include a few pathologically insignificant ones as well as some that are life threatening. The majority of these lesions do not have a characteristic radiographic appearance that enables us to determine the diagnosis from the radiograph alone. In fact, a diagnosis of a malignant tumor cannot be made until the pathologist, the clinician, and the radiologist have combined their findings. However, radiologists can detect the presence of lesions in bone and frequently can determine the

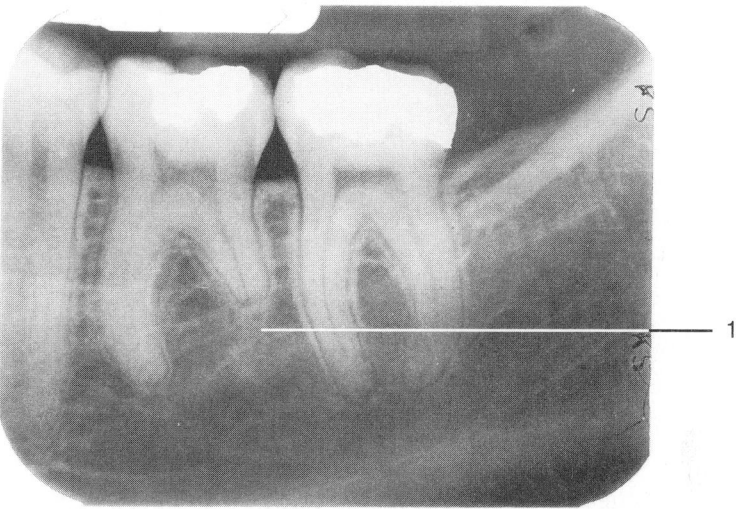

Figure 12–14. Radiograph of mandibular molar region shows **1** idiopathic resorption of the distal root of the first molar.

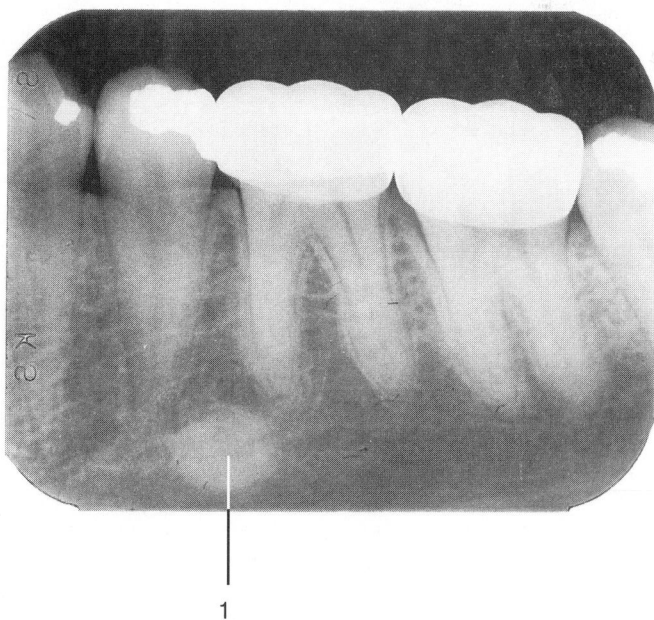

Figure 12–15. Radiograph of mandibular posterior region shows **1** radiopaque osteosclerosis, a hardening of the bone; the cause is unknown.

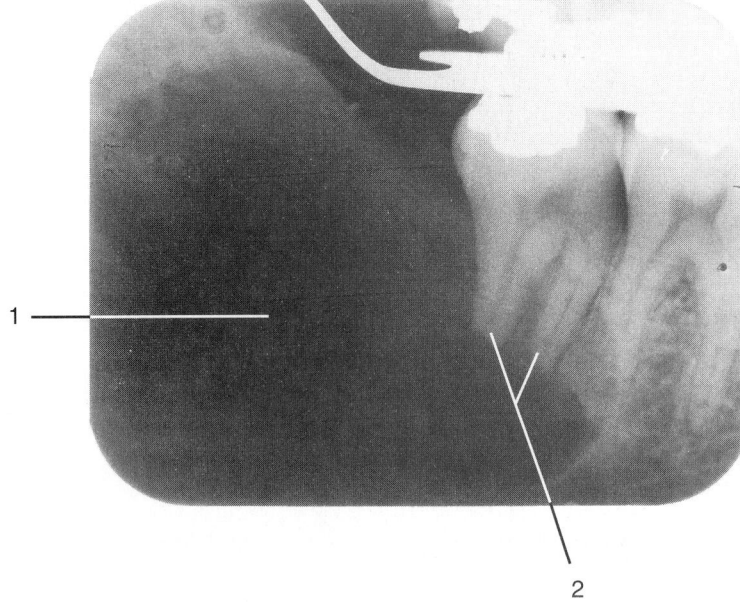

Figure 12-16. Radiograph of mandibular molar region shows **1** large radiolucent ameloblastoma and **2** resorption of the molar roots caused by pressure of the tumor.

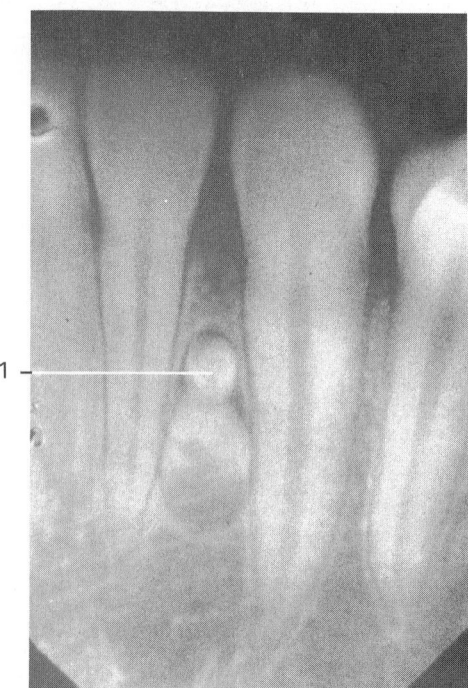

Figure 12-17. Radiograph of mandibular canine (cuspid) region shows odontoma consisting of small misshaped teeth located within a radiolucent fibrous capsule.

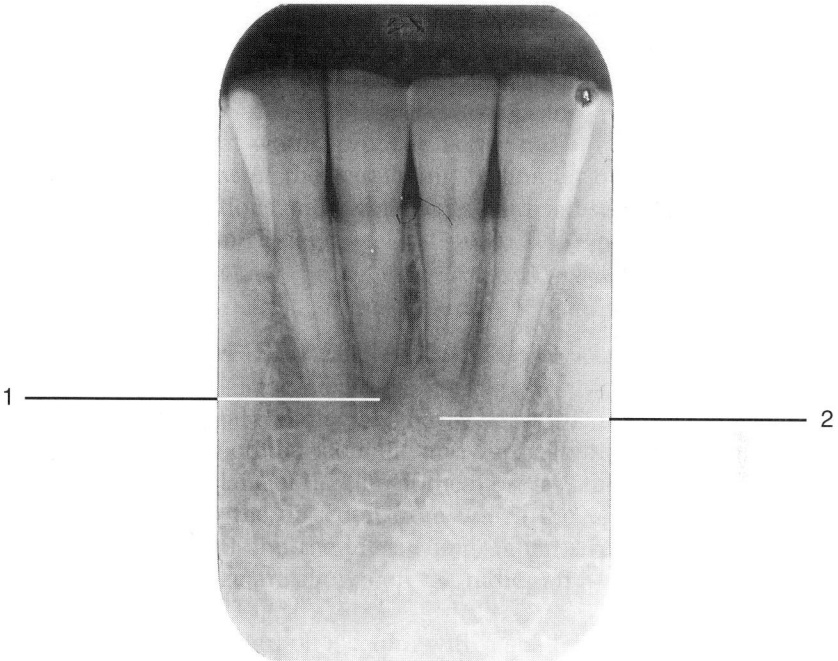

Figure 12–18. Radiograph of mandibular incisor region shows **1** early cementoma (radiolucent) and **2** cementoma in late stage of development (radiopaque). The teeth are vital.

nature of the lesion. As dental personnel we may on occasion be the first to detect malignancies and alert the patient.

Tumors are classed as **benign** (doing little or no harm) and **malignant** (very dangerous or life threatening). Fortunately most tumors that we see in the dental office are benign. Careful examination of the radiograph can often help to differentiate benign from malignant lesions.

Benign tumors may be either radiolucent or radiopaque. The cortex (outer layer) tends to remain intact, even though it may be thinned or expanded. The margins are usually well defined. Benign tumors do not metastasize (spreading of disease from one part of the body to another).

Malignant tumors tend to produce destruction of the cortex or elevation of the periosteum. They tend to have irregular margins and are less distinct, blending into the adjacent bone. Malignant tumors frequently metastasize.

Exostoses and tori are the most frequently encountered forms of benign tumors. An **exostosis** (plural exostoses) is a localized overgrowth of bone. The term **torus** (plural tori) is often used to describe an exostosis that occurs near the midline of the palate **(torus palatinus)** (Fig. 12–19) and on the lingual surface of the mandible **(torus**

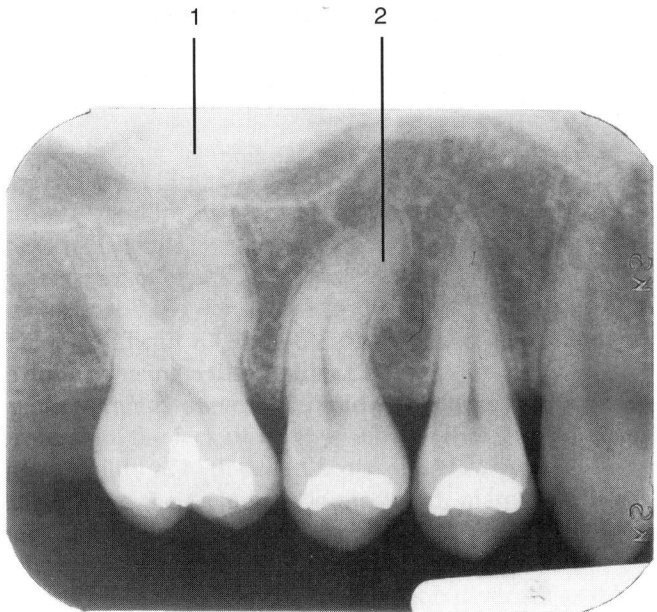

Figure 12–19. Radiograph of maxillary premolar (bicuspid) region shows **1** torus palatinus, a radiopaque overgrowth of bone on the midline of the palate, and **2** dilaceration, a sharp bend in the root of a tooth.

mandibularis) (see Figs. 11–23 and 11–26). Radiographically both appear as an area of increased radiographic density (radiopaque).

Another common benign tumor is the **osteoma,** a noninflammatory type of bone tumor that varies greatly in size and shape and is radiopaque.

Still another variety of benign tumor is a **giant cell tumor,** or granuloma, a radiolucent area of varying size that frequently can be observed anterior to the molars in children and young adults.

The two main types of oral malignancies are carcinomas and sarcomas. Both grow rapidly and spread into adjacent tissues.

Carcinomas are malignant tumors of epithelial origin. These are of many types and may arise from any organ in which there is epithelial tissue. The radiographic appearance is radiolucent with irregular and poorly defined borders.

Sarcomas are malignant tumors of connective tissue origin. Radiographically many of these appear as radiolucent, irregularly shaped, and diffuse destructions of bone, having a "patchy" appearance with no demarcation from normal surrounding bone. Some types may appear radiopaque because of excessive cartilage or bone formation in or on the bone. Such radiographs are vitally important in early detection because sarcomas produce changes in bone early in their development.

RADIOGRAPHIC APPEARANCE OF INJURIES

The two most common injuries are fractures of facial bones and teeth. **Fracture lines** are thin radiolucent lines that demarcate the region of bone or tooth separation. Radiographic evidence of healing may later show as a radiopaque line in the fracture area (Fig. 12–20); however, such evidence of union may take a long time and is generally not visible radiographically until long after the healing has taken place. Fractures may on occasion have a similar appearance to the nutrient canals described in Chapter 11.

The radiographic examination sometimes reveals **foreign bodies** in the jaws and soft tissues. The most common foreign body seen in the jaw is amalgam (Fig. 12–21). Most particles of amalgam are found in the edentulous areas of the mandible. Often amalgam is fractured during extractions and fragments fall into the root socket or under the gingival tissue. Amalgam situated under the gingival tissue may impart a bluish-purple color to the tissue called an **amalgam tattoo.**

Other foreign bodies of the jaws include cements, gutta-percha, and dental instruments such as files, broaches, and burrs (Fig. 12–22). Foreign bodies of the soft tissues are apt to be hypodermic needles, pins, birdshot, glass, sand, and metal objects from automobile and other accidents.

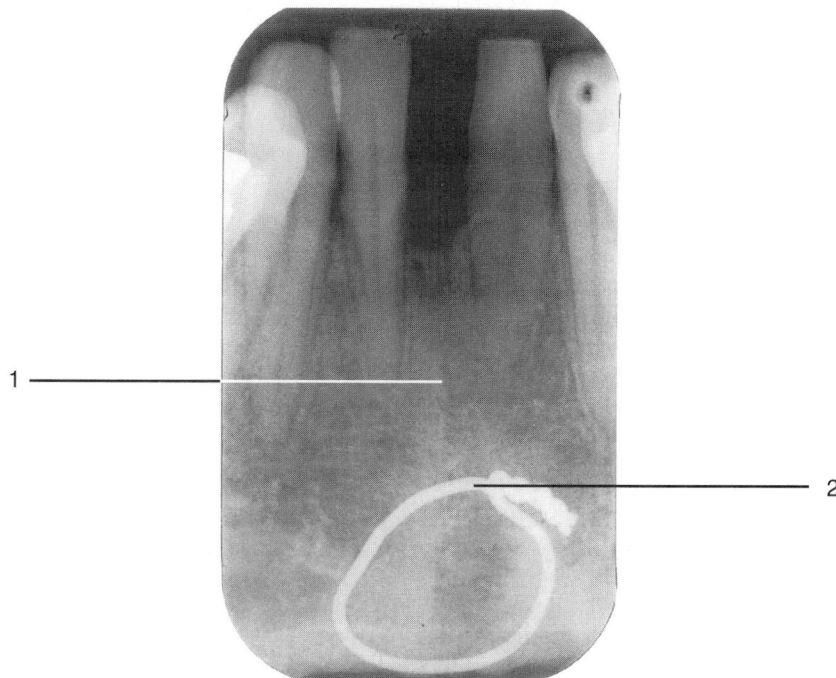

Figure 12–20. Radiograph of mandibular incisor region shows **1** old fracture line (radiolucent) and **2** wire used to reduce the fracture.

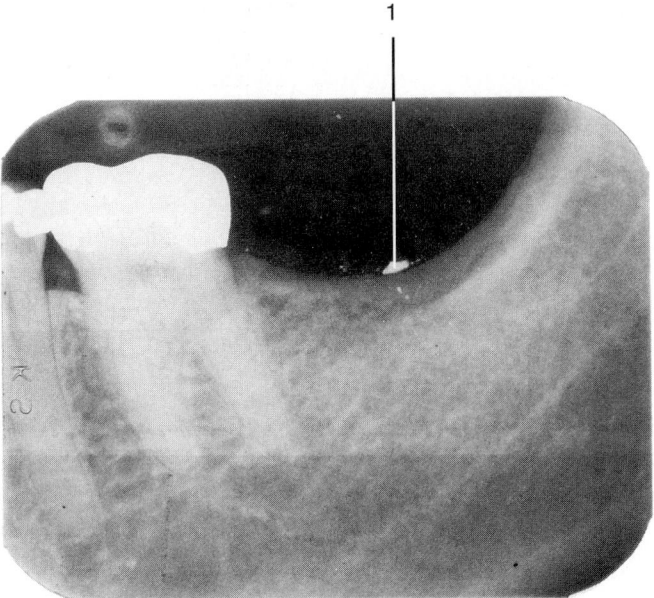

Figure 12–21. Radiograph of mandibular molar region shows fragments of amalgam under the soft tissue (pointer), probably left after an extraction. Clinically the gingiva appears bluish-purple and is called amalgam tattoo.

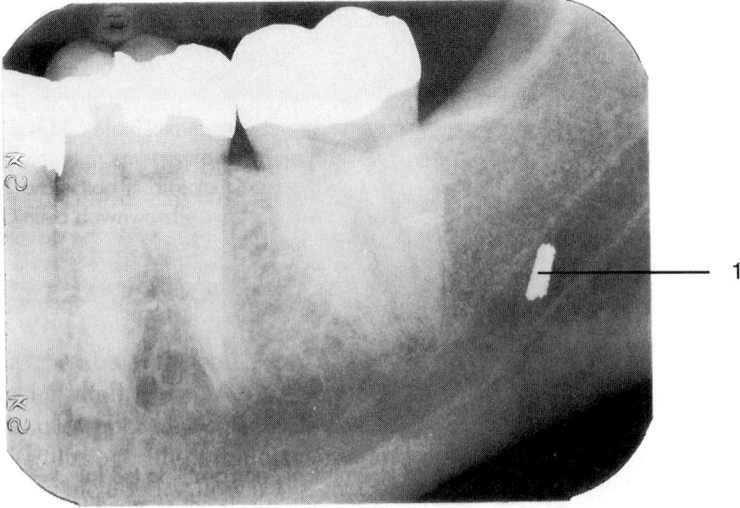

Figure 12–22. Radiograph of mandibular molar region shows **1** broken burr, which probably occurred when the third molar was removed.

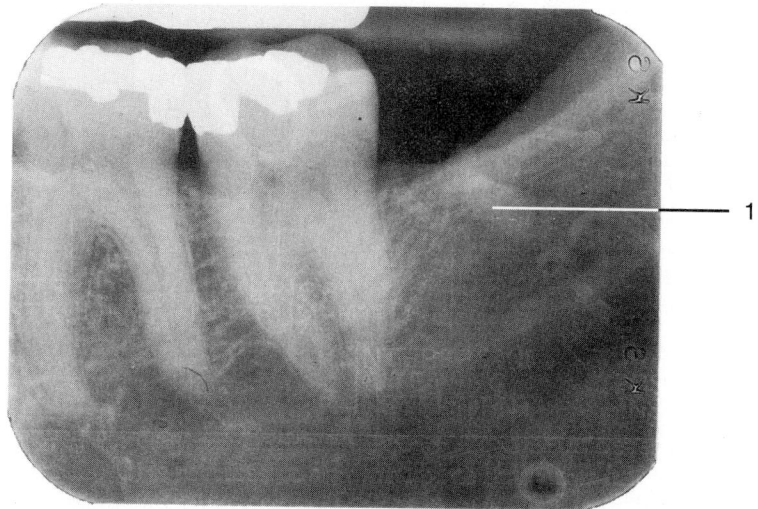

Figure 12–23. Radiograph of mandibular molar region shows **1** retained root.

Frequently encountered on radiographs are **retained roots,** which appear ra-diopaque (Fig. 12–23).

One other form of injury that is not often seen is **radio-osteosclerosis.** Generally limited to cancer patients, osteosclerosis is a devitalization of bone subjected to large doses of ionizing radiation.

A radiolucency that may involve large areas of bone is **osteomyelitis,** an inflam-mation of the bone marrow. Although not common, osteomyelitis may be either chronic or acute.

What has been described in this chapter is only a partial list of structures or le-sions that may be visible on radiographs; any attempt to describe them fully belongs in a text devoted entirely to radiographic interpretation. Furthermore, anyone who at-tempts to make a preliminary interpretation must constantly be aware that many of the lesions described look very similar and that a biopsy report may be required be-fore a final diagnosis can be attempted.

METHODS OF LOCALIZATION

When examining a radiograph it is generally not possible to determine whether a den-tal structure or a foreign object embedded within the maxilla or mandible is toward the front (facial or buccal) or behind (lingual) the teeth.

Several localization methods are currently in use. Each requires the exposure of an additional film; either the direction in which the tube points is shifted or the film is positioned at right angle to the position of the first film.

The oldest of these methods was first described by A. C. Clark **(Clark's rule).** Two

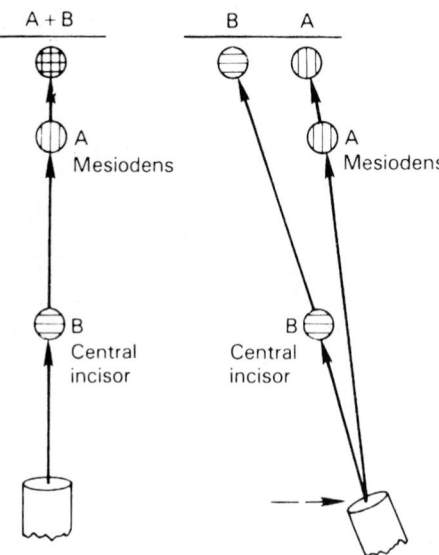

Tube Shift Localization Technique
(Clark's Rule)

Figure 12–24. In the tube shift localization technique (Clark's rule), the most lingual object (mesiodens in this case) will move in the same direction as shift of tube. *(Courtesy of Eastman Kodak Company, Rochester, NY, and Department of Dental Diagnostic Science, School of Dentistry, University of Texas at San Antonio. Reproduced with permission from Langland OE, Langlais RP, Morris CR: Radiographic localization techniques. Dent Radiogr Photogr 52(4):69–77, 1979.)*

periapical radiographs are positioned, one after the other, in the area of interest. Both exposures are made with the identical vertical angulation but the horizontal angulation is changed when the second exposure is made.

If the structure or object in question as seen on the second radiograph appears to have moved in the same direction as the horizontal shift of the tube, the structure or object is toward the lingual. Conversely, if the move is in the opposite direction to the shift of the tube, the structure or object must be toward the buccal or facial (Fig. 12–24).

Another method of localization, first suggested by Bosworth and later refined by Miller, shifts the position of the second film. Two periapical films are used; the first is a conventional radiograph of the area, which shows the superior–inferior relation of the object in question to the teeth and the alveolar crest; the second radiograph, positioned occlusally at a right (or 90-degree) angle to the first film, shows the buccal- (or facial-) to-lingual relationship. The occlusal technique is described in Chapter 17.

Still another method was suggested by A. G. Richards to determine the location of

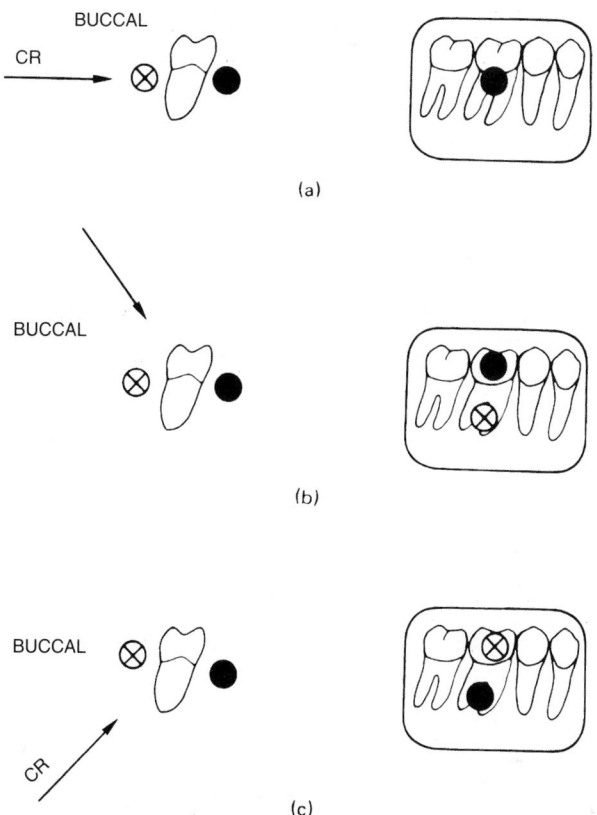

Figure 12–25. Buccal and lingual foreign bodies with a vertical shift of the x-ray beam of 20 degrees. **(a)** In the original radiograph, buccal and lingual objects are superimposed. **(b)** When the beam is directed inferiorly (positive vertical angulation is explained in Fig. 14–13), the buccal object appears to move down while the lingual object appears to move up. **(c)** When the beam is directed superiorly (negative vertical angulation is explained in Fig. 14–13), the buccal object appears to move up while the lingual object appears to have moved down. *(Courtesy of Eastman Kodak Company, and Department of Dental Diagnostic Science, School of Dentistry, University of Texas at San Antonio. Reproduced with permission from Langland OE, Langlais RP, Morris CR: Radiographic localization techniques.* Dent Radiogr Photogr *52(4):69–77, 1979.)*

the mandibular canal. This technique has been expanded by R. P. Langlais and O. E. Langland and is now known as the **buccal-object rule** (Figs. 12–25 and 12–26).

According to this rule, any buccal object will move when the angulation of the position indicating device (PID), is changed: up or down, right or left. As in the other methods described, two films are used. A 20-degree change of angulation in the desired direction is made when the second film is exposed.

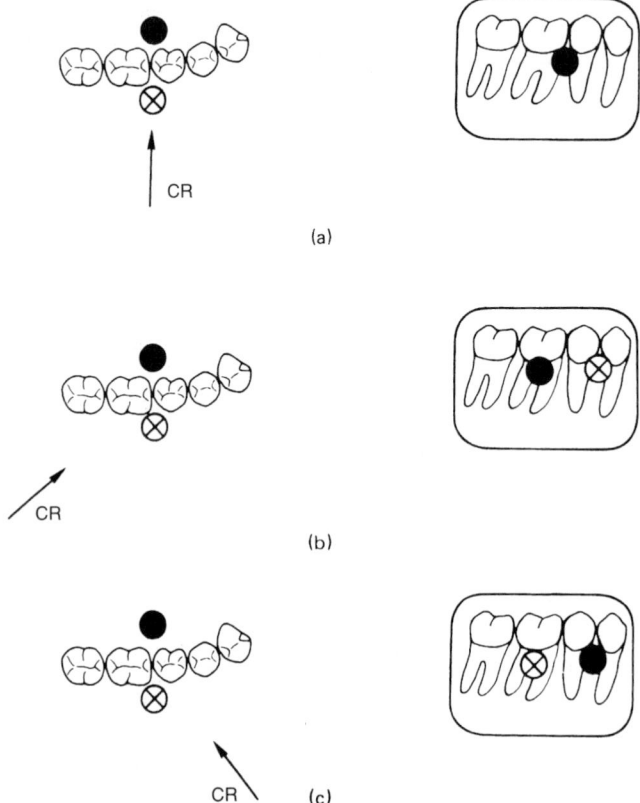

Figure 12–26. Buccal and lingual foreign bodies with a horizontal shift of the x-ray beam of 20 degrees. **(a)** In the original radiograph, buccal and lingual objects are superimposed. **(b)** When the beam is directed mesially, the buccal object appears to move mesially while the lingual object appears to move distally. **(c)** When the beam is directed distally, the buccal object appears to move distally while the lingual object appears to move mesially. *(Courtesy of Eastman Kodak Company, and Department of Dental Diagnostic Science, School of Dentistry, University of Texas at San Antonio. Reproduced with permission from Langland OE, Langlais RP, Morris CR: Radiographic localization techniques.* Dent Radiogr Photogr *52(4):69–77, 1979.)*

CHAPTER SUMMARY

The ability to read the radiograph is called interpretation. Some auxiliaries, by virtue of their training, are able to save the dentist time by preparing a preliminary interpretation. The final diagnosis, however, is based not only on the radiographs but also on a visual and digital inspection of the teeth, evaluation of clinical tests, and the patient's medicodental history. This task is reserved for dentists and is their sole responsibility.

Although never called upon to make a diagnosis, a skilled auxiliary should have little difficulty in differentiating between normal tooth structure and dental caries, calculus deposits, or granulomas. Other pathological conditions may be more difficult to identify. The auxiliary should also be able to recognize the radiographic appearance of gold, silver, gutta-percha, dental cement, silicate, acrylic resin, and porcelain. Some restorative materials are easy to identify; others can only be tentatively identified on a radiograph. For example, all metals have a similar radiopaque appearance, whereas silicates and acrylic resins have similar radiolucent appearance. Often a visual inspection is required to distinguish one from the other.

When viewing radiographs it is generally not possible to see whether a dental structure or foreign object is to the facial or to the lingual of the teeth. Two general methods of localization are in use: (1) the tube shift technique, or (2) exposing a second film position at a right angle to the first film. With the tube-shift technique, the object in question is to the lingual if it moves in the same direction as the horizontal shift of the tube. With the techniques in which two radiographs are at right angles to each other, one readily observes the location of the object in question.

KEY WORDS

Abscess

Amalgam tattoo

Ameloblastoma

Amelogenesis imperfecta

Ankylosis

Anodontia

Anomalies

Benign

Buccal-object rule

Calcification

Calculus

Caries

Cementoma

Cervical burnout

Clark's rule

Concrescence

Condensing osteitis

Cyst

Dens in dente

Dentinogenesis imperfecta

Diagnosis

Dilaceration

Exostosis

Follicular (eruptive) cyst

Foreign body

Fracture line

Fusion

Gemination

Giant cell tumor

Globulomaxillary cyst

Granuloma

Hypercementosis

Impacted tooth

Incisive canal cyst

Interpretation

Mach band effect

Macrodontia

Malignant

Malposed tooth

Mesiodens

Microdontia

Nonodontogenic cyst

Odontogenic cyst

Odontoma

Ossification

Osteoma

Osteomyelitis

Phlebolith

Pulp stone

Radicular cyst

Radiolucent

Radio-osteosclerosis

Radiopaque

Rarefying osteitis

Residual cyst

Resorption

Retained root

Rhinolith

Sarcoma

Sclerosis

Sialolith

Supernumerary tooth

Taurodontia

Torus

Tumor

REVIEW QUESTIONS

1. The competent dental auxiliary must be familiar with the more common abnormal or disease conditions in order to make a preliminary _____ of the radiograph.

2. The responsibility to finalize the diagnosis remains with the _____.

3. Which of these materials appears most radiolucent? (a) amalgam, (b) dental porcelain, (c) silicate, (d) acrylic resin.

4. Which of these appears radiopaque? (a) lamina dura, (b) oral mucosa, (c) pulp chamber, (d) residual cyst.

5. Which of these appears radiolucent? (a) impacted tooth, (b) chronic abscess, (c) calculus, (d) odontoma.

6. Radiographically it is not possible to accurately differentiate among a periapical abscess, a granuloma, or a cyst. (a) true, (b) false.

7. Two frequently observed radiolucencies that occasionally are mistaken for caries are (a) mental foramen and dentigerous cysts, (b) esthetic restorations in anterior teeth and cervical burnout, (c) incisive foramen and nutrient canals, (d) cementomas and nutrient canals.

8. All resorptive processes appear (a) in the mandible, (b) in the crown of the tooth, (c) radiolucent, (d) radiopaque.

9. Malignant tumors (a) have well-defined margins and do not metastasize, (b) have well-defined margins and metastasize, (c) have irregular margins that blend into adjacent bone and do not metastasize, (d) have irregular margins that blend into adjacent bone and metastasize.

10. According to Clark's rule for localization, (a) the object closest to the film appears to move in the same direction as the shift of the tube, (b) the object closest to the film appears to move in the opposite direction from the shift of the tube, (c) the object closest to the film does not appear to move in any direction.

BIBLIOGRAPHY

Farman AG, Nortje CJ, Wood RE: *Oral and Maxillofacial Diagnostic Imaging.* St. Louis, MO: CV Mosby, 1993

Goaz PW, White SC: *Oral Radiology Principles and Interpretation,* 3rd ed. St. Louis, MO: CV Mosby, 1994

Langlais RP, Kasle MJ: *Exercises in Oral Radiographic Interpretation,* 3rd ed. Philadelphia, PA: WB Saunders, 1992

CHAPTER 13

Identifying and Correcting
Faulty Radiographs

By the end of this chapter the student should be able to

1. Identify the types of radiographic errors caused by faulty exposure techniques.
2. Identify the types of radiographic errors caused by incorrect film positioning and angulation of the central ray.
3. Identify the types of radiographic errors caused by faulty processing techniques.
4. Identify the conditions that cause radiographs to be fogged.

IMPORTANCE OF IDENTIFYING FAULTY RADIOGRAPHS

It is important to be able to tell when a radiograph is inadequate and to understand why. Only clear, properly processed radiographs with minimal distortion of the image have diagnostic value to the dentist. Radiographs that fail to meet these standards must often be retaken. However, good common sense should be used in determining when a retake is absolutely needed. For example, a radiograph may show a major cone cut or artifact and yet show excellent quality of image at the root where an abscess is suspected. Such a radiograph, especially if it is a part of a full-mouth series in which the damaged film area is probably shown correctly on the neighboring film areas, should not be retaken. To do so would expose the patient to unnecessary radiation.

INADEQUACIES CAUSED BY FAULTY EXPOSURE TECHNIQUES

Many faulty radiographs are caused by errors in exposure technique, such as incorrect positioning of the film packet, incorrect positioning of the PID (position indicating device), or incorrect exposure factors. Of course, position errors may also mean that the patient's head moved after the film, tube head, and PID were in place or the patient allowed the film to slip. The radiographer must always caution patients not to move their head and to hold the film firmly.

Incorrect Positioning of the Film

1. *Absence of Apical Structures* (Figs. 13–1 and 13–10)
   Probable cause: Film was not placed high enough or low enough in the patient's mouth. Ideally, there should be approximately a 1/4-in. (6.4-mm) margin above or below the crown of the tooth. When the paralleling technique is used, this error may also be caused by the film not being parallel to the long axes of the teeth.

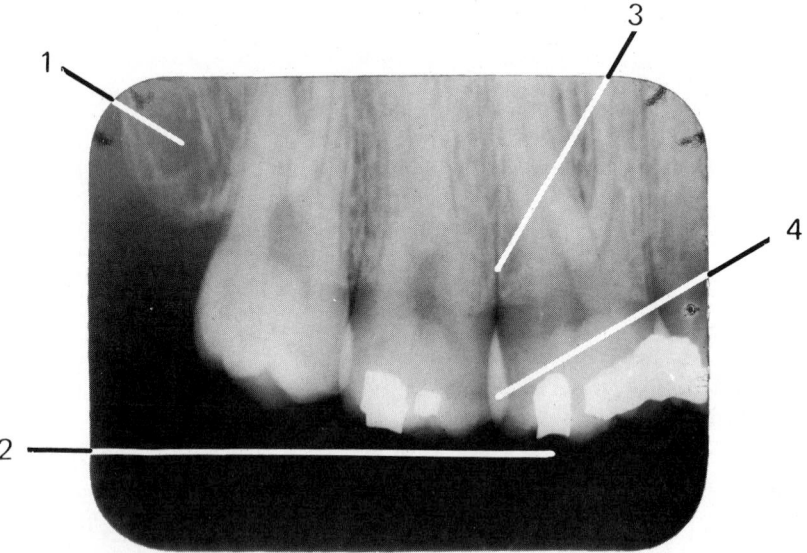

Figure 13–1. Radiograph of maxillary molar: **1** radiograph too dark; it was overexposed or overdeveloped; **2** excessive occlusal margin with resultant absence of the complete apical structures caused by film being placed too low in mouth; **3** tooth structures are elongated because the vertical angulation was insufficiently steep (too low); **4** overlapping in the proximal areas because in horizontal angulation the central beam was not directed through the interproximal spaces.

Correction: In maxillary areas, raise the film in the patient's mouth. In mandibular areas, lower the film in the patient's mouth. When paralleling, verify that film and axes are parallel.

2. *Absence of Coronal Structures* (Fig. 13–2)

Probable cause: Film was not placed high enough or low enough in the patient's mouth. Ideally there should be a 1/4-in. (6.4-mm) margin above or below the crown of the tooth. When the paralleling technique is used, this error may also be caused by the film not being parallel to the long axes of the teeth.

Correction: In maxillary areas, lower the film in the patient's mouth. In mandibular areas, raise the film in the patient's mouth. When paralleling, verify that film and axes are parallel.

3. *Absence of Mesial Structures*

Probable cause: Film was placed too far back in the patient's mouth.

Correction: Move the film mesially (toward the front of the mouth).

4. *Absence of Distal Structures*

Probable cause: Film was placed too far forward in the patient's mouth.

Correction: Move the film distally (toward the back of the mouth).

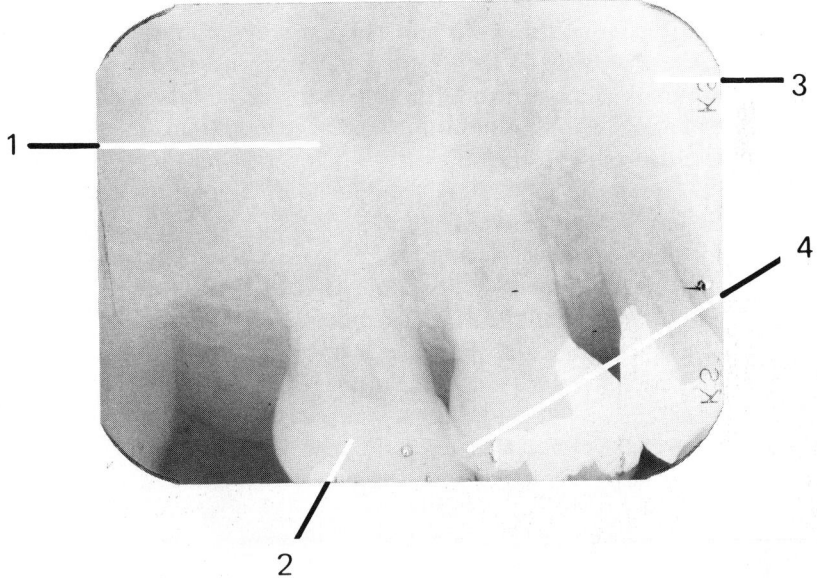

Figure 13–2. Radiograph of maxillary molar area: **1** light image caused by underexposure or underdevelopment; **2** absence of occlusal margin or all coronal structures—film was placed too high in mouth, not parallel to long axis of the teeth, and vertical angulation was too steep (too high); **3** cone cut—an unexposed area caused by faulty centering of the PID; **4** overlap in interproximal area traceable to faulty horizontal angulation.

5. *Slanting or Diagonal Instead of Straight Occlusal Plane* (Fig. 13–3)
   Probable cause: Edge of the film was not parallel with the incisal or occlusal plane of the teeth, or film holder was not placed flush against occlusal surfaces. When this error occurs in bitewing radiographs, it is usually caused by the top edge of the film contacting the lingual gingiva or curvature of the palate.
   Correction: Straighten the film packet. The use of a cotton roll between the film and the tooth may make this easier.
6. *Vertical Instead of Horizontal Film Placement in Posterior Areas*
   Probable cause: Film was placed with its longest dimension vertically. This is seldom desirable in posterior areas.
   Correction: Rotate the film so that the widest dimension is placed horizontally and the film edge is parallel with the occlusal plane.
7. *Horizontal Instead of Vertical Film Placement in Anterior Areas*
   Probable cause: Film was placed with its widest dimension horizontally.

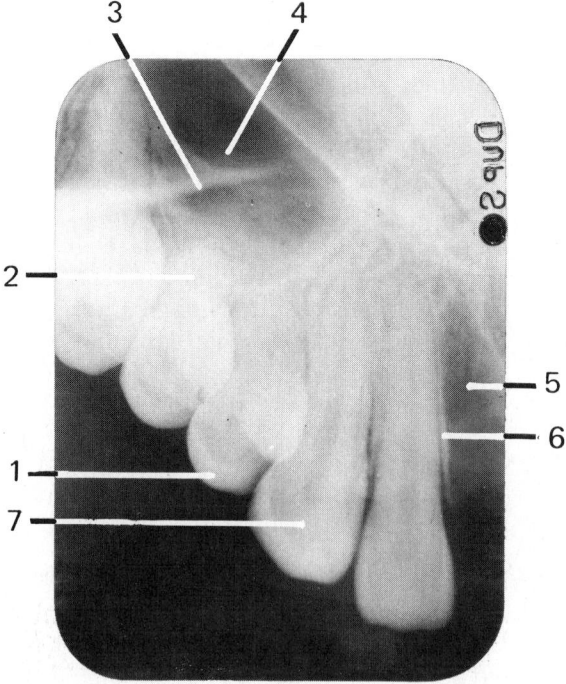

Figure 13–3. Radiograph of maxillary canine area shows **1** slanting or diagonal occlusal plane caused by improper positioning of the film packet; **2** extreme foreshortening caused by a combination of excessive vertical angulation and faulty film position; **3** distortion of image caused by film bending; **4** maxillary sinus; **5** recent extraction site; **6** lamina dura; and **7** canine is not properly centered in film.

Such placement is undesirable and produces major dimensional distortion of the image; furthermore, these anterior teeth are sometimes longer than the narrow dimension of the film.

Correction: Rotate the film so that the longest dimension is placed vertically. The short edge of the film should be placed parallel to the incisal edges of the anterior teeth.

8. *Bent Film Packet* (Fig. 13–4)

Probable cause: Curvature of the palate or lingual arch and strong finger pressure on film.

Correction: Place a cotton roll behind the teeth in the area of greatest curvature and ask the patient to reduce finger pressure. Consider the use of a film holder and narrower film.

9. *Diamond or Herringbone Pattern* (Fig. 13–5)

Probable cause: Film was reversed and the back side was facing teeth and the radiation source.

Correction: Turn the film so that the tube side faces toward the teeth and the radiation source.

10. *Incorrect Position of Identification Dot*

Probable cause: Dot positioned in apical area.

Correction: Position the dot in incisal or occlusal area.

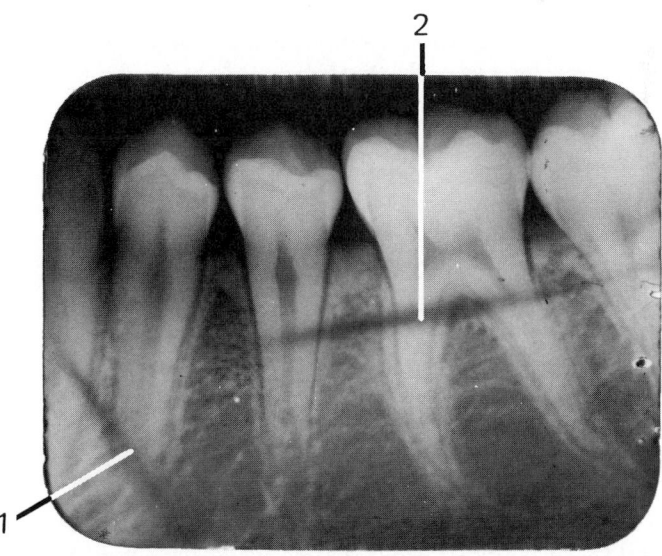

Figure 13–4. Radiograph of mandibular posterior area shows **1** distortion caused by bending the lower left film corner and pressure mark (thin radiolucent line); and **2** long radiolucent streak—a pressure mark caused by bending or by careless handling with excessive force.

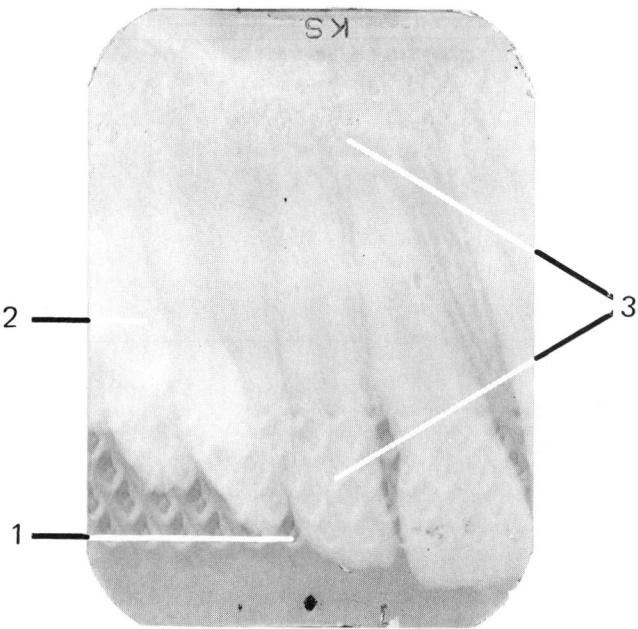

Figure 13–5. Radiograph of maxillary anterior area shows **1** film not correctly centered, occlusal plane not straight, **2** foreshortening of images of the premolar and canine caused by a combination of excessive vertical angulation and faulty film placement, **3** light image and two bars of herringbone (diamond) pattern showing that the film was accidentally reversed during placement in the mouth. The image is light because the x-rays were partially absorbed by the lead foil.

Incorrect Positioning of the Tube Head or PID

1. *Elongation of the Image* (Fig. 13–1)
   Probable cause: Insufficient vertical angulation of the PID.
   Correction: Increase the vertical angulation. Also check the position of the film and the patient's head.
2. *Foreshortening of the Image* (Fig. 13–3)
   Probable cause: Excessive vertical angulation of the PID.
   Correction: Decrease the vertical angulation. Also check the position of the film and the patient's head.
3. *Overlapping of the Image* (Figs. 13–1, 13–2, and 13–6)
   Probable cause: Incorrect rotation of the tube head and PID in the horizontal plane. Superimposition of the images of proximal surfaces occurs when the central beam is not directed perpendicularly toward the film through the interproximal spaces. The two common errors are **mesiodistal** and **distomesial projections.** When the angle of projection in the horizontal plane is from mesial to distal, the mesiobuccal root of maxillary molars appears to be superimposed over the lingual root, and the areas of overlapping

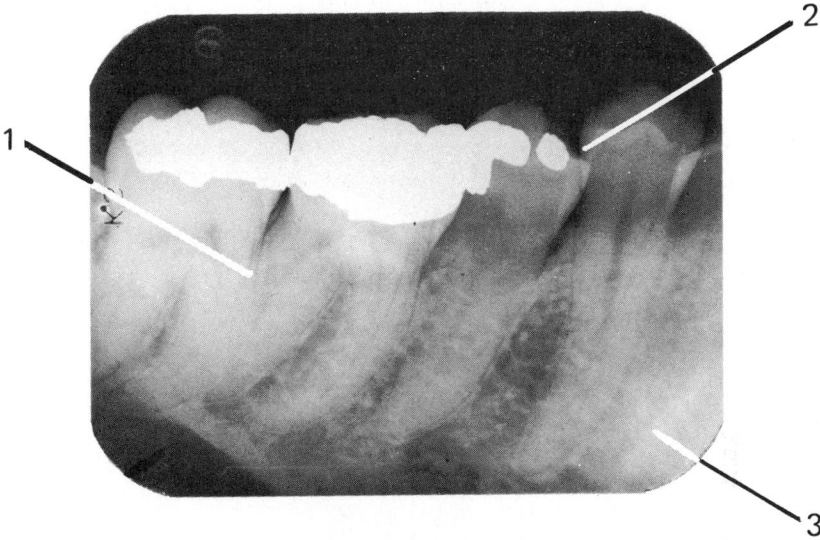

Figure 13–6. Radiograph of mandibular premolar area shows **1** distorted image and poor definition caused by movement of the patient, the film, or the tube head during the time of exposure, **2** overlapping of adjacent tooth structures caused by error in horizontal angulation, and **3** distortion of image caused by bending of the film packet during placement in the mouth.

contacts are larger in the posterior part of the radiograph. Conversely, when the angle of projection is from distal to mesial, the distobuccal root of maxillary molars appears to be superimposed over the lingual root, and the areas of overlapping contacts are larger in the anterior part of the radiograph.

Correction: Unless there is also elongation or foreshortening, maintain the vertical angulation. To compensate for mesiodistal angulation, change the direction of the PID so that the central ray is projected more to the mesial; to compensate for distomesial angulation, change the direction of the PID so that the central ray is projected more to the distal.

4. *Cone Cut* (Figs. 13–2 and 13–7)
   Probable cause: The primary beam of radiation was not directed toward the center of the film and did not completely expose all parts of the film.
   Correction: Maintain horizontal and vertical angulation and move the tube head either up, down, mesially, or distally, depending on which area of the radiograph shows a clear unexposed area.

Exposure Factors

1. *Light (Thin) Image* (Figs. 13–2 and 13–5)
   Probable cause: Insufficient exposure time in relation to milliamperage, kilovoltage, and distance selected. Also timer inaccuracy or faulty switch.

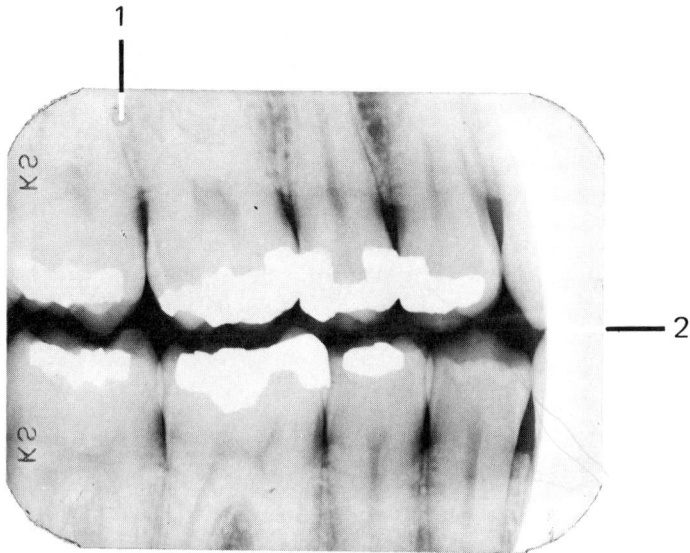

Figure 13–7. Premolar bitewing film shows **1** identification dot, and **2** cone cut caused by not directing the central ray toward the middle of the film. The white circular area was beyond the range of the x-ray beam and thus was not exposed.

May also be caused by insufficient time in developer, weak or oxidized developer, or reversed film.

Correction: Increase the exposure time, the milliamperage, the kilovoltage, or a combination of these factors. If the problem persists, check the accuracy of the timer or switch for possible malfunction.

2. *Dark Image* (Fig. 13–1)

Probable cause: Overexposure (excessive mAs, kVp, or time). Alternate cause: too long in the developer.

Correction: Decrease the exposure time, the milliamperage, the kilovoltage, or a combination of these factors.

3. *Absence of Image*

Probable cause: Failure to turn on the line switch or to maintain firm pressure on the activator button during the exposure. Alternate causes: electrical failure, malfunction of the x-ray machine, or processing errors (placing the film in fixer first or having the emulsion dissolve in warm rinse water).

Correction: Turn on the x-ray machine and maintain firm pressure on the activator button during the entire exposure period. On newer machines, listen for the audible tone that indicates that x-rays are being made.

Miscellaneous Errors in Exposure Technique

1. *Poor Definition* (Fig. 13–8)

Probable cause: Movement during exposure. Caused by patient movement, film slippage, or vibration of the tube head.

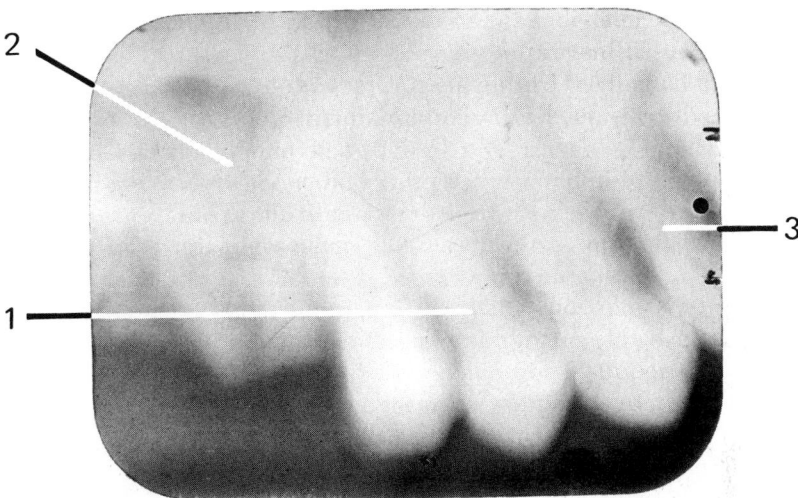

Figure 13–8. Radiograph of maxillary premolar area shows **1** poor definition caused by excessive movement of patient, film, or the tube head, **2** chemical fog caused by overage or contaminated processing solutions, and **3** film was positioned too far forward in the mouth.

Correction: Steady the tube head before starting exposure. Ask the patient to maintain steady pressure on the film and not to move.

2. *Double Image*
   Probable cause: Accidentally exposing the same film twice.
   Correction: Place the exposed film in the film safe immediately.

3. *Superimposed Image*
   Probable cause: Failure to first examine the mouth and remove any appliances such as removable bridges, partial or full dentures, and space maintainers.
   Correction: Look in the patient's mouth and remove any appliance.

4. ***Pressure Marks*** (black streaks) (Fig. 13–4)
   Probable cause: Bending or excessive pressure that causes the film emulsion to crack.
   Correction: Avoid excess pressure on the film. Do not bend the film except for minimal softening of corners to avoid hurting the patient with the sharp edges of the film packet.

5. *Wrapping Paper Stuck to Film*
   Probable cause: Break in wrapping by rough handling enabled saliva to penetrate to the emulsion. Moisture softened the emulsion, causing the black paper to stick to the film.
   Correction: Careful handling prevents a break in the seal of the film packet. Always blot moisture from the film packet after removing it from the mouth.

INADEQUACIES CAUSED BY FAULTY PROCESSING TECHNIQUES

Another major cause of faulty radiographs can be traced to errors in the processing technique. Many of these, such as misreading the temperature on the thermometer, forgetting to wind or set the timer, setting the timer incorrectly, failure to remove the film from the developer when the timer rings, and damage to the emulsion by handling or by chemical contamination, can be blamed on haste or carelessness.

Failure to Follow the Suggested Time–Temperature Cycle

1. *Light Image* (Fig. 13–2)
   Probable cause: Underdevelopment—film not left in developer for long enough time. The colder the developer, the longer the time required. Alternate causes: weakened developer, underexposure, or fixer contamination of the developer.
   Correction: Check the temperature of the developer and consult the time–temperature chart before placing the film in developer. If necessary, fill the inserts with fresh solutions.
2. *Dark Image*
   Probable cause: Overdevelopment—film left in developer for too long a time. The warmer the developer, the less time is required. Alternate cause: overexposure to radiation.
   Correction: Check the temperature of the developer and consult the time–temperature chart before placing the film in developer.
3. *Absence of Image*
   Probable cause: Film was placed in fixer before being placed in developer, or emulsion may have dissolved in warm rinse water. Alternate cause: film may not have been exposed.
   Correction: Place the film in developer first and promptly remove the film at the end of the washing period.

Faulty Handling of the Film

1. *Smudged Film*
   Probable cause: Fingermarks on the dry film or on the soft wet emulsion.
   Correction: Avoid contact with the surface of the radiograph. Handle films carefully and by the edges only. Hands should be clean and free of moisture.
2. *Thin Black Lines*
   Probable cause: Static electricity was produced when the film was pulled out of the wrapping too fast.
   Correction: Pull the film out of the wrapping slowly.
3. *White Lines or Marks* (Fig. 13–9)
   Probable cause: Soft film or emulsion was scratched by a sharp object

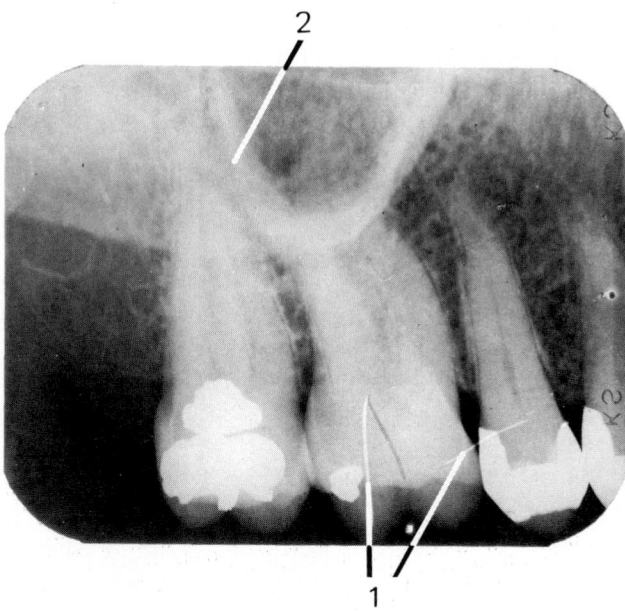

Figure 13-9. Radiograph of maxillary posterior area shows **1** white streak marks where the softened emulsion was scratched off the film during processing, and **2** U-shaped radiopaque band of dense bone shows the outline of the zygoma.

such as a film clip or film hanger. Scratching removes the emulsion from the base.

Correction: Be careful when inserting a second film hanger into an insert. Avoid contact with other films or hangers.

4. *Black Image*

Probable cause: Film was accidentally exposed to white light or exposed for a long period in warm developer.

Correction: Turn off all light in the darkroom except the proper safelight before unwrapping the film. Lock the door or warn others to stay out by turning on the "in-use" sign.

5. *Partial Image*

Probable cause: Level of the developer was too low to cover the entire film.

Correction: Replenish the processing solutions to the proper level or fasten the films to lower clips on the hanger.

6. *Clear Areas on Film*

Probable cause: Films stuck together in developer, so developer was not able to act on both sides of the film emulsion. Alternate cause: Attaching two films to a clip through failure to separate films in two-film packets.

Correction: Agitate films gently when inserting into the developer; make certain that films do not touch those on other hangers.

7. *Dark Areas on Film* (Fig. 13–10)

Probable cause: Films stuck together in fixer. The fixer was not able to remove the undeveloped silver halide crystals or to neutralize the developer in those areas, and development continues partially.

Correction: Agitate films gently when inserting into the fixer; make certain the films do not come in contact with those on other hangers.

8. *Reticulation*

Probable cause: Temperature of processing solutions is too hot, or there is too great a difference between the temperature of the processing solutions and the rinse water. Temperature differences of 10 degrees Fahrenheit may cause the film to become pitted and reticulated through the softening and melting of the emulsion.

Correction: Determine that the temperature in the processing solutions is approximately the same as that of the rinse water. Do not begin to process the film until the circulating water has cooled or warmed the developer and fixer. In manual processing, temperatures in excess of 80 degrees Fahrenheit (26.7 degrees Celsius) should be avoided.

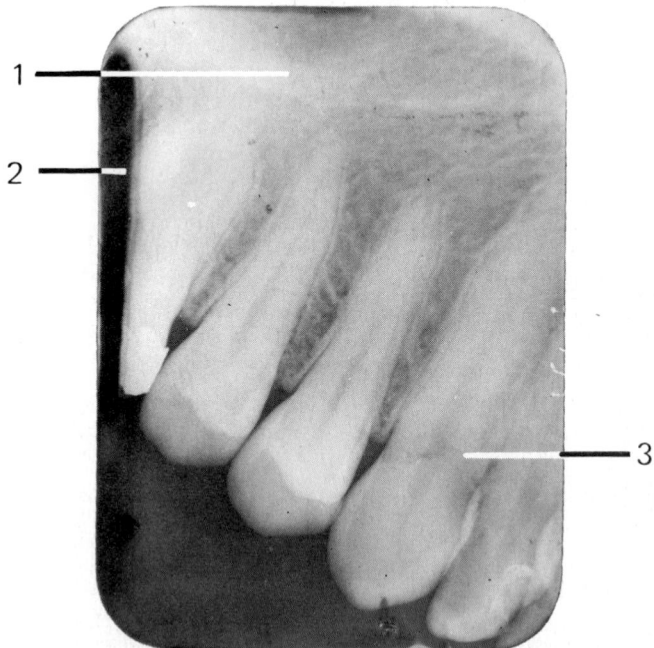

Figure 13–10. Radiograph of maxillary canine area shows **1** rusty or brown stain covering entire radiograph caused by improper washing after fixing, **2** thin dark area along side of film caused by two films touching in fixer with failure to stop the action of the developer, and **3** positioning error—canine not in center of film, with resultant loss of apical structure and a diagonal occlusal plane.

9. *Curled Films*

Probable cause: too rapid drying of the film through the use of heat.

Correction: Slower, more gradual drying. Avoid prolonged drying in the electric dryer.

10. *Scratched Film* (Fig. 13–9)

Probable cause: Failure to protect the dried radiograph.

Correction: Careful handling of processed radiographs. Mount the radiographs promptly and enclose in a protective envelope.

Chemical Contamination

1. *White Spots on Film*

Probable cause: Premature contact with fixer—drops of fixer may have been splashed on the workbench.

Correction: Clean the workbench and place a clean towel on the work area before opening the film packet.

2. *Dark Spots on Film* (Fig. 13–11)

Probable cause: Premature contact with developer—drops of developer may have been splashed on the workbench.

Correction: Clean the workbench and place a clean towel on the work area before opening the film packet.

3. *Iridescent Stain*

Probable cause: Oxidation and exhaustion of developer.

Correction: Replace the developer with fresh solution.

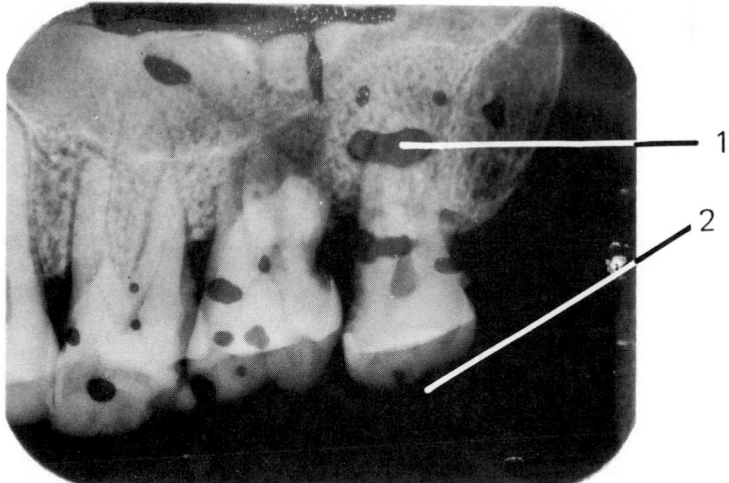

Figure 13–11. Radiograph of maxillary molar area shows **1** dark spots on radiograph caused by premature contact of film surface with developer splashed on workbench (bench should always be clean), and **2** uneven occlusal margin caused by poor film positioning.

4. *Dark Brown or Gray Film*
   Probable cause: Oxidation and exhaustion of fixer.
   Correction: Replace the fixer with fresh solution.
5. *Brownish-Yellow Stains*
   Probable cause: Insufficient or improper washing of the film.
   Correction: Rinse in circulating water for at least 20 minutes, preferably 30. Always return the film that was taken out for "wet-reading" for completion of fixing and washing.

INADEQUACIES CAUSED BY FOG ON THE FILM

Still another cause of inadequate radiographs is the formation of a thin, cloudy layer that fogs the film surface. **Fog** diminishes contrast and makes it difficult and often impossible to interpret the radiograph. Fog on radiographs is produced in many ways and can occur before or after the film is exposed or during processing. Most fogged radiographs have a similar appearance, and it is difficult to determine the cause unless one knows, for example, that the film was outdated; in that case one would suspect it to be age fog.

Fog Caused During Storage

1. *Age Fog* (Fig. 13–12)
   Probable cause: Overage film was used.
   Correction: Watch the date on film boxes. Use the oldest film first. Do not overstock film.
2. *Storage Fog*
   Probable cause: Film stored in warm, damp area or in vicinity of fume-producing chemicals.
   Correction: Store in cool, dry, fume-free area.

Fog Caused Before or After Exposure

1. *Radiation Fog*
   Probable cause: Film not properly protected before or after exposure.
   Correction: Store film at safe distance from the source of x-rays or protect it by placing it in a lead-lined dispenser. Never take more than one film out of the dispenser at a time, and place the film in the film safe after exposure is made.

Fog Caused During Processing

1. *Safelight Fog*
   Probable cause: Incorrect size of safelight bulb or prolonged exposure to the safelight. Also scratched filter or incorrect filter for type of film used.

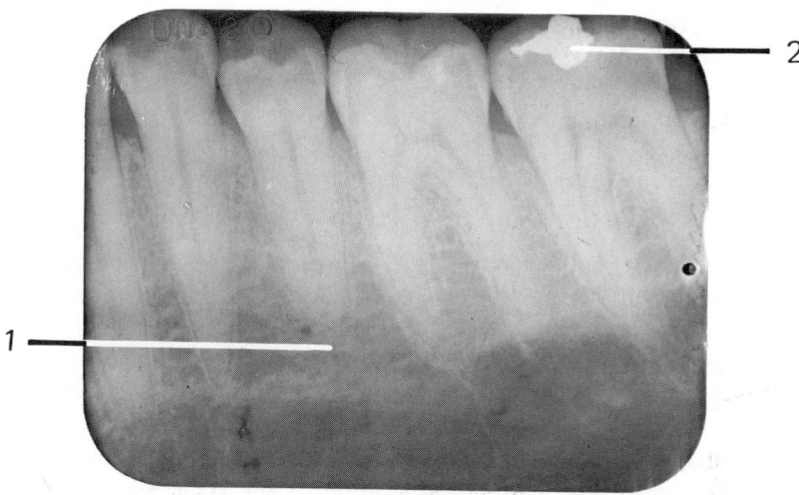

Figure 13–12. Radiograph of mandibular premolar area shows **1** entire radiograph fogged, with a resultant lack of contrast (fog may be caused by overage film [as in radiograph shown], storage, exposure to radiation or light, contaminated chemicals, or numerous other causes), and **2** metallic restoration.

Correction: Check the size of the safelight bulb. Minimize exposure to the safelight. Replace scratched filter. Follow film manufacturer's recommendations on type of filter to use with type of film used.

2. *White Light Fog*

   Probable cause: Light leak around the door of the darkroom or a minute break in the wrapping of the film. Scratched or cracked safelight filter.

   Correction: Check the darkroom for white light leaks. Check the filter for cracks and scratches. Avoid rough handling or bending of the film packet.

3. *Processing Contamination Fog* (Fig. 13–9)

   Probable cause: Contamination of processing chemicals.

   Correction: Avoid contamination of processing chemicals. Always replace the tank cover in the same way and rinse the film to remove developer before moving the film hanger into the fixer insert.

4. *Chemical Fog*

   Probable cause: Development for too long a time or at too high a temperature.

   Correction: Develop at recommended time–temperature cycle.

5. *Cigarette Fog*

   Probable cause: Smoking in the darkroom. The glow of the cigarette is sufficient to fog the film.

   Correction: Do not smoke in the darkroom.

CHAPTER SUMMARY

The dental auxiliary should be able to identify what type of error was made in handling, exposing, or processing any radiograph and should be aware of what must be done to avoid repetition of the same mistake.

Faulty radiographs are traceable to many causes. Frequently several different errors may cause similar-looking defects. The well-trained auxiliary handles film carefully and develops neat work habits. The price of good diagnostic radiographs is expertise and meticulous attention to details in all stages.

Most unsatisfactory radiographs can be attributed to faulty film handling, using incorrect exposure factors, failure to project the central ray toward the center of the film in both the horizontal and vertical planes, failure of the film to remain where placed, and poor processing techniques. Only clear, properly processed radiographs with minimal distortion that show the entire intended areas have real diagnostic value.

Processing errors cause absence of image, partial image, light image, dark image, scratched film, curled film, reticulation, smudged areas, black lines, brown and opaque spots, and so forth. Each error can usually be attributed to one of several possibilities. Being aware of the cause helps the operator to prevent repeating the mistake. The goal should always be to do it right the first time.

The majority of errors made at chair-side during exposure can be avoided if the operator is well-trained, skillful, and dedicated. The production of radiographs of high quality with high diagnostic yield should always be the goal of each operator.

KEY WORDS

Cone cut

Distomesial projection

Elongation

Fog

Foreshortening

Horizontal angulation

Mesiodistal projection

Overlapping

Pressure mark

Reticulation

Vertical angulation

REVIEW QUESTIONS

1. What should be done with the film when a previous radiograph of the maxillary molar area did not show the third molar? (a) raise in the mouth, (b) lower in the mouth, (c) move forward in the mouth, (d) move backward in the mouth.

2. What does a diamond or herringbone pattern on the processed radiograph indicate? (a) overage film, (b) underexposed film, (c) reversed film, (d) overdeveloped film.

3. Which of these conditions is caused by insufficient vertical angulation? (a) elongation, (b) overlapping, (c) foreshortening, (d) cone cutting.

4. A radiograph of the maxillary molar area shows that the mesiobuccal root is superimposed over the lingual root. What correction is needed? (a) increase the vertical angulation, (b) change the direction of horizontal angulation toward the mesial, (c) decrease the vertical angulation, (d) change the direction of the horizontal angulation toward the distal.

5. What error was made when the area of overlapped contacts is much larger in the second molar area than in the first premolar area? (a) excessive vertical angulation, (b) insufficient vertical angulation, (c) mesiodistal projection of horizontal angulation, (d) distomesial projection of horizontal angulation.

6. Which of these conditions results from a failure to direct the central ray toward the middle of the film packet? (a) cone cut, (b) overlapping, (c) elongation, (d) foreshortening.

7. Which of these indicates that the radiograph was overexposed? (a) light image, (b) reticulation, (c) dark image, (d) thin black lines.

8. Which of these indicates that the film was not properly washed? (a) light image, (b) fogging, (c) brownish-yellow stains, (d) white spots.

9. Which of these conditions indicates that the level of the developer in the tank insert was too low? (a) partial image, (b) cone cut film, (c) light image, (d) reticulation.

10. Which of these is not a cause of fogging of the radiograph? (a) exposure to scatter radiation, (b) use of overage film, (c) underexposure, (d) chemical-fume contamination of film.

BIBLIOGRAPHY

Eastman Kodak: *Exposure and Processing for Dental Radiography*. Rochester, NY: 1993

Goaz PW, White SC: *Oral Radiology Principles and Interpretation,* 3rd ed. St. Louis, MO: CV Mosby, 1994

Eastman Kodak: *Successful Intraoral Radiography*. Rochester, NY: 1990

CHAPTER 14

Intraoral Radiographic Procedures

By the end of this chapter the student should be able to

1. Identify the three basic intraoral procedures.
2. Compare the principles of the paralleling and bisecting techniques.
3. Locate the points of entry on the face.
4. Differentiate between the methods used to obtain proper horizontal and vertical angulation.
5. Identify the advance preparations required before radiographs are exposed.

INTRAORAL PROCEDURES

Intraoral radiography consists of methods of exposing dental x-ray films within the oral cavity. It includes positioning the patient in the chair, selecting a film packet of suitable size, determining how the film is to be positioned and held in place while the exposure is made, aiming the position indicating device (PID), and setting the control devices correctly to make the exposure. All these steps need careful planning. Techniques described in this chapter will help the dental auxiliary make good radiographs.

There are three common types of intraoral examinations. Each uses a slightly different film and technique, and each has a different objective. The first of these is the **periapical examination,** the fundamental purpose of which is to show the apices of the teeth and the structures that surround them. The second, the **bitewing examination,** is to show the coronal portions of the teeth and the alveolar crests of bone of both the maxillae and mandible of a given area on one film. The third type is the **occlusal examination.** Its purpose is to show the entire maxillary or mandibular arch (or a portion thereof) on a single film.

We have mentioned previously the two basic techniques employed in intraoral radiography—**bisecting** and **paralleling.** Either technique can be modified to meet special conditions and requirements. Each gives good results if one exercises care and remembers the fundamental principles of the technique. Paralleling is the technique of choice.

The first and earliest technique is called either the **bisecting,** the **bisecting-angle,** or the **short-cone technique.** The second and newer technique, now taught in all dental schools, is variously referred to as the **paralleling,** the **right-angle,** the **extension-cone,** or **long-cone technique.** To avoid confusion, these techniques are described as the bisecting and paralleling techniques in this text.

In 1904 Dr. W. A. Price suggested the basics of both the bisecting and paralleling methods. As others were working on the same problems and were unaware of Price's contributions, the credit for developing angulation techniques went to others.

The concept of the bisecting technique originated in 1907 through the application of a geometric principle known as the **rule of isometry.** This theorem states that two triangles having equal angles and a common side are equal triangles (Fig. 14–1). Be-

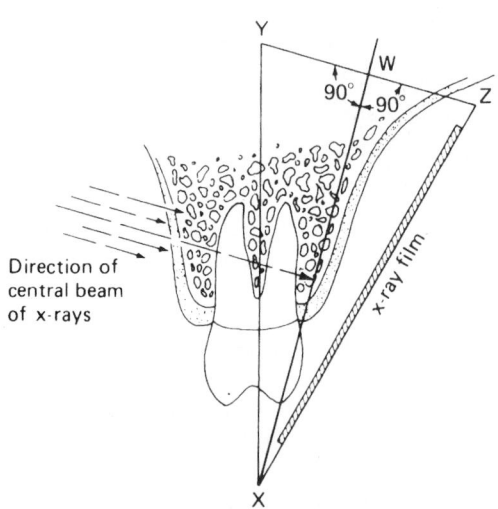

Figure 14–1. Isometric triangle applied to the bisecting technique. Line XY passes through the long axis of a maxillary first premolar while the film is positioned along line XZ. The central beam of radiation is directed perpendicularly through the apical area of the tooth toward the bisector XW. Because triangles WXY and WXZ are equal, the shadow image cast on the film will be approximately equal to the length of the film, provided that the bisector line is correctly estimated. Most errors in foreshortening and elongation are traceable to incorrectly estimating the location of the bisector line.

cause this theory was first suggested by A. Cieszynski, a Polish engineer, it became known as Cieszynski's rule of isometry.

This was the only method used for many years. However, since many radiographers experienced difficulties and obtained unsatisfactory results, the search for a less complicated technique that would produce better radiographs more consistently resulted in the development of the paralleling technique by Franklin McCormack in 1920. Technique modifications and refinements were subsequently made by Dr. Gordon Fitzgerald, Dr. William Updegrave, Dr. Donald T. Waggener, and many others.

FUNDAMENTALS OF SHADOW CASTING

The basic objective of dental radiology is to direct the PID toward the patient's face so that the central rays pass both horizontally and vertically through the tissues to be examined to the recording plane of the film at the most favorable angle. The film must be placed in relation to both the direction from which the x-ray photons originate (the source being on the target) and the intervening dental structures, so that all parts of the resulting shadow image are shown on the radiograph with a minimum of distortion.

Remember: (1) the radiograph is a film with a shadow image; (2) the source of the x-ray photons is the focal spot on the target of the x-ray tube; and (3) the function of the film is to record the shadow image.

When a hand is placed between a nearby light source such as an electric bulb and a flat object such as a tabletop, the shadow of the hand becomes magnified and fuzzy when the distance between it and the tabletop is increased. This fuzziness or partial shadow is called **penumbra.** The same happens in dental radiography, where the tooth is the object and the film is the recording plane. To obtain a sharp and accurate shadow image, the two should be as close together as possible. The image can also be sharpened by increasing the distance between the light source and the object.

There are five basic rules for casting a shadow image.

(1) The smallest possible source (focal spot) of radiation should be used.
(2) The object (tooth) should be as far as practical from the source.
(3) The object (tooth) and the recording plane (film) should be as close to each other as possible.
(4) The object (tooth) and the recording plane (film) should be parallel to each other.
(5) The radiation (central ray) must strike both the object (tooth) and the recording plane (film) at right angles.

Neither of the intraoral techniques completely meets these five requirements for accurate shadow casting. In the bisecting method, the object and film are not parallel to each other and the radiation does not strike the object and the film at right angles; in the paralleling method, the distance between the object and the film is greater than ideal in most film placement areas.

PRINCIPLES OF THE PARALLELING TECHNIQUE

The paralleling technique was developed to solve some of the problems of the bisecting technique. In the paralleling technique, the film is placed as nearly parallel to the long axes of the teeth as mouth anatomy permits. The central rays are directed at right angles to both the teeth and film (Fig. 14–2).

Normally, the target–film distance used in paralleling is 16 in. (41 cm). The accepted rule is that the distance between the target and the tooth should be as long as is practical with the equipment used. It is also necessary to increase the distance between the crowns of the teeth and the film, because oral structures, particularly the curvature of the palate, make it difficult to place the film parallel to the long axes of the teeth. This can best be done by using a **film holder.**

Historically, three things prevented rapid acceptance of the paralleling technique by the dental profession: the lack of x-ray machines that could operate at higher kilovoltages, the unavailability of high-speed films, and the absence of easy-to-use and accurate film holders. Once the technique is mastered, many find it easier than the bisecting technique, and the results are superior. Film placement is simpler, and one need not locate the bisector.

As discussed in Chapter 4, the beam of radiation diverges as it becomes more distant from its source and fans out like the spokes of a wheel. To prevent penumbra (the production of a fuzzy shadow around the outline of the image) and magnification of the image, the target–object distance must be as long as possible so that only the most central and parallel rays are directed at the tooth structures and film. The use of longer target–object distances diminishes the intensity of the radiation according to the inverse square law (see Fig. 4–3). When greater penetrating power of the rays is needed, higher kilovoltage is desirable. When the target–object distance is increased, the kilovoltage, milliamperage, exposure time, or a combination of these factors must be increased. The most common practice is to increase the exposure time by a factor of four when the target–object distance is doubled. Such prolonged exposures could not be safely and routinely made until films with very fast emulsion speed became available.

Films may be positioned in several ways. Biteblocks of various lengths can be used, or the film can be placed between the beaks of a hemostat. More advanced and

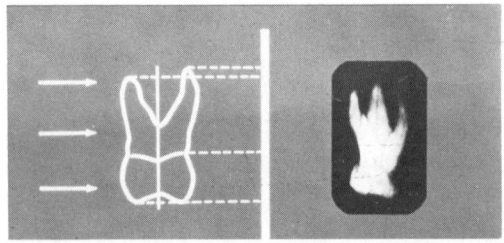

Figure 14–2. Principle of the paralleling technique. The x-ray beam is directed perpendicular to the recording plane of the film, which has been positioned parallel to the long axis of the tooth. *(Courtesy of Rinn Corporation, Elgin, IL.)*

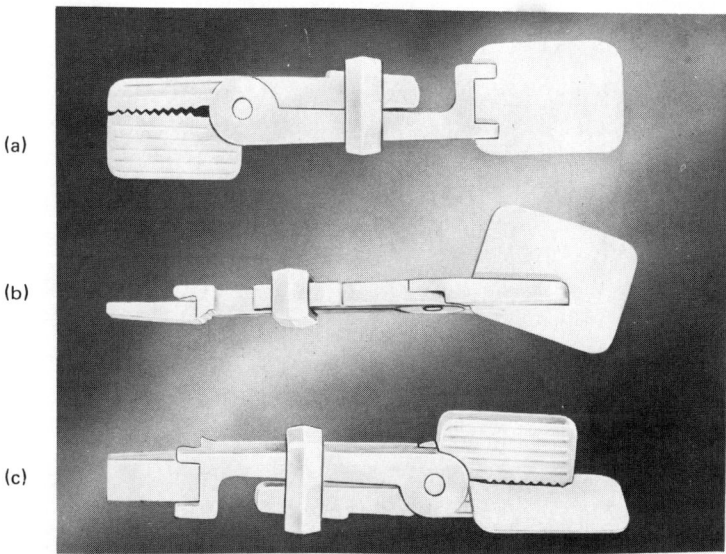

Figure 14–3. The Rinn EEZEE-GRIP film holder. This versatile film holder provides an excellent and simple method of standardizing the technique for intraoral radiography. The film is positioned to x-ray **(a)** the anterior areas, **(b)** the mandibular third molar area, and **(c)** the posterior areas. *(Courtesy of Rinn Corporation, Elgin, IL.)*

sophisticated film holders have made the paralleling technique easy. The newest film holders vary from simple disposable biteblocks that require no sterilization to complex devices that indicate the correct angle for directing the PID in relation to the teeth and film (Figs. 14–3, 14–4, and 14–5). Little trouble should arise in choosing a suitable holder to produce good results.

An advantage of the paralleling technique is that it takes less time to direct the rays perpendicular to the tooth than at a hard-to-locate bisector. A further advantage is that the image has only minimal dimensional distortion when compared with the bisecting technique.

PRINCIPLES OF THE BISECTING TECHNIQUE

When the bisecting principle is applied to casting a shadow of a tooth on a film, the angle formed by the long axis of the tooth and the plane of the film must be bisected, and the beam must be directed perpendicularly through the apex of the tooth toward the bisecting line (Fig. 14–1). One must first imagine a line, called the **bisector,** and then direct the radiation beam to it instead of to the long axis of the tooth or the film plane. This procedure is necessary because the irregularities of the oral tissues and the curvature of the palate seldom allow the film to lie parallel to the tooth when it is held with the finger against the oral structures.

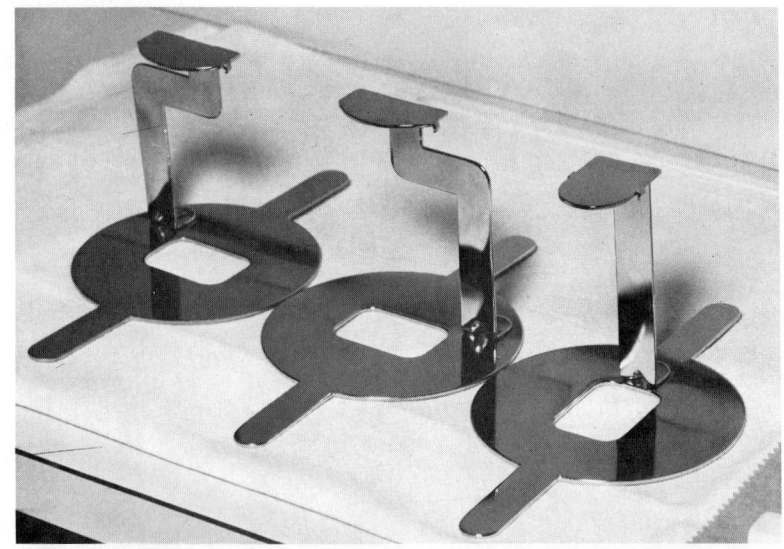

(a)

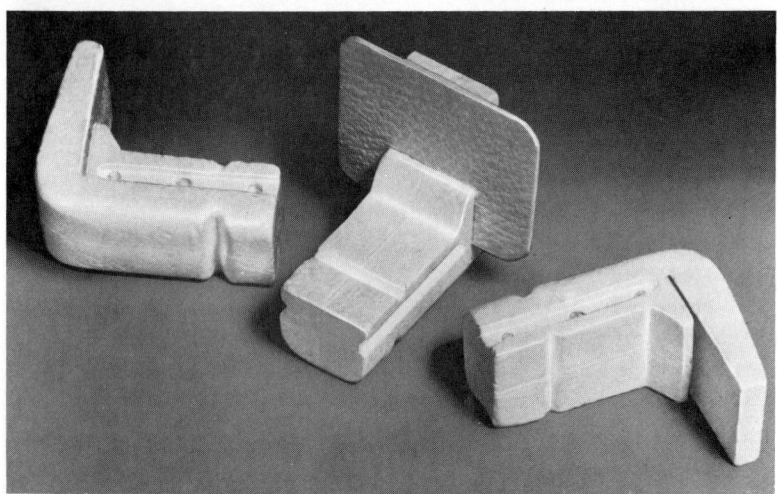

(b)

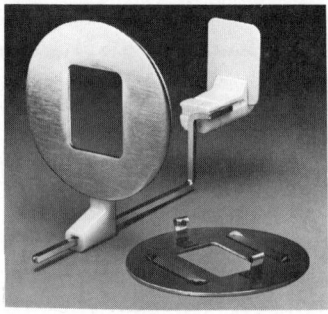

(c)

Figure 14–4. (a) Set of "Precision" instruments featuring metal collimating shield that restricts the x-ray beam to the size of the opening, providing just enough radiation to expose the film properly. *(Courtesy of Isaac Masel Company, Philadelphia, PA)* **(b)** Disposable XCP bite blocks. **(c)** A new stainless-steel collimation device that can be substituted for the plastic aiming device used in the BAI and XCP instruments. This reduces the amount of radiation the patient receives. BAI, bisecting angle instruments; XCP, extension cone paralleling. *(Courtesy of Rinn Corporation, Elgin, IL.)*

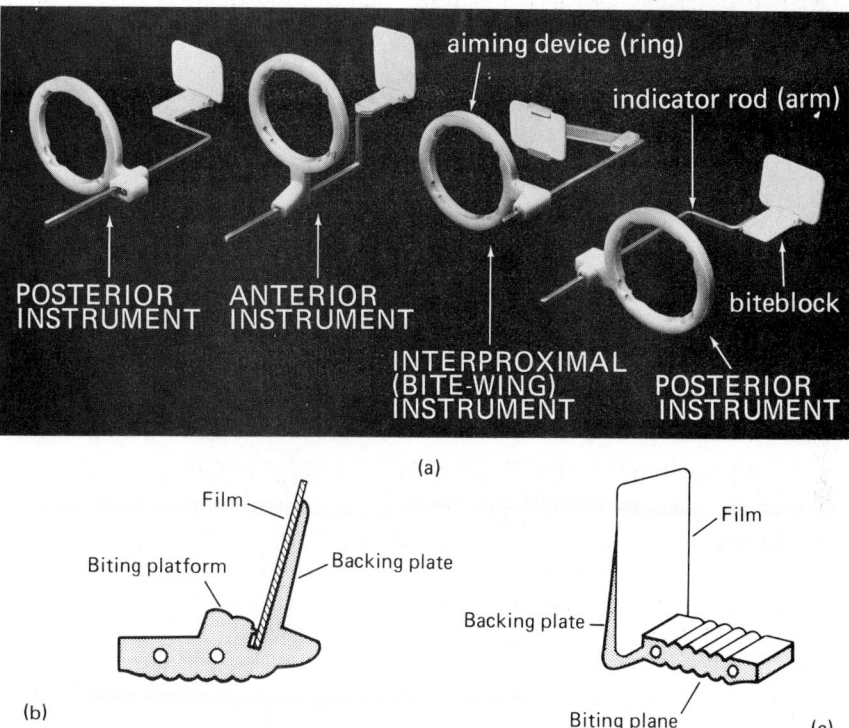

Figure 14–5. (a) XCP (extension cone paralleling) instruments for aligning and holding x-ray film packets. The instruments automatically indicate the correct horizontal and vertical angle. The complete kit includes one anterior instrument, right and left posterior instruments, and optionally, a bitewing instrument. The difference between the XCP and the BAI (bisecting angle) instruments are the periapical biteblocks. On the XCP, the backing plates are at a 90-degree angle, whereas on the BAI, the backing plates are at a 105-degree angle. **(b)** Anterior biteblock of BAI. The raised platform on which the patient bites is close to the backing plate. The 105-degree angle of the backing plate keeps the film close to the lingual surface of the tooth. **(c)** Anterior biteblock of XCP. The biting plane is at a right angle with the backing plate. The patient bites down far enough back on the biting plane to keep film and teeth parallel. *(Courtesy of Rinn Corporation, Elgin, IL.)*

Theoretically, two isometric triangles (triangles having equal measurements) are formed when the central ray is directed perpendicularly toward the bisector, and the film image that results should be the same size as the tooth. However, in practice this does not always happen. The image is usually satisfactory for diagnostic purposes, but some dimensional distortion is inherent in the bisecting technique.

One of the disadvantages of the bisecting technique is that many operators have trouble estimating the direction of the bisector. Thus, they may misdirect the central rays and cause the resulting image to be either elongated or foreshortened. Another

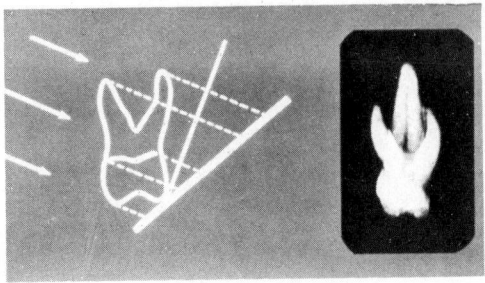

Figure 14–6. Principle of the bisecting technique. The x-ray beam is directed perpendicular to the imaginary line that bisects the angle formed by the recording plane of the dental x-ray film and the long axis of the tooth. *(Courtesy of Rinn Corporation, Elgin, IL.)*

disadvantage is that the divergence of the rays in the beam causes the image to appear slightly magnified. To cover the entire area of the film, the rays have to diverge more when the target–object distance is short. This divergence of the rays increases the closer the target is positioned to the object; thus a degree of magnification is inevitable when a target–film distance less than 8 in. (20.5 cm) is used. However, this is not the only cause of magnification. Because all teeth and surrounding bone structures have depth besides length and width, the degree of magnification on any x-ray film is unequal. For example, the buccal roots of a maxillary molar show more magnification than the lingual root, which is located closer to the film.

Still another disadvantage is that dimensional distortion occurs when the three-dimensional tooth and bone structures are projected on the two-dimensional recording plane of the film. This means that structures farther from the film appear more elongated than those closer to the film (Fig. 14–6). Also the steeper angle of vertical projection of the beam necessitated by directing the rays perpendicularly to the bisector instead of the tooth causes a shadow of the zygoma to be superimposed over the molar roots in the maxillary areas.

However, the bisecting technique can be useful. The film can be held by finger pressure when a suitable film holder is not available. Although using a film holder is preferable to having the patient hold the film, the anatomical restrictions of the mouth or the patient's state of mind occasionally restrict its use.

SHADOW CASTING IN THE TWO TECHNIQUES

Because most modern x-ray machines meet the requirements of either technique and the size of the effective focal spot is the same in both, the degree of image distortion is affected by the distances and angles one selects (Fig. 14–7).

As we have seen, distances differ in the two techniques. The shorter 8-in. (20.5-cm) target–film distance is generally, but not necessarily, used in the bisecting method. In the paralleling method, a longer target–film distance is preferred to compensate for the

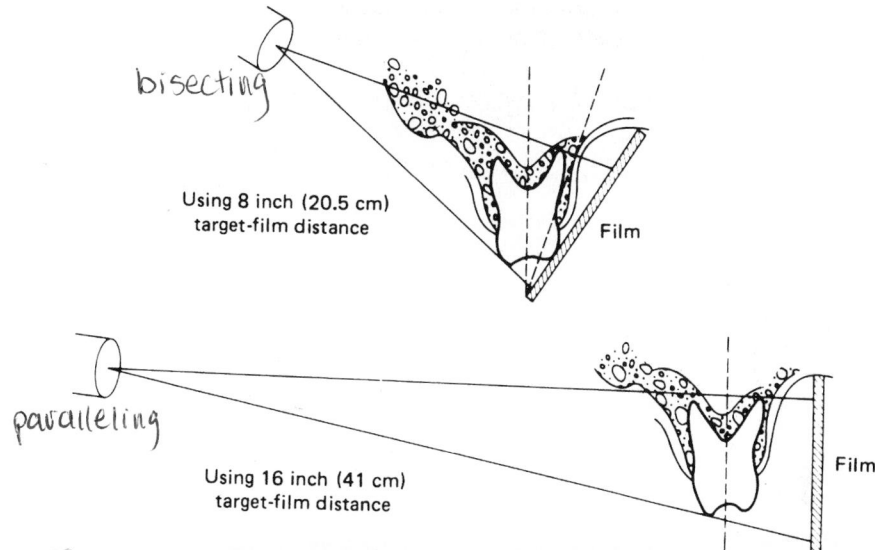

bisecting

Using 8 inch (20.5 cm)
target-film distance

Film

paralleling

Using 16 inch (41 cm)
target-film distance

Film

obj 4 .90

Figure 14–7. Comparison of the bisecting and paralleling methods. In the bisecting angle method, the film is positioned adjacent to the tooth structure, and the target–film distance is approximately 8 in. (20.5 cm). In the paralleling method, the film is positioned near the center of the oral cavity, where it must be retained in a position parallel to the long axes of the teeth, and the target–film distance is approximately 16 in. (41 cm). *(Courtesy of Rinn Corporation, Elgin, IL.)*

greater object–film distance. The use of a 16-in. (41-cm) target–film distance with the bisecting technique will improve the quality of the image. The 8-in. (20.5-cm) target–film distance is the minimum distance one should use with the paralleling technique. With the exception of the mandibular molar areas, where film placement is almost identical in both techniques, a shorter object–film distance is used in bisecting procedures. The film is placed as close to the teeth as possible, thus forming an angle between the long axes of the teeth and film. In paralleling procedures, the film must be placed farther from the teeth in order to get the film and teeth parallel.

A further difference is in the angle at which the radiation strikes the tooth structures and the film plane. In the bisecting method, the central rays are aimed perpendicularly to the bisector, whereas in the paralleling method, they are directed perpendicularly to both the long axes of the teeth and to the film plane. Thus, the bisecting method produces more dimensional distortion (Fig. 14–8).

Using the bisecting method, patients may either hold the film with their finger or bite on a film holder; with the paralleling method, they must bite on a film holder. Unless special holders that indicate PID positions are used in the bisecting technique, patients are usually seated upright with their head straight. This position is necessary for consistent results in determining the best horizontal and vertical angulations of the x-ray beam. Head positions and angulations are described in the next section. In the

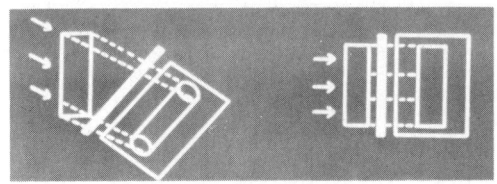

Figure 14–8. The figure on the left shows dimensional distortion such as found in the bisecting technique. It occurs when a three-dimensional object is projected on a two-dimensional surface, creating an angular relationship between the object and the film. The part of the object farthest from the film is projected in an incorrect relationship to the parts closest to the film. Such distortion is eliminated in the paralleling technique, shown in the figure on the right. The film is positioned parallel to the object, so that all parts of the object are in their true relationship to one another. *(Courtesy of Rinn Corporation, Elgin, IL.)*

paralleling technique, the patient's head can be in any position, so the patient can easily be placed horizontally in a contour chair. The horizontal angulation is determined in the same manner in both techniques. The vertical angulation necessarily differs because the rays are directed at the bisector instead of at the long axes of the teeth.

The final difference is in results. Bisecting images may not be anatomically accurate. Longer target–object distances and a more parallel relationship between the film and the tooth structures improve the quality of the radiographic image (Fig. 14–9).

Proficiency should be developed in both techniques. The dentist's preference may determine which technique is used. An operator using the paralleling technique may

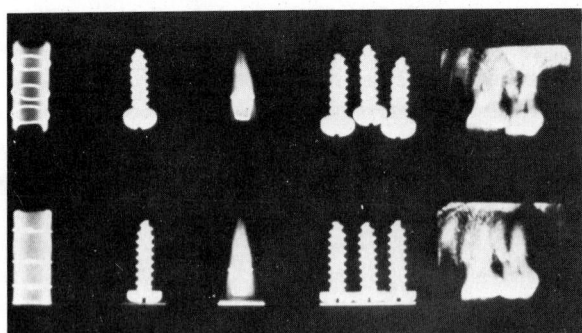

Figure 14–9. The superior radiographic quality of the paralleling technique is readily demonstrated when results are compared. Radiographs produced by the bisecting technique **(top)** are not anatomically accurate in most instances, since obvious dimensional distortion is inherent in this technique. This kind of distortion does not occur with the paralleling technique **(bottom)** in which objects are reproduced in their normal size and relationship. *(Courtesy of Rinn Corporation, Elgin, IL.)*

change to the bisecting method for one or two exposures during a full-mouth series because of anatomical limitations such as heavy muscle attachments or the shape of the palate.

POINTS OF ENTRY

The **point of entry** is the spot on the surface of the face at which the center of the end of the PID (the central ray) is directed (Fig. 14–10). Points of entry are most useful when film-holding instruments are not used (bisecting technique). With most film-holding instruments, the aiming ring will determine the point of entry by its predetermined relationship to the film packet.

Points of entry are located at the level of the apices of the teeth. Chapter 11 referred to anatomical landmarks that can be used to determine the location of the apices of the teeth. When the patient is seated in the conventional position, the apices of the maxillary teeth are located along an imaginary line drawn from the ala of the nose to the tragus of the ear.

The following landmarks are helpful in determining the point of entry. For maxillary teeth these are located along an extension of the ala–tragus line as follows: (1) the tip of the nose for the incisors, (2) the depression formed by the ala of the nose for the canines, (3) a point below the pupil of the eye for the premolars, and (4) a point below the outer canthus of the eye for the molars.

A point directly below the same landmarks and approximately 1/2 in. (1.3 cm) above an imaginary line parallel to the lower border of the mandible is used to locate

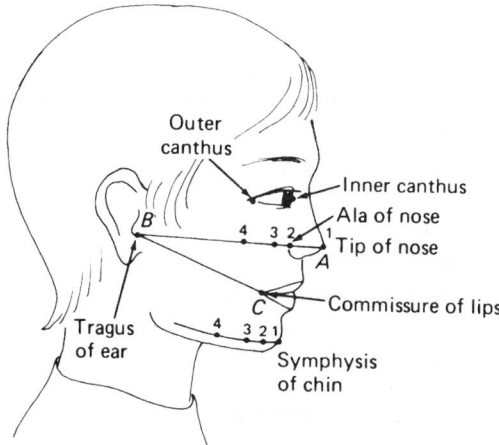

Figure 14–10. The term **points of entry** refers to the facial landmarks that provide the radiographer with a quick reference for the positioning of the PID and the directing of the central beam of radiation. Unless special film holders that eliminate the need for positioning are used, the patient is seated upright with the midsagittal plane perpendicular to the floor.

the point of entry for the corresponding mandibular teeth. These points of entry are only approximations.

With a little practice, the point of entry (Fig. 14–10) for each maxillary and mandibular tooth position can be determined at a glance. In some cases, particularly where third molars are involved, these points are located farther distally. The truest image is produced when the central rays are directed through the point of entry toward the apices of the roots. However, the increased use of smaller beam diameters and film holders with collimating devices that limit the size of the beam makes it preferable to direct the central rays through the middle of the teeth instead of through the apices. After the tube head and PID are in approximately correct horizontal and vertical alignment, the end of the PID should almost touch the face with its midpoint centered over the point of entry. Failure to project the central ray through this point and toward the middle of the film packet results in cone cutting. Before making the exposure, a final check of the patient's head position, film position, and angulation is made, and the patient is cautioned not to move.

HORIZONTAL AND VERTICAL ANGULATION PROCEDURES

One of the most difficult procedures for the beginner to learn is how to determine the correct direction of the central beam in the horizontal and vertical planes.

Although an experienced radiographer can expose radiographs with the patient either upright or supine, the use of predetermined head positions is recommended for the beginner. This makes it possible to standardize the procedure. As the contour chair has become increasingly popular, many dental professionals are learning to make exposures with the patient in a supine position. The conventional position, particularly when bisecting, is to seat the patient upright and adjust the headrest so that the plane of occlusion for the jaw being examined is parallel to the floor, and the midsagittal plane that divides the patient's head into a right and left side is perpendicular to the floor (Fig. 14–11). This procedure requires periodic changes in the headrest position because there are two planes of occlusion when the mouth is open. One is the occlusal plane of the maxillary and the other of the mandibular teeth. The only time when both planes are the same is during the exposure of bitewing films, when the patient's mouth is closed when biting on the bitetab. One must also realize that the occlusal plane is not a straight line but is usually curved. For this reason, the headrest position may have to be changed several times while exposures are being made on each jaw.

Immediately after the head position is adjusted and the film placed, the tube head and PID must be adjusted in both horizontal and vertical planes (angulation) and the tip of the PID brought as close as possible to the face at the predetermined point of entry. Angulation is defined as the procedure by which the tube head and PID are aligned to obtain the optimum angle at which the radiation is to be directed toward the film.

The angulation is changed by rotating the tube head horizontally and vertically. The x-ray machine is constructed with three swivel joints to support the yoke and tube

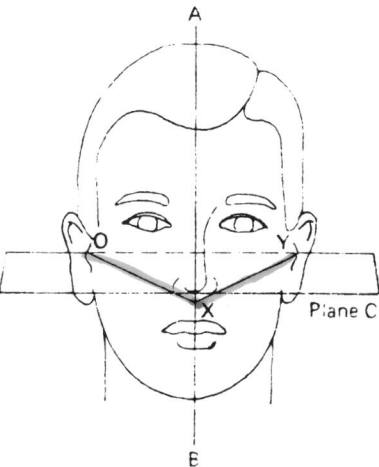

Figure 14–11. Head divided by midsagittal plane A–B and occlusal plane C. The midsagittal plane must always be perpendicular to the floor, and the occlusal plane must be parallel with the floor unless special film-holding devices are used. The O–X is the line of orientation for the maxillary teeth. It is also known as the **ala–tragus** line. The apices of the roots of the maxillary teeth are located close to this line. *(Reproduced with permission from Ennis LM, Berry. HM, Phillips JE:* Dental Roentgenology, *6th ed. Philadelphia, PA: Lea & Febiger, 1967.)*

head. One of these, located at the top and center of the yoke where it attaches to the extension arm, permits horizontal movement of the tube head to control the antero-posterior dimensions. The other two swivel joints are located at either side of the yoke. These permit the tube head to be rotated up or down in a vertical direction to control the longitudinal dimensions of the resulting image.

Horizontal angulation may be explained as a procedure used to direct the central rays perpendicularly (at a right angle) toward the film surface in a horizontal plane (Fig. 14–12). Identical steps are followed in the bisecting and paralleling methods. To change direction, swivel the tube head from side to side. As the direction of the film position is known, a visual sighting along the front of the tube head serves as a guide. If the flat surface along the front of the tube head is parallel with the film packet, the direction of the central ray should be perpendicular to the mean tangent of the teeth being radiographed. The objective is to permit the central rays to pass directly through the interproximal spaces. Any anatomical or tooth irregularity may make this difficult if not impossible. Incorrect alignment in the horizontal plane through deviation of the angulation toward the mesial or the distal results in an overlapping of the tooth structures shown on the radiograph.

Vertical angulation may be described as a procedure used to direct the central rays perpendicularly toward the film surface in a vertical plane. Because the film position, with the exception of the mandibular molar area, is not the same in bisecting and paralleling, the technique procedures differ. The direction of the central ray is changed

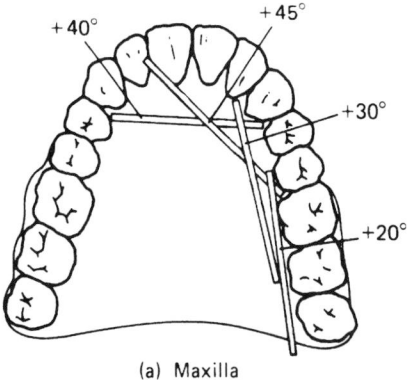
(a) Maxilla

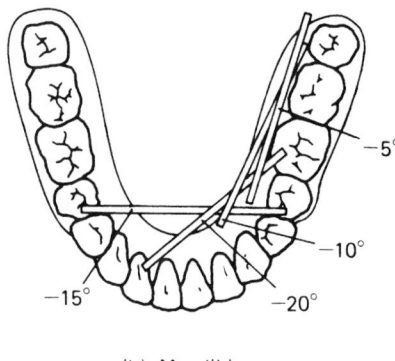
(b) Mandible

Figure 14–12. The horizontal angulation is determined by directing the x-ray beam perpendicularly to the mean tangent of the teeth being radiographed, which is also the corresponding position of the film. The beam passes directly through the interproximal spaces. Standard #2 film is shown; however, the narrow #1 film is recommended for the incisor and canine region. The average vertical angulation is also shown on **(a)** the maxilla, in positive (+) degrees and **(b)** the mandible, in negative (−) degrees.

by swiveling the tube head vertically so that the tip of the PID is raised or lowered (Fig. 14–13). Vertical angulation is customarily described in degrees. On most x-ray machines the vertical angles are scaled in intervals of 5 degrees on both sides of the yoke where the tube head is connected.

The vertical angulation of the tube head and the PID begins at zero. In that position the PID is parallel to the plane of the floor. All deviations from zero in which the tip of the PID is tilted toward the floor are called **positive** (plus) **angulations.** Those in which the PID is tipped upward toward the ceiling are called **negative** (minus) **angulations.**

When the bisecting technique is used, the central ray—in the vertical plane—must be directed through the roots of the teeth perpendicularly toward the bisector (Fig. 14–1). When the patient's head is in the conventional position, predetermined vertical angulations can often be used. Obviously, such angulations will vary from patient to patient. The average vertical angulations listed below are intended only as a guide and should not replace good judgment:

Maxillary incisors	plus 40 degrees
Maxillary canines	plus 45 degrees
Maxillary premolars	plus 30 degrees
Maxillary molars	plus 20 degrees
Mandibular molars	minus 5 degrees
Mandibular premolars	minus 10 degrees
Mandibular canines	minus 20 degrees
Mandibular incisors	minus 15 degrees

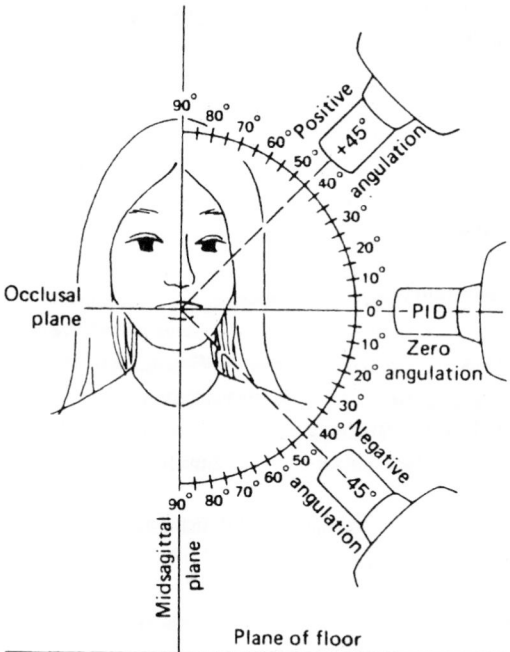

Figure 14–13. Diagram showing patient sitting in the preferred position upright in dental chair with midsagittal line perpendicular and occlusal plane parallel with the floor. Zero angulation is achieved when the long axis of the PID is directed parallel to the floor. All vertical angulations above the occlusal plane are called **positive** or **plus (+) angulations;** these are used for all maxillary and bitewing exposures. Vertical angulations below the occlusal plane are **negative** or **minus (–) angulations;** these are used for all mandibular exposures. Average vertical angulations are used when the film is held by the patient, as in the bisecting technique. Film holders that automatically indicate the correct horizontal and vertical angulations can be used, thus eliminating the necessity for numerically setting the angulations and for placing the patient's head in a predetermined position.

Many prefer to minimize guesswork by using some form of film holder, as shown in Figure 14–5.

When the paralleling technique is employed, the central ray—in the vertical plane—must be directed perpendicularly (at right angle) through the roots of the teeth toward the film packet (refer to Fig. 14–2).

Regardless of which technique is used, there will be situations that defy the operator's best effort. Crowded arches with malpositioned teeth, tight muscle attachments, or anatomical abnormalities often make it impossible to position the film properly or direct the central ray ideally. When this occurs it may be necessary to "increase" or to "decrease" the vertical angulation. For example, a change from +40 to +50 degrees or from –10 to –20 degrees is called an increase in vertical angulation; the reverse, a change from +50 to +40 degrees or from –20 to –10 degrees, is called a decrease in vertical angulation.

The operator should be alert to observe anatomical variations and to understand what change in angulation is required in each instance. For example, the table of average angulations presented above suggests that the average vertical angulation for the maxillary molars is about +20 degrees. Changes are indicated when the patient's vault (palate) is high or low; depending on the degree of the deviation from normal, a change of at least 5 degrees is called for. Therefore when the vault is high, the angulation is decreased to +15 degrees or less because the film packet now lies in a more vertical plane in the mouth. Conversely, when the vault is low, an increase to +25 degrees or more should be made, since the film packet now assumes a more horizontal position. In the mandibular region, if the floor of the mouth is shallow or the teeth are facially inclined, the vertical angulation should be increased by 5 to 10 degrees. It should be decreased by 5 to 10 degrees when the floor of the mouth is very deep or the teeth incline lingually.

As already indicated, the degree of vertical angulation controls the longitudinal dimension of the image produced. When the vertical angle is correctly estimated and the rays are directed perpendicularly to the bisector, no appreciable distortion results. Excessive angulation, so that the direction of the rays is increased, or steepened, foreshortens the image. Insufficient angulation, so that the direction of the rays is decreased, or flattened, elongates the image. It must always be considered that the tube head moves in both the horizontal and vertical planes. These movements must be coordinated if an accurate image is to be produced. It is seldom possible to position the tube head and PID correctly in both planes in one movement. The beginner, especially, should first determine the correct angulation in one plane and then in the other, being careful not to tilt the angulation that has already been established out of position. One should not make the exposure until satisfied that the angulation is properly coordinated in both planes in relation to the teeth and the film.

PRELIMINARY PREPARATION FOR RADIOGRAPHY

Unless the x-ray machine is located in the main operatory and the radiograph is to be exposed during dental procedures, advance preparations should be made. These save the time of both the patient and the operator.

First sanitize the entire area (see Chapter 7). Then turn on the x-ray machine and check that the dials work. Prepare film holders. Always check the film dispenser to see if it contains an adequate supply of various sizes of films, including films with bite-wing tabs. Remember to wash your hands thoroughly before donning gloves.

Secure the patient's cooperation before any procedures are begun. New patients or young patients may be concerned with pain, and some patients are worried about safety. A few words of explanation generally relieves the patient's anxiety. Explanations, of course, depend on the patient's understanding. As a rule, confidence allays the patient's fears, while hesitation increases them.

Whatever their understanding of radiation, patients need to know that modern equipment and high-speed films have reduced radiation exposures to safe levels and that radiographs are essential for making an adequate diagnosis. In simple language, tell the patients how they benefit from the timely discovery of incipient decay, unsuspected impacted teeth, deep calculus formations, the location of unerupted teeth, and numerous other unsuspected conditions. Informed and cooperative patients always make the task of producing good radiographs easier.

Eyeglasses and large earrings (which might get in the way of the PID) should be removed and put aside in a safe place. Check the mouth for dentures or removable bridgework. These should generally be removed because the clamps of partial dentures and removable bridges will be superimposed on the image of the teeth. Dentures, too, may be dislodged. The only time an appliance should be left in the mouth is when it is needed to stabilize the film holder or to bite on a tab.

After determining the age, general physique, and health of the patient, and completing the oral inspection for unusual conditions, one must decide whether the planned technique must be changed. During the oral examination observe (1) the position of the teeth, (2) the length of the crowns, (3) edentulous areas, (4) the thickness of the bone structures, (5) the general shape of the floor of the mouth and the palate, (6) the presence of lesions, unusual structures, loose teeth, or swelling, (7) the size of the tongue and oral opening, and (8) the flexibility of the lips and cheek muscles.

Adjust the headrest to whatever position the technique requires and drape the patient with a protective lead apron. Then show the patient how to hold the film with the film holder, or if by digital, either with positive pressure of the thumb (maxillary areas) or index finger (mandibular areas). Caution the patient to hold still while the exposure is made, so that the film will not be blurred or the relationship between film and the angulation of the PID lost.

Use the exposure chart to set the proper kilovoltage, milliamperage, and time. Be sure that patients know what is expected before placing the film in their mouth. Always position the film firmly and carefully; otherwise a gag reflex may begin. Gagging is a frequent problem and may be caused by apprehension or by hypersensitivity of the oral tissues, particularly at the back of the mouth. One way to avoid or lessen gagging is to complete the exposure rapidly and remove the film immediately. Another is to premedicate the patient. This is extremely effective with children and extremely nervous patients. Still another method is to desensitize the nerve endings of the delicate mucosa by having the patients hold some ice water in their mouth for a short time before film placement. In rare instances, a topical anesthetic can be applied to the sensitive areas.

After each exposure, inspect the film for moisture and blot off excess saliva. When finished, be sure to return all appliances, eyeglasses, and earrings to the patient.

Final procedures include (1) identifying the films and taking them to the darkroom, (2) turning off the x-ray machine, and (3) sanitizing the room and equipment in preparation for the next patient.

CHAPTER SUMMARY

The three common types of intraoral radiographic procedures are the periapical, bitewing, and occlusal surveys. Each of these examinations differs in purpose, and a variety of film sizes may be used to achieve the desired result. Both the paralleling and bisecting techniques are used to produce a shadow image of the tooth on the exposed radiograph. The paralleling technique produces superior results. Neither of these completely satisfies all the requirements for accurate shadow casting. Both are based on the principle of aligning the central ray in both its horizontal and vertical planes in such a manner that it will be projected perpendicularly toward the center of the film packet, the essential difference being in the relationship that the film has to the x-ray beam that is directed toward it. Each technique has its advantages and disadvantages. The skilled operator, within the limits of the equipment available, must select the technique that fits the occasion.

Although an experienced operator can achieve good results with either technique, it is generally conceded that less image distortion is likely when the target–film distance is increased from 8 to 16 in. (20.5 to 41 cm) and when a film-holding device is used to place the film parallel to the teeth. All dental schools are now teaching the newer paralleling method. Horizontal angulation is achieved in the same manner in both techniques. The central ray is directed perpendicularly to the film in the horizontal plane. The technique for vertical angulation differs in that, in bisecting, the central ray is aimed perpendicularly in the vertical plane at the bisector rather than at the film. The method of positioning and holding the film also differs. In bisecting, the film is positioned closer to the teeth and is sometimes held by digital pressure; in paralleling, the film is farther from the teeth, and the use of a film holder is mandatory. Unless special film-holding devices that indicate the correct angulation are used, care must be taken to seat the patient so that the occlusal plane is parallel with the floor and the median line perpendicular to it.

A definite routine of advance preparations should be followed before exposures are made. This includes (1) checking to see that the area is sanitized, (2) securing the patient's cooperation by explaining what is to be done and why, (3) answering the patient's questions on radiation safety if needed, (4) seating the patient, draping a lead apron over the patient, and adjusting the headrest, (5) explaining to the patient how the film is held, (6) making an oral inspection to determine whether any unusual conditions exist, (7) regulating the controls and positioning the tube head, (8) positioning the film, (9) adjusting the horizontal and vertical angulation as needed, and (10) making a final check to make sure that the patient or tube head has not moved.

After making the exposure, (1) blot moisture from the film packet, (2) turn off the x-ray machine, (3) dismiss or return the patient to the operatory, (4) identify the film before taking it to the darkroom, and (5) sanitize the equipment and immediate area in preparation for the next patient.

KEY WORDS

Angulation

Bisecting technique

Bisector

Biteblock

Film holder

Horizontal angulation

Negative angulation

Paralleling technique

Penumbra

Point of entry

Positive angulation

Vertical angulation

Zero angulation

REVIEW QUESTIONS

1. Which of these is not an intraoral survey? (a) bitewing, (b) occlusal, (c) panoramic, (d) periapical.

2. Who first described the rules of the bisecting technique? (a) Roentgen, (b) Coolidge, (c) Updegrave, (d) Cieszynski.

3. What term describes the imaginary line between the long axis of the tooth and the film plane? (a) tangent, (b) median, (c) bisector, (d) midsagittal.

4. Which of these target–film distances is generally used in the paralleling technique? (a) 7 in. (18 cm), (b) 8 in. (20.5 cm), (c) 12 in. (30 cm), (d) 16 in. (41 cm).

5. Which term describes the formation of a fuzzy shadow around the outline of the image on the radiograph? (a) penumbra, (b) delineation, (c) definition, (d) reticulation.

6. What is the effect on the radiographic image if the vertical angulation is 15 degrees greater than necessary? (a) overlapping, (b) cone cutting, (c) elongation, (d) foreshortening.

7. What is the result of incorrect horizontal angulation? (a) adumbration, (b) cone cutting, (c) reticulation, (d) overlapping.

8. What change in angulation should be made when a patient has an unusually low vault? (a) horizontal angulation is shifted mesially, (b) horizontal angulation is shifted distally, (c) vertical angulation is increased, (d) vertical angulation is decreased.

9. In the paralleling technique, the tooth and the ___Film___ must be parallel to each other.

10. The ___Paralleling___ technique produces superior radiographs.

11. ___Gloves___ should be worn when taking dental x-rays to prevent skin contact with blood, saliva, or mucous membranes.

BIBLIOGRAPHY

Eastman Kodak: *X-rays in Dentistry.* Rochester. NY: 1985

Goaz PW, White SC: *Oral Radiology Principles and Interpretation,* 3rd ed. St. Louis, MO: CV Mosby, 1994

Langland OE, Sippy FH, Langlais RP: *Textbook of Dental Radiology,* 2nd ed. Springfield, IL: Charles C Thomas, 1984

Rinn Corporation: *Intraoral Radiography with Rinn XCP/BAI Instruments.* Elgin, IL: 1983

CHAPTER 15

The Periapical Examination

OBJECTIVES

By the end of this chapter the student should be able to

1. Select the type and number of films required to make a complete **periapical survey.**
2. Identify and be able to assemble and position film holders for the paralleling and bisecting-angle techniques.
3. Differentiate between the method of positioning the film packet when using the paralleling and the bisecting methods.
4. Differentiate between conventional periapical film placement and endodontic film placement techniques.

FILM REQUIREMENTS

A full-mouth series of periapical radiographs can provide the dentist with much valuable information about the patient's teeth and the bone structures that surround them. Individual radiographs focus attention on conditions that require treatment and serve as a guide in making the diagnosis and plan of treatment.

The **periapical examination,** frequently called the **full-mouth survey,** can be made with any of the three periapical film sizes (#0, #1, #2) or any combination of these films. Film size depends on (1) the age of the patient, (2) the size of the mouth opening, (3) the shape of the dental arches, (4) the presence or absence of unusual conditions or anatomical limitations, (5) the film holder and technique used, and (6) the patient's ability to tolerate the film.

Normally, a minimum of 14 films is used to cover the following tooth areas: (1) one film each for the maxillary and mandibular incisor area, (2) one film in each of the

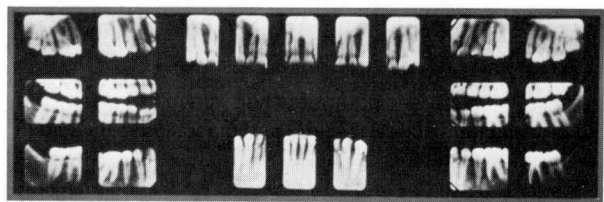

Figure 15–1. The complete radiographic series shown includes four bitewing films in addition to the eight anterior and eight posterior periapical films. Although all of the exposures may be made with the standard #2 films when space permits, it is suggested that the narrow #1 film be used in all the anterior areas to assure patient comfort and easier placement without distortion. By using five narrow films in the maxillary anterior areas and three in the mandibular anterior areas, maximum accurate periapical and interproximal coverage can be obtained. *(Courtesy of Rinn Corporation, Elgin, IL.)*

four canine (cuspid) areas (two in the maxillary and two in the mandibular arches), (3) one film in each of the four premolar (bicuspid) areas (two in the maxillary and two in the mandibular arches), and (4) one film in each of the molar areas (two in the maxillary and two in the mandibular arches). More films may be required for unusual conditions or for narrow arches requiring small films. The general rule is to use the largest film that can readily be positioned. Doing so minimizes the number of exposures.

Many dentists choose to use the narrow #1 film routinely instead of the standard #2 film for exposures of the anterior teeth. Two film combinations are often used when the narrow #1 film is employed: (1) five films for the maxillary anterior teeth—one each for the canines, one each for the laterals, and one film centered at the midline over the central incisors—and three films for the mandibular arch where the teeth are smaller—one film centered on each of the canines and the third film centered over the incisors (Fig. 15–1); or (2) four films for the maxillary anterior teeth and four for the mandibular anterior teeth—the films centered over each of the canine and the central-lateral incisor regions.

Usually the standard #2 film is used to make the posterior periapical exposures. When space is limited, other film sizes may be used posteriorly.

PLACEMENT OF THE FILM PACKET

Regardless of which technique is used or how the film is held in place, correct placement of the film packet is important to prevent the film from bending or moving during exposure, thus causing distortion. Movement of the film, the patient, or the tube head will blur the radiograph or fail to show the intended teeth.

With few exceptions, all films for the anterior areas are placed with the longest dimension of the film vertically (described as **vertical placement**) and the films for the posterior areas are placed with the widest dimension horizontally (described as **horizontal placement**). The edge of the film packet is placed parallel to, and protrudes 1/8 to 1/4 in. (3 to 6 mm) above or below, the incisal or occlusal edges of the teeth.

One should develop a standard film placement for each region to be radiographed to ensure that comparable serial radiographs can be made later. The tube side of the film is placed behind the teeth. Place films gently to prevent tissue irritation or gagging. Slight bending or rolling of the film corners toward the lingual makes it easier to place the film and increases the patient's comfort. However, excessive bending of the film results in creases, streaks, and distortion.

Most film manufacturers show the location of the identification dot by a small circle or dot on the **back side** of the film. The identification dot is always positioned toward the occlusal or incisal edges where it is least likely to interfere with diagnostic information.

It is always best to keep the film surface as flat as possible. A film holder with a backing plate on the biteblock makes this almost automatic. However, when the film is held by finger pressure (digital method), some additional support may be needed to keep it from bending in the middle. One means of support is to insert one or two cotton rolls between the film packet and the lingual surfaces of the teeth. Such a technique is particularly effective in the anterior regions and when the mandible has very sharp curvature. Besides minimizing film bending, the use of cotton rolls between teeth and film may produce a more parallel relationship and increase patient comfort.

SEQUENCE OF FILM POSITIONING

Opinions differ as to which region should be exposed first in making a full-mouth survey. Some operators prefer to make the first exposure in the right maxillary molar region and continue in sequence to the left maxillary molar region, then drop down to the left mandibular molar region, finishing in the right mandibular molar region. Others prefer a similar sequence but with the directions reversed, while still others begin with the anterior exposures, on the theory that the patient is less liable to gag when a film is placed in this region than when it is placed in the upper molar region where the tissues are more sensitive. Gagging is frequently psychological. If the first few films produce no discomfort, the patient will become used to the feel of the film and will accept it.

With an experienced operator who can place the film skillfully and rapidly, it probably makes little difference which area is exposed first. But the same system of film placement should always be followed to make sure that all regions are exposed.

Because the paralleling technique produces superior radiographs, most schools now begin by teaching the paralleling methods first and devote minimal time to bisecting procedures. Because of this trend, the paralleling technique is described first.

FILM RETENTION FOR PARALLELING PROCEDURES

As previously indicated, a **film holder** is needed with the paralleling technique. The simplest are wood, plastic, or styrofoam **biteblocks** with a backing plate and slot for film retention. The film can be inserted either vertically for the anteriors or horizontally for the posteriors. Slightly more complex is the EEZEE-GRIP (formerly the Snap-A-Ray holder shown in Figure 14–3), a double-ended instrument that holds the film

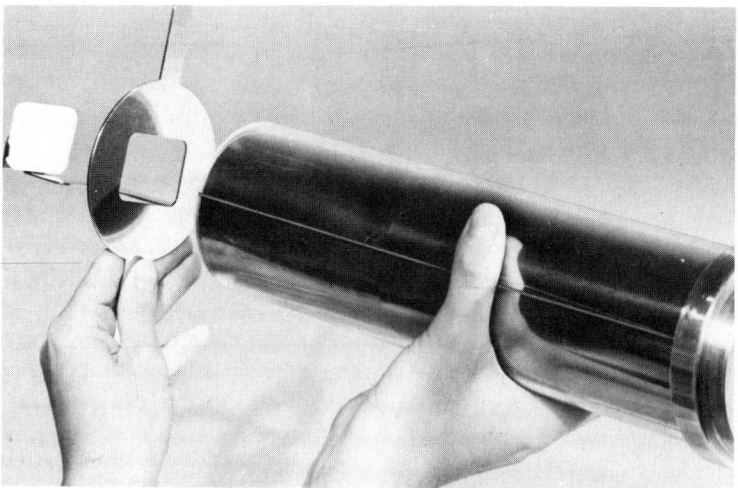

Figure 15–2. Metal Precision posterior x-ray film holder for use with long, round, metal-type PID. The metal collimating shield, combined with the lead-lined cone, restricts the size of the x-ray beam and reduces tissue radiation. Precision instruments are available for anterior, posterior, and bitewing radiography in adult and child sizes. *(Courtesy of Isaac Masel Company, Philadelphia, PA.)*

between two plastic jaws that are locked in place. The plastic jaw serves as a bite plane in the posterior areas. The other end of the instrument is a backing plate with a slot that holds the film during anterior exposures. More complex still are the metal "Precision" film holders (Fig. 15–2), which have a metal facial shield attached to an arm on which the patient bites. At the end of the arm a backing plate supports the film and holds it parallel to the shield. The XCP instruments (Fig. 15–3) and the rectangular collimated instruments (Fig. 15–4) function in a similar manner. These instruments must be assembled prior to use and have separate components for anterior and posterior positioning. The XCP instruments were developed in an attempt to simplify paralleling procedures and minimize dimensional distortion. These instruments are simple to position and highly adaptable, in that the patient may be in any position.

Because it is not practical to describe the technique for the use of each of the many available film holders, the descriptions and illustrations for the following sequence of tooth regions are based on the use of the XCP instruments. Other instruments require slight changes in technique.

MANDIBULAR PERIAPICAL EXPOSURES: PARALLELING TECHNIQUE

To make an exposure of the **mandibular incisor** region, follow these steps:

1. Place the patient's head in any comfortable position within convenient reach of the position indicating device (PID).

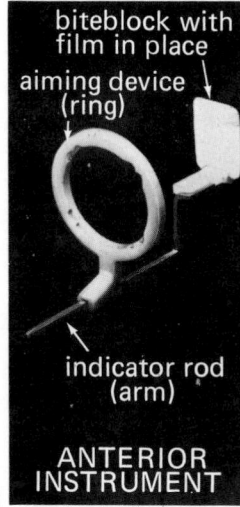

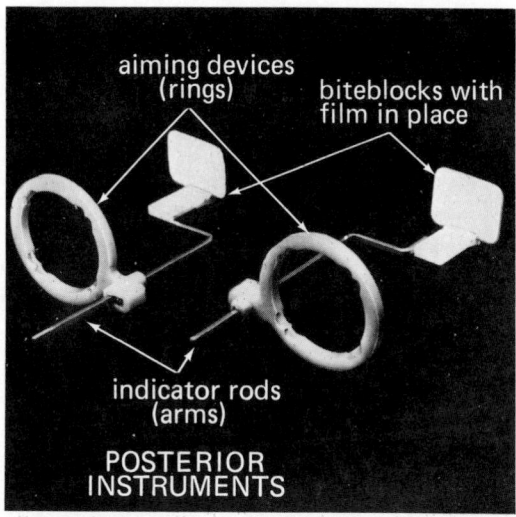

Figure 15–3. The assembled Rinn XCP instruments are intended for use with the paralleling technique using the 16-in. (41-cm) target–film distance. Each instrument consists of an indicator rod (arm), and aiming device (ring), and a biteblock. By substituting a 105-degree biteblock for the 90-degree biteblock shown here, these instruments become the BAI instruments suitable for use with the bisecting technique. **(a)** The assembled anterior XCP instrument with film positioned vertically in the biteblock. **(b)** The posterior instruments with the films positioned horizontally in the biteblocks. One instrument is used for exposure on the maxillary right and the mandibular left, while the other is used for exposure on the maxillary left and on the mandibular right. BAI, bisecting-angle instrument; XCP, extension cone paralleling. *(Courtesy of Rinn Corporation, Elgin, IL.)*

2. Insert the film vertically into the slot of the film holder with the tube side of the film toward the lingual of the teeth. Although the #2 film is occasionally used, the narrow #1 film is preferred for all anterior exposures. Place a cotton roll between the biteblock and the maxillary teeth and ask the patient to close firmly on the block.
3. Insert the film and holder by directing the lower edge of the film toward the floor of the mouth and against the frenum of the tongue. Do this by first turning the film holder so that the film is parallel with the floor and then gradually raising the holder so that the film assumes a vertical position in the mouth. If resistance is encountered, ask the patient to first raise and then relax the tongue.
4. Place the film holder back far enough to achieve parallelism and center the film on the midline or between central and lateral incisors if right and left exposures are to be made.
5. Slide the **aiming ring** to about 1/2 in. (12 mm) from the skin surface and align the PID with both **indicator rod** and ring on vertical and horizontal planes.
6. Make the exposure.

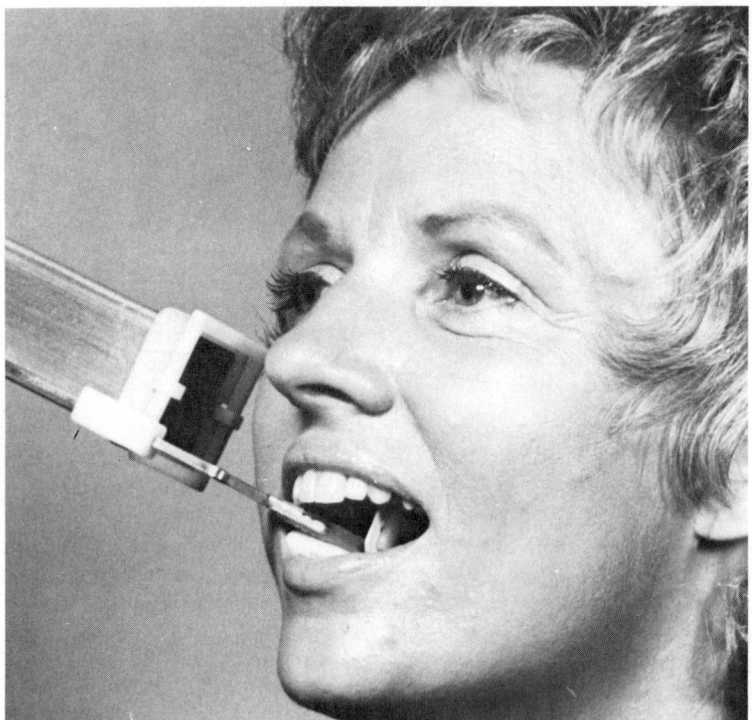

Figure 15–4. Rectangular instrumentation for reduced tissue exposure. Lead-lined rectangular PID limits the size of x-ray beam. Slots on the PID align with studs on the placement holder. Both the XCP and the BAI instruments can be modified by substituting the rectangular aiming device for the circular one. The use of a lead-lined collimating device makes possible reductions of 50 percent or more in tissue exposure area. *(Courtesy of Rinn Corporation, Elgin, IL.)*

To make an exposure of the **mandibular canine** (cuspid) region, follow these steps:

1. Use the same film placement procedure as for the mandibular incisor but center the film over the canine.
2. Instruct the patient to close on the block and slide the aiming ring near to the skin surface. Align the PID with both rod and ring on horizontal and vertical planes.
3. Make the exposure.

To make an exposure of the **mandibular premolar** (bicuspid) region (Fig. 15–5), follow these steps:

1. Use the larger #2 film and place it with its widest dimension horizontally. If the teeth are too long to show the root apices, place the film vertically. This is seldom necessary.

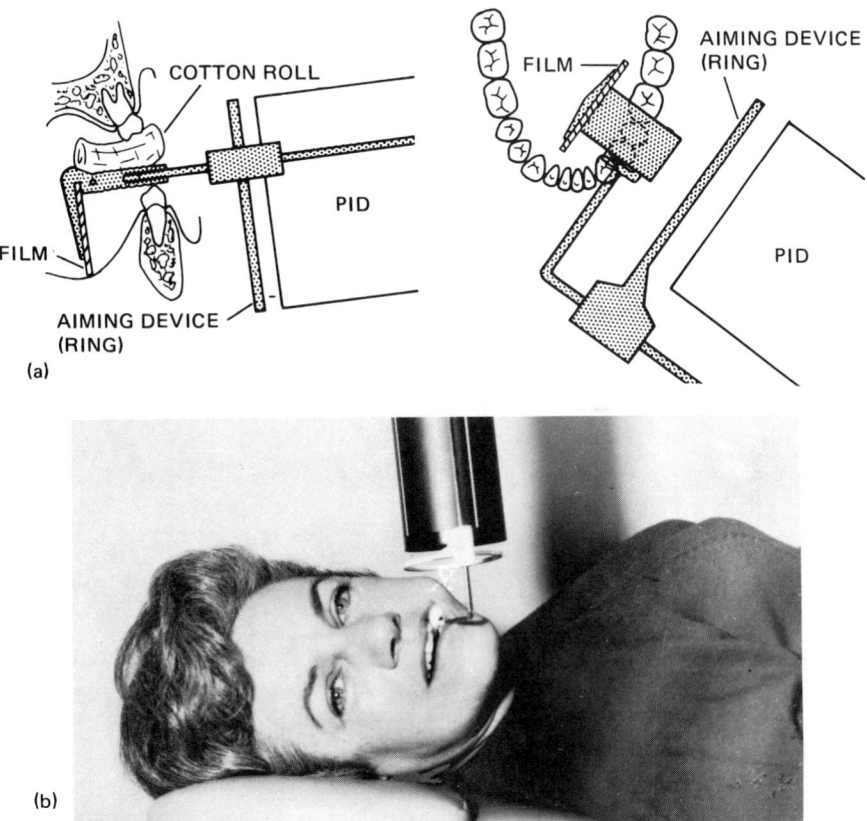

Figure 15–5. The mandibular premolar area. **(a)** Diagram shows the relationship of film, XCP instrument, and PID. Film is positioned with widest dimension horizontally in posterior areas and parallel to teeth. A cotton roll should be between the opposing teeth and the biteblock, causing the opposing teeth to force the biteblock firmly against the biting surfaces of the teeth to be x-rayed. **(b)** Photograph showing patient in reclined position. When using BAI and XCP instruments, the necessity for definite head positioning with respect to occlusal and sagittal alignment is eliminated, regardless of the type of chair employed. The patient may be reclined at any angle or seated upright. BAI, bisecting-angle instrument; XCP, extension cone paralleling. *(Courtesy of Rinn Corporation, Elgin, IL.)*

2. Position the film in the mouth centered over the second premolar. The anterior edge of the film should include the distal half of the canine. The long edge of the film should be parallel to the buccal surfaces of the premolars to prevent overlapping of interproximal contact areas. Soften the lower front corner of the film packet if necessary for easier placement.
3. Instruct the patient to close on the block and slide the locator ring to about 1/2 in. (12 mm) from the skin. Align the PID with both rod and ring on horizontal and vertical planes.
4. Make the exposure.

To make an exposure of the **mandibular molar** region, follow these steps:

1. Use the same placement procedures as for the mandibular premolar regions but place the anterior film border to include the distal half of the second premolar. The center of the film is between the first and second molars. In this region the film slides into the sulcus between the teeth and the tongue and close to the teeth. The long edge of the film should be parallel to the buccal surfaces of the molars to prevent overlapping of interproximal contact areas.
2. Instruct the patient to close on the block and slide the aiming ring to about 1/2 in. (12 mm) from the skin surface. Align the PID with both rod and ring on horizontal and vertical planes.
3. Make the exposure.

MAXILLARY PERIAPICAL EXPOSURES: PARALLELING TECHNIQUE

To make an exposure of the **maxillary incisor** region (Fig. 15–6), use the following steps:

1. Place the patient's head in any comfortable position within convenient reach of the PID.
2. Insert the film vertically into the slot of the film holder with the tube side of the film toward the lingual of the teeth.
3. Insert the biteblock far enough into the mouth (about 1 in. [25 mm]) so that the upper edge of the film contacts the palate in the first molar area and is parallel to the long axes of the incisors. Depending on the number of films to be exposed in the incisor area, center the film at the midline or between the central and lateral incisors.
4. Rest the biteblock on the incisal edges and insert a cotton roll between the block and the mandibular teeth. Ask the patient to close firmly.
5. Slide the aiming ring down the indicator rod to about 1/2 in. (12 mm) from the skin and align the PID with both rod and ring on vertical and horizontal planes.
6. Make the exposure.

For the **maxillary canine** (cuspid) region, follow these steps:

1. Use the same film placement as for the incisors, with some minor changes. Depending on the number of films to be exposed in the anterior area, either center the film over the canine or center the film between the lateral incisor and the canine.
2. Instruct the patient to close on the block and slide the locator ring down the indicator rod to about 1/2 in. (12 mm) from the skin. Align the PID with both rod and ring on horizontal and vertical planes.
3. Make the exposure.

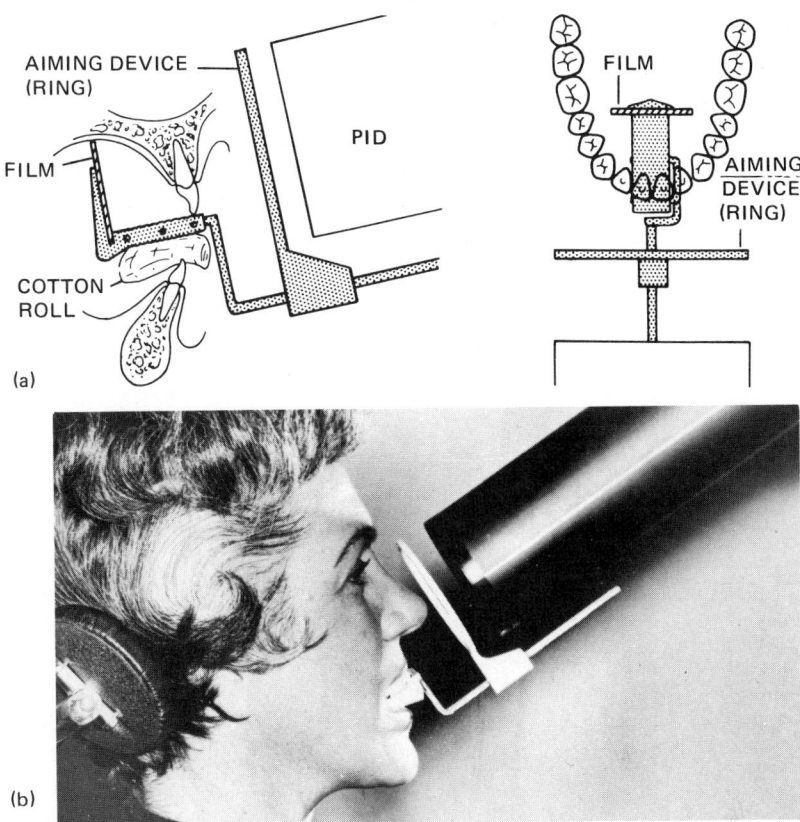

Figure 15–6. The maxillary incisor area. **(a)** Diagram shows relationship of film, teeth, XCP instrument, and PID. As in all anterior areas, film is positioned with longest dimension vertically. Film is parallel to teeth with the block inserted to its full length to position the film back toward the region of the first molars. **(b)** Photograph of patient showing position of XCP instrument and long, circular, open-type PID. *(Courtesy of Rinn Corporation, Elgin, IL.)*

For the **maxillary premolar** (bicuspid) region, follow these steps:

1. Use the larger #2 film and place it with its widest dimension horizontally. Insert the biteblock far enough into the mouth so that the upper edge of the film contacts the palate near the midline. Center the film over the second premolar so that the anterior border of the film covers the distal half of the canine. The widest edge of the film should be parallel to the buccal surfaces of the molars to prevent overlapping of the interproximal contact areas. Softening the upper front corner of the film packet makes positioning easier.
2. Instruct the patient to close on the block and slide the aiming ring down the indicator rod to about 1/2 in. (12 mm) from the skin. Align the PID with both rod and ring on horizontal and vertical planes.
3. Make the exposure.

For the **maxillary molar** region, use the following steps:

1. Use film placement very similar to that for the premolar region. Center the film over the embrasure between the first and second molars so that the anterior film border covers the distal portion of the second premolar. The widest edge of the film should be parallel to the buccal surfaces of the molars to prevent overlapping of the interproximal contact areas. Place the film farther posterior if the center of interest is the third molar.
2. Instruct the patient to close on the block and slide the aiming ring down the indicator rod to about 1/2 in. (12 mm) from the skin. Align the PID with both the rod and ring on horizontal and vertical planes.
3. Make the exposure.

FILM RETENTION FOR BISECTING PROCEDURES

The bisecting technique is a good method to know but is not recommended except when anatomical irregularities require its use. Whenever the digital method is used, the film is positioned and the patient is instructed to use the thumb to hold the film in all maxillary areas and to use the index finger in all mandibular areas. The left hand holds the film on the right side and vice versa. All fingers except the one holding the film must be kept out of the path of the x-ray beam.

As already mentioned in Chapter 14, a variety of holders, ranging in complexity from plastic biteblocks to the bisecting-angle instruments (BAIs), may be selected. The BAIs are assembled and used in the same manner as the XCP instruments, the only difference being that the biting platform is set at a 105-degree angle. When correctly used, these instruments reduce errors of judgment by automatically indicating correct horizontal and vertical angulation.

Make a final inspection to be sure that the patient's head is still in the conventional position (see Fig. 14–11) and that the film packet or film holder has not shifted before bringing the PID as close to the face as possible; then finalize the adjustments in horizontal and vertical angulation.

To avoid repetition of instructions for each of the eight usual areas of film placement, it will be assumed that, unless a special film holder is used, the digital method is described, that the patient's head is in the conventional position, and that the tube side of the film faces the source of the radiation. This should not be mistaken for a recommendation to use the digital method.

MANDIBULAR PERIAPICAL EXPOSURES: BISECTING TECHNIQUE

The **mandibular incisor** region is shown in Figures 15–7 and 15–8. If the #2 film is used, it is centered at the midline, and all four incisors will be shown on the radiograph. Number 1 film may either be centered at the midline or to the right or left of the

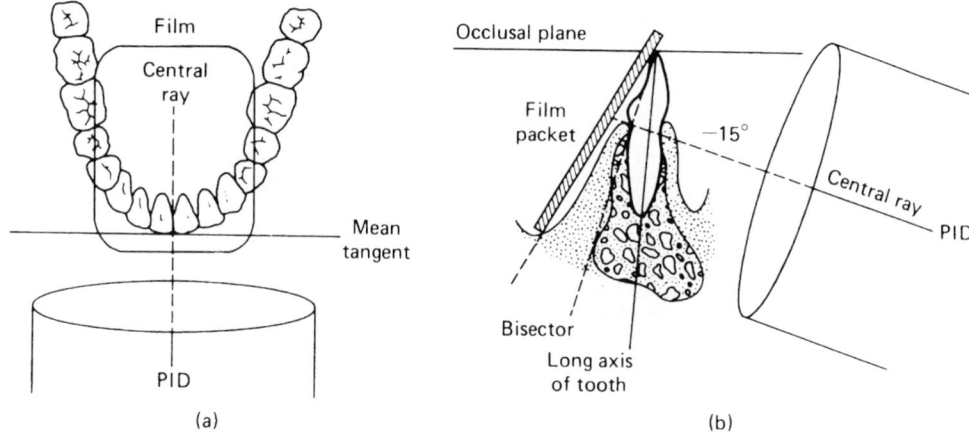

(a)   (b)

Figure 15–7. Mandibular incisors—film packet and PID position. **(a)** Horizontal projection is through midline embrasure and perpendicular to mean tangent; **(b)** vertical projection is directed perpendicular to bisector at approximately −15 degrees with PID tilted upward.

midline, so that the center of the film is between the central and lateral incisors. To make this exposure, the following steps are suggested:

1. Check the patient's head position and make a mental note of abnormal occlusion or other irregularities.
2. Grasp the film packet along the narrow edge between the index finger and the thumb. Position the film vertically and allow it to extend about 1/4 in. (6 mm) above the incisal edges. If resistance is encountered, ask the patient to first raise and then relax the tongue.
3. Instruct the patient to hold the film with the index finger of either hand by exerting a slight pressure against the upper middle of the film. A cotton roll may be placed between the film and the tooth to avoid bending the film and shaping it to the arch.
4. Establish the horizontal angulation by directing the **central rays** through the embrasures either between the central incisors or between the central and lateral incisors perpendicularly toward the film.
5. Establish the vertical angulation by determining the location of the bisector (halfway between the long axis of the tooth and the film plane). In most instances this will be between −15 and −20 degrees.
6. Center the PID over the **point of entry,** a point on the chin about 1 in. (25 mm) above the lower border of the mandible. Adjust the tip of the PID so that it almost touches against the skin.
7. Make the exposure.

To make exposures in the **mandibular canine** (cuspid) region, follow the same basic procedures but make the following changes (Fig. 15–9).

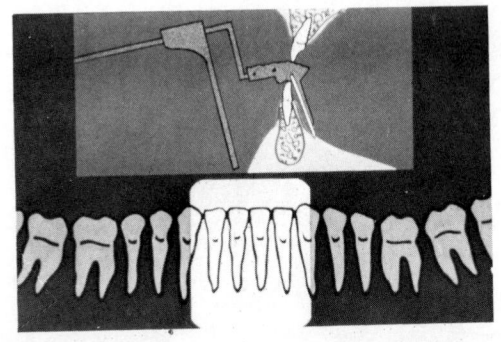

(a)

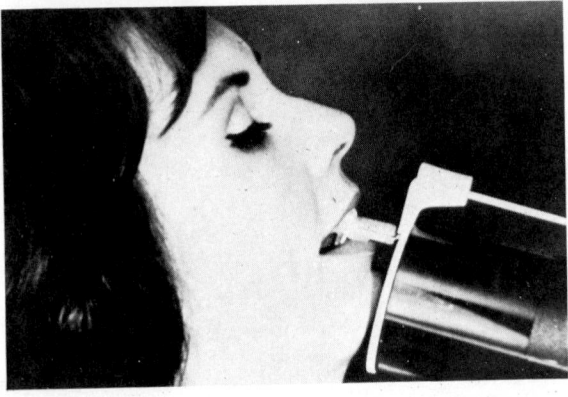

(b)

Figure 15–8. The mandibular incisor area. **(a)** Diagram showing positioning of x-ray film using BAI. In this illustration, a standard #2 film is shown. Generally a narrow #1 film is preferred. **(b)** Photograph showing position of BAI and open-ended PID with patient. BAI, bisecting-angle instrument. *(Courtesy of Rinn Corporation, Elgin, IL.)*

1. Place the film as for the preceding exposure but center it vertically over the canine. Allow 1/4 in. (6 mm) to protrude over the incisal edges.
2. Change the horizontal angulation so that the central ray passes through the embrasure between the canine and the first premolar.
3. Change the vertical angulation to about –20 degrees.
4. Change the point of entry to the center of the root of the canine, about 1 in. (25 mm) above the inferior border of the mandible.
5. Make the exposure.

To make exposures in the **mandibular premolar** (bicuspid) region, follow the same basic procedures but make the following changes (Fig. 15–10):

1. Place the film as before with minor modifications. Grasp the film at the corner and insert it horizontally. Use the index finger of the opposite hand to press the film against the lingual. Center the film over the premolar area and move the film forward enough so that the front edge covers the distal

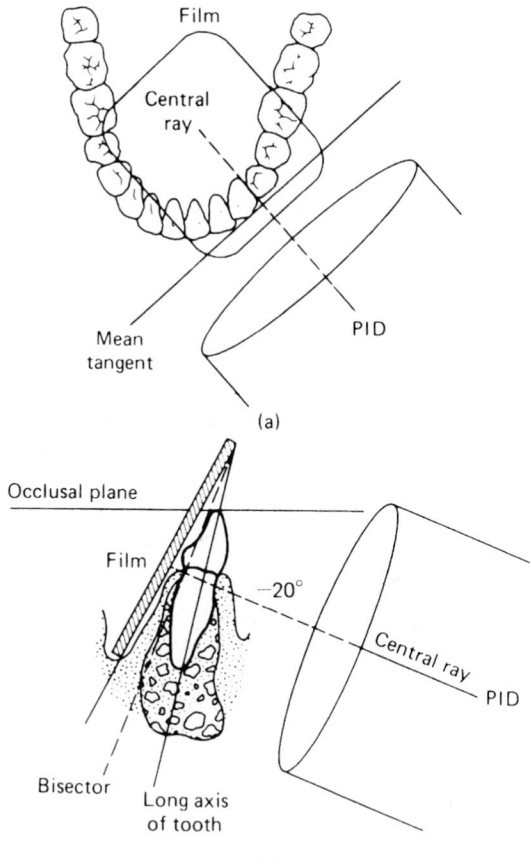

Film

Central ray

Mean tangent

PID

(a)

Occlusal plane

Film

−20°

Central ray

PID

Bisector

Long axis of tooth

(b)

Figure 15-9. Mandibular canine—film packet and PID position. **(a)** Horizontal projection is through embrasure between canine and first premolar and perpendicular to mean tangent. **(b)** Vertical projection is directed perpendicular to bisector at approximately −20 degrees with PID tilted upward.

half of the canine. Allow about 1/8 in. (3 mm) of the film to protrude above the occlusal surfaces of the teeth.

2. Change the horizontal angulation so that the central ray passes through the embrasure between the second premolar and first molar.

3. Change the vertical angulation as needed, usually between −10 to −15 degrees.

4. Center the PID over the point of entry slightly below the pupil of the eye and about 1/2 in. (12 mm) above the lower border of the mandible.

5. Make the exposure.

To make an exposure in the **mandibular molar** region, follow the same basic procedures but with the following changes (Fig. 15–11):

1. Make adjustments in the occlusal plane because this often curves in the molar area. Place the film in the same manner as before but center the film between the first and second molars. Unless the main interest is in the

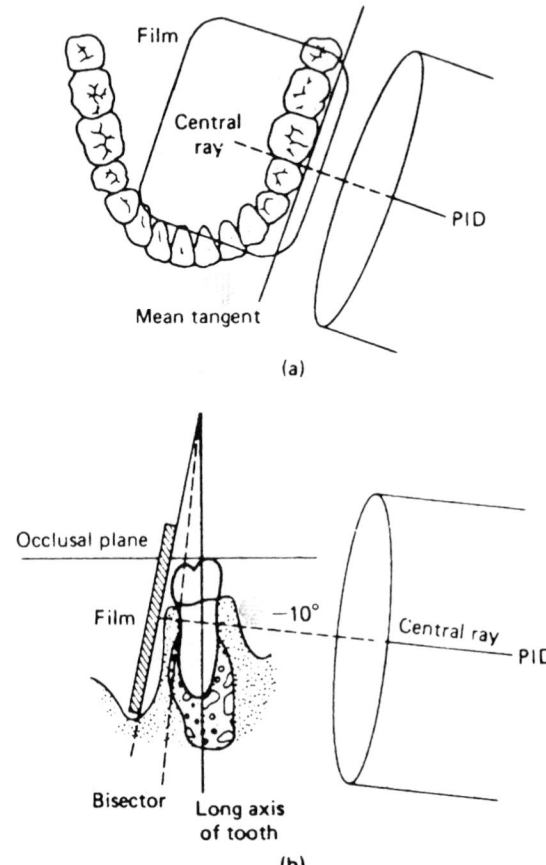

Figure 15-10. Mandibular premolar—film packet and PID position. **(a)** Horizontal projection is through embrasure between the premolars and perpendicular to mean tangent. **(b)** Vertical projection is directed perpendicular to bisector at approximately −10 degrees with PID tilted upward.

third molar area, place the film forward far enough to cover the distal half of the second premolar. Allow a 1/8-in. (3-mm) margin above the occlusal edge.

2. Change the horizontal angulation so that the central ray passes through the embrasure between the first and second molar.
3. Change the vertical angulation to about −5 degrees.
4. Center the PID over the point of entry slightly below the outer canthus of the eye and about 1/2 in. (12 mm) above the lower border of the mandible (farther back for third molar exposures).
5. Make the exposure.

MAXILLARY PERIAPICAL EXPOSURES: BISECTING TECHNIQUE

In the **maxillary incisor** region (Fig. 15–12), if the #2 film is used, it is centered at the midline, and both central and lateral incisors are shown on the same film. If the expo-

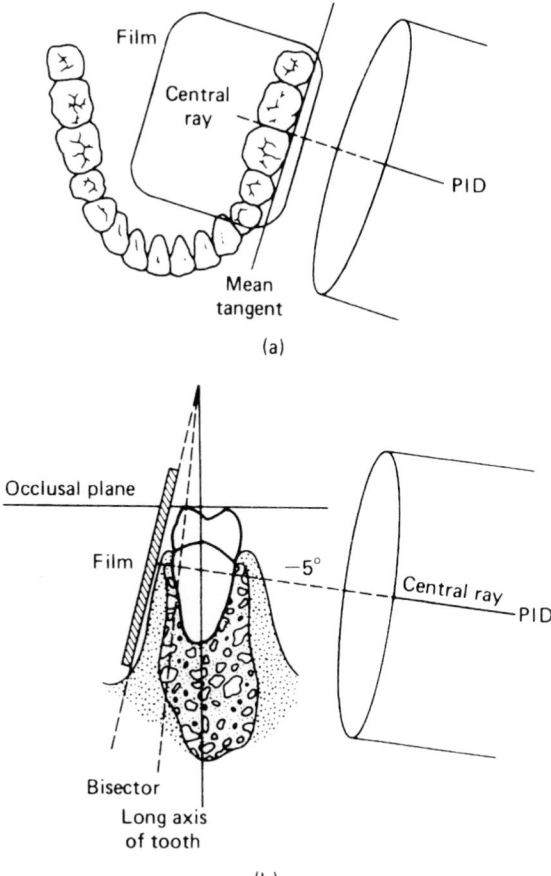

Figure 15–11. Mandibular molars—film packet and PID position. (a) Horizontal projection is through the embrasure between first and second molar and perpendicular to mean tangent. (b) Vertical projection is directed perpendicular to bisector at approximately –5 degrees with slight upward tilt of PID.

sure is made with the narrower #1 film, less of the lateral incisors will be shown. Many operators prefer to center the narrower film between the central and lateral incisors. This requires a film for the right and left sides. To make this exposure, the following steps are suggested:

1. Position the film vertically and allow about 1/8 in. (3 mm) to extend below incisal edges.
2. Instruct the patient to hold the film with the thumb by exerting a slight pressure against the lower middle part of the film. Either thumb may be used if the film is centered at the midline; otherwise, ask the patient to use the hand opposite to the side on which the film is placed.
3. Establish the horizontal angulation by directing the central rays through the embrasure either between the central incisors or between the central and lateral incisors perpendicularly toward the film.
4. Establish the vertical angulation by determining the location of the bisector. In most instances this will be between +40 and +45 degrees.

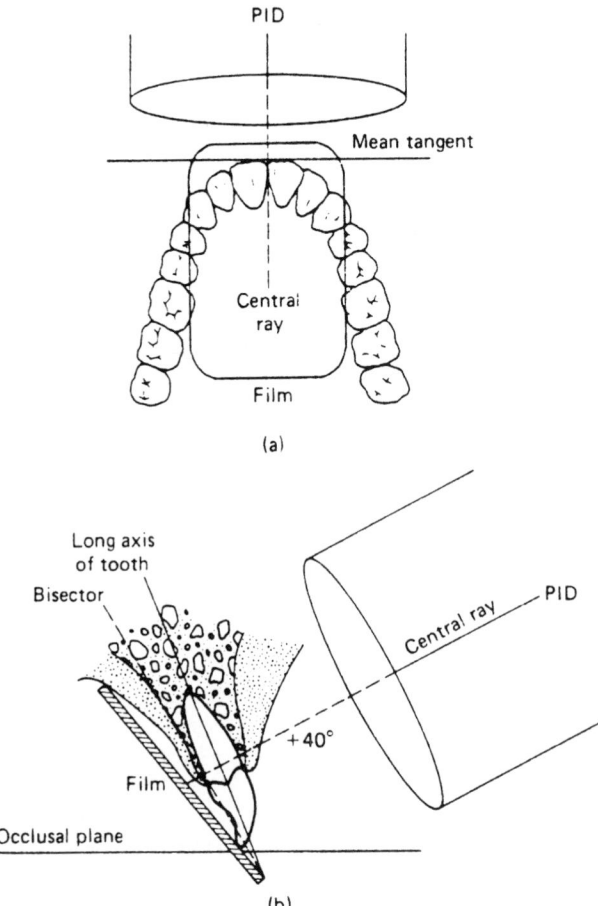

Figure 15–12. Maxillary incisors—film packet and PID position. **(a)** Horizontal projection is through midline embrasure and perpendicular to mean tangent. **(b)** Vertical projection is directed perpendicular to bisector at approximately +40 degrees with PID tilted downward.

5. Center the PID over the point of entry near the tip of the nose. Adjust the PID so that its end almost touches the patient's skin.
6. Make the exposure.

To make the exposure of the **maxillary canine** (cuspid) region (Fig. 15–13), follow these steps:

1. Use essentially the same procedures for film placement as for the central incisors. Position the film vertically so that the canine is in the center and the lateral is included. Allow an incisal margin of about 1/8 in. (3 mm).

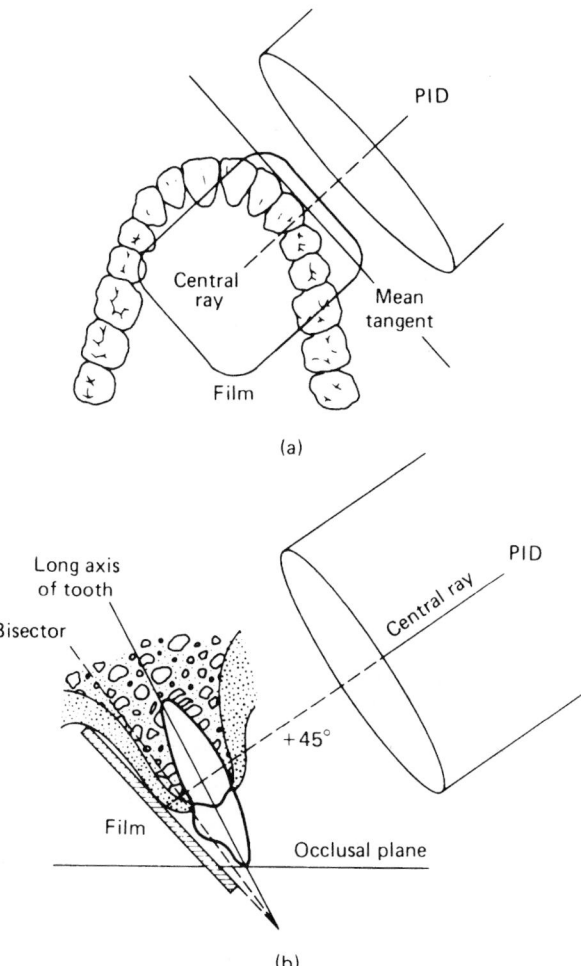

Figure 15–13. Maxillary canine—film packet and PID position. **(a)** Horizontal projection is through canine and perpendicular to mean tangent. **(b)** Vertical projection is directed perpendicular to bisector at approximately +45 degrees with PID tilted downward.

2. Change the horizontal angulation so that the central ray passes through the distal of the canine, perpendicularly to the **mean tangent** of the film.
3. Change the vertical angulation to about +45 degrees.
4. Center the PID over the point of entry near the center of the root of the canine, at the ala of the nose.
5. Make the exposure.

To make exposures in the **maxillary premolar** region (Fig. 15–14), follow the same basic procedures, but make these changes:

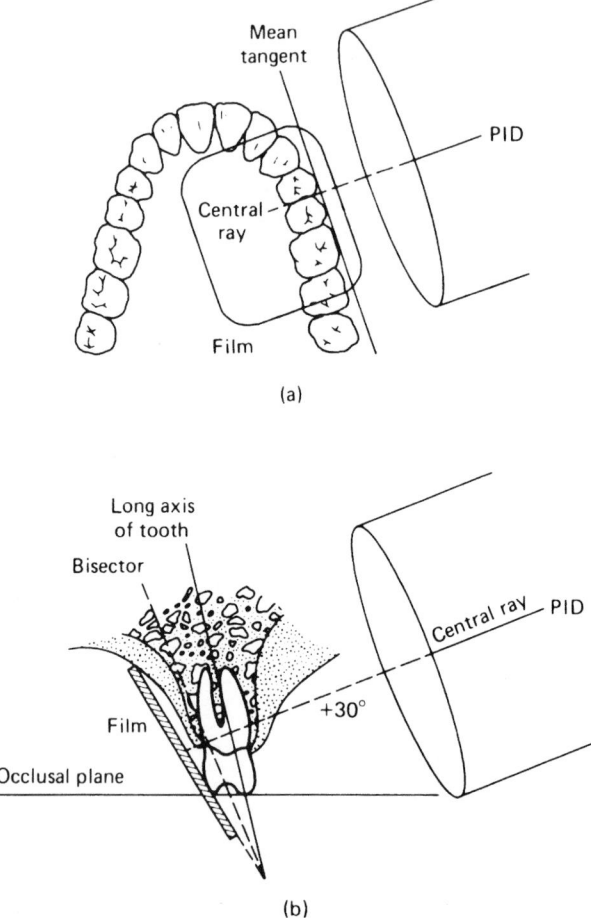

Figure 15–14. Maxillary premolars—film packet and PID position. **(a)** Horizontal projection is through embrasure between premolars and perpendicular to mean tangent. **(b)** Vertical projection is directed perpendicular to bisector at approximately +30 degrees with PID tilted downward.

1. Grasp the film at the corner and insert it horizontally. Use the thumb of the opposite hand to press the film toward the palate. If necessary, slightly soften the upper film corners to conform with the shape of the palate. Center the film over the premolar area and position it so the distal half of the canine is included. Allow a 1/8-in. (3-mm) occlusal margin.
2. Change the horizontal angulations so that the central ray passes through the embrasure between the premolars.
3. Change the vertical angulation to about +30 degrees.

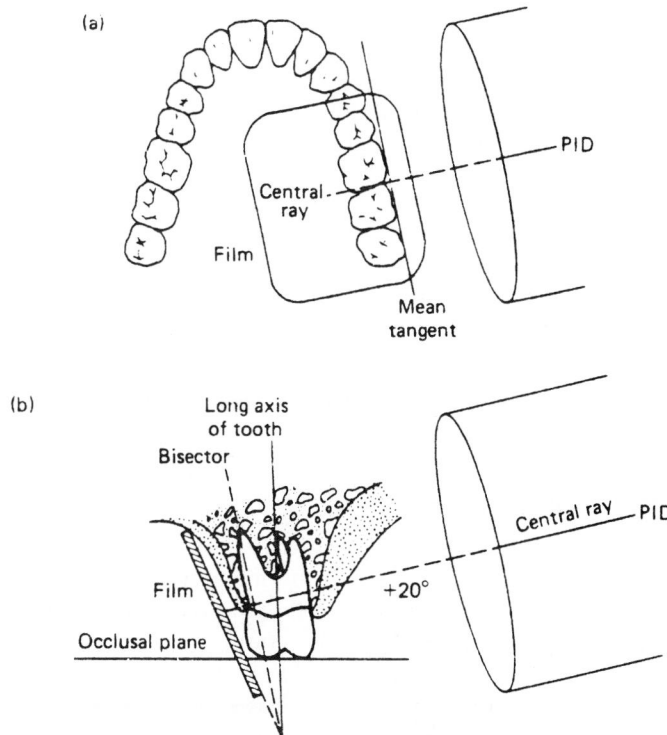

Figure 15–15. Maxillary molars—film packet PID position. **(a)** Horizontal projection is through embrasure between first and second molars and perpendicular to mean tangent. **(b)** Vertical projection is directed perpendicular to bisector at approximately +20 degrees with PID tilted downward.

4. Center the PID over the point of entry, located on the ala–tragus line directly below the pupil of the eye.
5. Make the exposure.

To make an exposure of the **maxillary molar** region (Fig. 15–15), follow these steps:

1. Adjust the headrest as necessary to parallel the occlusal plane with the floor. Center the film horizontally over the molar area and let the front edge of the film cover the distal half of the second premolar. Occasionally, it may be desirable to position the film farther back to include erupting third molars.
2. Change the horizontal angulation so that the central ray passes through the embrasure between the first and second molars.
3. Change the vertical angulation as needed, usually to between +20 and +25 degrees. Depending on whether third molars are impacted or not, the ver-

tical angulation required may be as steep as +55 degrees. Direct the central rays horizontally through the embrasure between the first and second molars perpendicularly toward the film.

4. Center the PID over the point of entry on the ala–tragus line, directly below the outer canthus of the eye. When unerupted or impacted third molars are suspected, direct the center of the PID about 1/2 in. (12 mm) farther back and higher.

5. Make the exposure.

VARIATIONS

Because of anatomical limitations, rotation of the teeth, variations in the height of the palate, the presence of unerupted third molars, or excessive root lengths, one must occasionally depart from the usual procedures. Such changes include horizontal or vertical angulation and film placement.

1. Frequently the embrasures between the molars are not at right angles to the plane of a film that is parallel to the mean tangent of the buccal surfaces of the teeth. Consequently, overlapping of the contact areas results. One can overcome this by a slight alteration of the film placement so that the anterior border of the film is closer to the lingual than the posterior.

2. Often a conventionally positioned film that shows the tuberosity region reveals a coronal portion of a third molar to be at the level of apices of the second molar. In this case, one places the film as far back as anatomy and patient comfort permit. Drastic changes in both vertical and horizontal angulations may be required. This varies according to the location of the imbedded tooth.

3. Absolute parallelism between the film and the long axes of the teeth is difficult to accomplish in patients with low palatal vaults. If the discrepancy from parallelism does not exceed 15 degrees, the radiograph is generally acceptable. In many instances, one can solve the problem of low vault by using two cotton rolls, one on each side of the bite block. These may parallel the film with the long axes adequately but will reduce periapical coverage. Occasionally, especially when the roots are longer than average, one can increase periapical coverage by making the vertical angulation 5 to 15 degrees greater than indicated.

Bone and tissue density vary with the age and physical structure of the patient. Moreover, in most persons the bone structures are thinnest in the mandibular incisor region and densest in the maxillary molar region. Thus, for the best radiographs, it may be desirable to make minor changes in exposure time or milliamperage to vary the film density, or to make changes in kilovoltage to alter the contrast. However, many operators prefer a given exposure time for a film of a given sensitivity (film speed), slightly increasing it for the maxillary molars and decreasing it for the mandibular incisors. Obviously, exposure time must be decreased for children and edentulous patients. As experience is gained, most operators learn to make variations based on age, size, and estimated density of the bone structures.

ENDODONTIC RADIOGRAPHY TECHNIQUE

The interest in endodontia (from the Greek words *endon*, meaning "within," and *odontos*, meaning "tooth") has risen steadily. **Endodontia** is best defined as that branch of dentistry that deals with the cause, diagnosis, prevention, and treatment of diseases of the dental pulp. Treatment is generally accomplished by removing the nerves and tissues of the pulp cavity and replacing them with some form of filling material. The technique is often described as **pulp canal** or **root canal treatment.** More patients than ever before are now availing themselves of endodontic services.

Although most of the periapical procedures described can be applied in endodontic radiographic exposures, there are some differences. These differences add to the difficulty of obtaining radiographs of high quality.

Many of the exposures, particularly those made in the posterior areas of the mouth, are made under poor visual conditions. The placement of the film and holder is further complicated by the coverage of the area with a rubber dam and by the reamers, broaches, files, or the silver or gutta-percha points, which of necessity must be left in place while the film is exposed.

A series of films on the same tooth is needed for the dentist to evaluate various stages of endodontic treatment. The initial film is exposed to determine the preoperative condition and to make a diagnosis. Additional radiographs are made as the work progresses to determine the length of the root; the position of a reamer, broach, or file in the canal; or the position of the sealer and point or points (the tooth may have several canals). And finally a posttreatment radiograph is needed to make sure that the canal or canals are obturated (closed) satisfactorily. Periodic follow-up radiographs may be needed.

The avoidance of distortion or magnification of the image is a major concern in endodontic treatment because the length of each canal must be accurately measured. Therefore the paralleling technique—which consistently produces the least distortion—should be used whenever possible. Although preoperative and postoperative radiographs are made in the usual manner, some technique modifications are required for the "working" radiographs that are exposed with the rubber dam and instruments in place.

The XCP or the disposable biteblocks should be used where possible. However, compromises must often be made when exposing working films. It may become necessary to use methods that rely heavily on visual alignment of the PID with the film while it is held in place either by the patient's finger (least satisfactory), the hemostat, the tongue depressor with cotton rolls attached, or the EEZEE-GRIP holder.

The preferred method for radiographing the anterior regions of the mouth is the paralleling principle (Fig. 15–16a). The next best procedure is to Scotch-tape two large cotton rolls to a film and tape both to a tongue depressor or have the patient hold the film-cotton roll combination against the area of interest. The cotton rolls position the

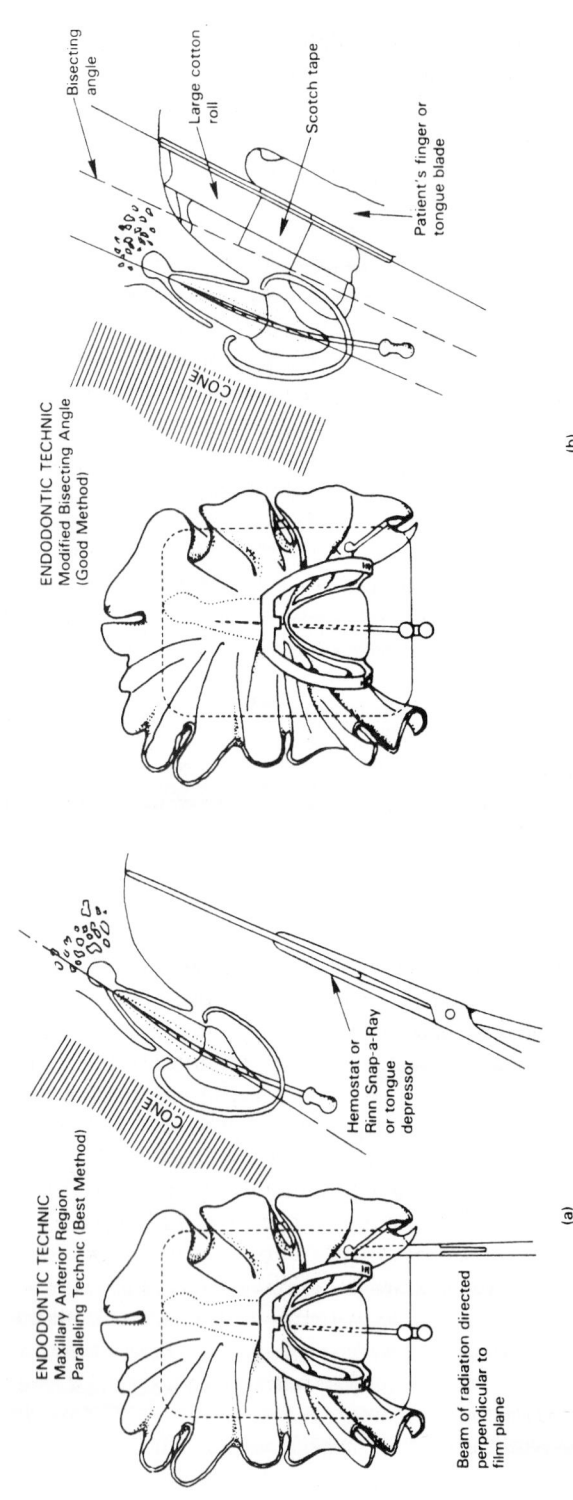

Figure 15–16. Endodontic technique for maxillary anterior region. **(a)** Preferred paralleling method. **(b)** Modified bisecting-angle method. *(Courtesy of John W. Preece, DDS, Department of Dental Diagnostic Science, School of Dentistry, University of Texas at San Antonio.)*

ENDODONTIC TECHNIC
Maxillary Anterior Region
Paralleling Technic (Best Method)

Beam of radiation directed perpendicular to film plane

CONE

Hemostat or Rinn Snap-a-Ray or tongue depressor

(a)

ENDODONTIC TECHNIC
Modified Bisecting Angle
(Good Method)

CONE

Bisecting angle

Large cotton roll

Scotch tape

Patient's finger or tongue blade

(b)

film farther away from the crown of the tooth and permit, at least partially, placing the film more nearly parallel to the long axis of the tooth. The beam of radiation is then directed perpendicularly to the film plane, or perpendicularly to a plane bisecting the long axis of tooth and film (Fig. 15–16**b**).

Obviously, severe space restrictions may occasionally require some experimentation with less-acceptable methods. With minor changes, the technique for exposing the mandibular anterior regions is the same.

If true paralleling is not possible when exposing the posterior teeth (maxillary or mandibular), a 20-degree compromise technique often produces good or acceptable results. Film-holding methods similar to those described for the anterior regions can be used, but the film is placed as parallel as possible (within 20 degrees) to the long axis of the tooth, and the beam of radiation is directed perpendicularly to the film.

It often happens that when multirooted teeth, such as the maxillary first premolar, are radiographed, the buccal and lingual roots appear superimposed. This can be remedied by a shift of the tube head and PID. (Refer to the buccal-object rule in Chapter 12.) For example, the buccal root can be separated from the lingual root if a second exposure is made and the tube head is moved toward the mesial. If that is done, the lingual root canal will appear to move in the direction of the tube shift (mesial position in relation to the buccal canal), and the buccal canal will appear to move in a direction opposite to the tube shift.

CHAPTER SUMMARY

The full-mouth radiographic survey of an adult patient is normally made with a minimum of 14 standard-sized films—more if narrow films are used in the anterior areas or if bitewing films are included. Exposures are made in the incisor, canine, premolar, and molar areas of the mandible and maxilla. Every effort should be made to center the film over the area of interest, to avoid excessive bending of the film packet, and to make a final check to determine that the horizontal and vertical angulations are correct in relation to the film and the teeth.

When the bisecting technique is used, the film may be held in position by the patient's finger or by a film-holding device. Because the film is positioned farther from the teeth in the paralleling technique, some form of film-holding device is always required. Modifications or variations in film placement or exposure techniques may be required when the mouth is small, when anatomical abnormalities exist, or when the patient is uncooperative. Some technique modifications may be necessary when taking endodontic radiographs.

The paralleling technique produces radiographs with the least dimensional distortion. It is the technique of choice.

KEY WORDS

Aiming ring
Bisector
Biteblock
Central ray
Endodontia
Film holder
Horizontal placement

Indicator rod (arm)
Mean tangent
Occlusal plane
Periapical radiograph
Point of entry
Survey
Vertical placement

REVIEW QUESTIONS

1. What is the normal film requirement for the adult periapical survey when standard-sized film packets are used? (a) 12, (b) 14, (c) 16, (d) 18.

2. Which of these factors does not need to be considered when deciding which film size to use when making the full-mouth survey? (a) age of the patient, (b) shape of the dental arches, (c) previous accumulated exposure, (d) patient's ability to tolerate the film packet.

3. How wide should the margin above or below the occlusal edge be on posterior radiographs? (a) 1/16 in. (1.5 mm), (b) 1/8 in. (3 mm), (c) 1/4 in. (6 mm), (d) 3/8 in. (9 mm).

4. Which part of the film packet should face the lingual surface of the teeth and the source of radiation? (a) the narrow edge, (b) the printed side, (c) the widest edge, (d) the tube side.

5. In what location should the identification dot be on a correctly placed film? (a) toward the midline, (b) toward the incisal or occlusal, (c) toward the palate or floor of the mouth, (d) toward the distal.

6. Which of these is not a part of the assembled XCP holder? (a) aiming ring, (b) biteblock, (c) extension tube, (d) indicator rod.

7. In which of these tooth areas is it often necessary to make a large deviation from average vertical angulation? (a) mandibular premolar, (b) mandibular molar, (c) maxillary third molar, (d) maxillary premolar.

8. In which of these areas is it occasionally advisable to position the film vertically instead of horizontally? (a) mandibular premolars, (b) mandibular third molar, (c) maxillary premolars, (d) maxillary third molars.

9. The avoidance of radiographic distortion or magnification is a major concern in endodontic treatment because: (a) the tooth is to be extracted, (b) the length of the canal must be accurately measured, (c) the canal may already be filled, (d) the canal may be too large.

BIBLIOGRAPHY

Del Rio CE, Canales ML, Preece JW: *Radiographic Technique for Endodontics.* San Antonio, TX: University of Texas Dental School at San Antonio, 1982

Eastman Kodak: *X-rays in Dentistry.* Rochester, NY: 1985

Langland OE, Langlais RP: *Projection Techniques.* San Antonio, TX: University of Texas Dental School at San Antonio, 1981

Rinn Corporation: *Intraoral Radiography with Rinn XCP/BAI Instruments.* Elgin, IL: 1983

CHAPTER 16

Bitewing Examination

OBJECTIVES

By the end of this chapter the student should be able to

1. Select the type and number of films required to make the bitewing survey.

2. Compare the difference between periapical and bitewing radiographs.

3. Compare the methods of holding the bitewing film in position.

4. Identify the positions of the film placement and the vertical and horizontal angulations normally used.

FUNDAMENTALS OF BITEWING RADIOGRAPHY

The **bitewing (interproximal) examination** is made either in conjunction with the complete periapical examination (usually repeated at intervals of from 2 to 6 years) or alone at the time of the 6-month or annual regular checkup if it is deemed necessary and if, in the judgment of the dentist, it would benefit the patient.

Dental caries frequently begin in the interproximal areas of the teeth and periodontal disturbances near the gingival line. Thus, bitewing radiographs that show the crowns and alveolar crests of both the maxillary and mandibular teeth on the same film are ideal for identifying these problems.

An advantage of the bitewing over the periapical film is that it can be positioned near and almost parallel to the teeth of both arches when the patient's jaws are closed. This often makes it possible to see decay and the height of the alveolar crests better than on periapical films of the same area, because the film is closer to the teeth and the

277

central ray can be directed at a more ideal angle. One of the great values of the **bite-wing radiograph** is that it reveals caries in the earliest stages. This is particularly important in the premolar and molar regions, where small carious lesions are often concealed by the wide bucco-lingual diameters of these teeth. Such lesions are frequently unnoticed in a visual inspection. A disadvantage of the bitewing radiograph is that it does not show apical conditions or lesions.

The bitewing survey can be made with two to eight films, using any size from #0 through #3, or any combination of these. Many factors must be considered by the operator when deciding what size film to select. For example, the preferred size for the deciduous and mixed dentition bitewing survey is the standard #2 film, but often tissue sensitivity or anatomical limitations make it advisable to select a smaller film. A good rule to remember is to use the largest-sized film that will do the job without causing discomfort to the patient. Exposures can be made in both the anterior and posterior areas of the mouth. Anterior exposures are not often made because they seldom show anything not shown on properly positioned periapical films. Moreover, caries are much easier to detect by mirror and explorer examination and strong transillumination in the anterior than in the posterior.

Manufacturers package most film sizes with **bitetabs** attached to them. If such special films are not stocked in the office, it is easy to paste a bitetab to the tube side of the selected periapical film or to slide the film into a bite **loop,** thus converting it into a bitewing film. For posterior use, fasten the tab or slide the film into the loop so that the film can be positioned in the mouth with its longest dimension horizontal.

The length and curvature of the posterior arches vary in all individuals. A single small film placed on each side of the mouth often provides adequate coverage for all areas of interest in a small child or young adult. On most adults, four #2 films (two on each side) are generally preferred; however, some dentists routinely make the posterior survey with one #3 (extra-long) film on each side. When compared with the standard #2 film, the longer film has two serious disadvantages. One is that in most dental arches there are two slightly divergent pathways of the posterior teeth, one for the premolars and the other for the molars. As the central rays pass through these divergent embrasures, some of the interproximal structures **overlap** on the radiograph. The other is that the long film is too narrow to reveal all of the periodontal bone level.

The horizontal angulation for bitewing exposures is the same as that used for periapical ones of the same area. The vertical angulation is +5 to +10 degrees. The point of entry for the central ray for all bitewing exposures is on the level of the incisal or occlusal plane (near the lip line) at a point opposite the center of the film and through the interproximal spaces of the teeth being x-rayed.

METHODS OF HOLDING THE BITEWING FILM PACKET IN POSITION

Several methods are used to stabilize the film; all of them make use of some type of **bitetab, film loop,** or **biteblock.** Because anterior films must be placed vertically in the mouth, bitetabs that can be fastened to the tube side with adhesive are easiest to use.

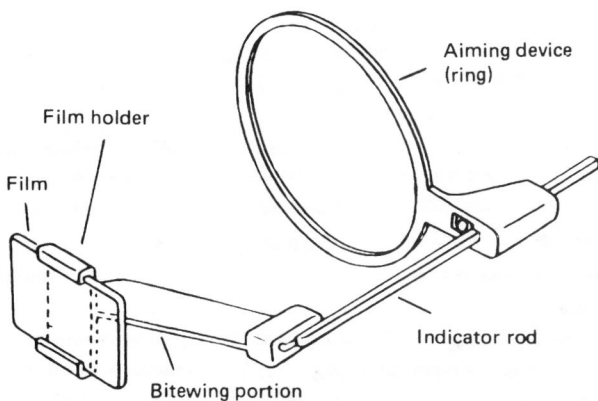

Figure 16–1. The Rinn bitewing instrument consists of a plastic biteblock with a thin biting portion that supports the film-holding device at one end and a receptacle for insertion of the metal indicator rod at the other end. A ring slides over the rod. The instrument is also available with a rectangular aiming device for use with the collimated rectangular PID. *(Courtesy of Rinn Corporation, Elgin, IL.)*

The film loop, into which the film can be slid with the tube side facing the tab, and bite planes are most often used for posterior exposures.

Another film holder is the combination metal and plastic bitewing instrument (Fig. 16–1). This instrument is similar in appearance to the XCP instruments described in Chapters 14 and 15. It differs in that the indicator rod is straight and short and the plastic block has two slots between which the film is inserted with the exposure side (tube side) facing the thin biting plane of the block. Either the conventional round locator ring or the newer rectangular placement holder can be used with the long or short position indicating device (PID) to align the central beam vertically and horizontally at the most advantageous angle.

The metal or metal-and-plastic film holders are easy to disinfect, assemble, and position. By eliminating the necessity for numerical angulation or specific head positioning, many of the common errors such as cone cutting, closed interproximal spaces, overlapping crowns, and diagonal occlusal planes can be reduced when film holders are used. Specific instructions are available from the various manufacturers. The exposure techniques that follow are based on the use of bitetabs or film loops. Because the overwhelming majority of bitewing films are exposed in the premolar and molar regions, the techniques for the posterior exposures are described first.

POSTERIOR BITEWING EXPOSURES

Unless special film holders are used, it is generally best to seat the patient upright in the conventional position. If two exposures are to be made on each side, position one film in the molar and the other in the premolar region. Otherwise, center a single film behind the molars and premolars (Fig. 16–2). Although vertical angulations may vary slightly from patient to patient, the average vertical angulation used is +8 degrees. Regardless of the technique used, the horizontal angulation is directed perpendicularly through the embrasures toward the film.

Extreme care must be exercised when positioning the PID in the horizontal plane because if the central ray is not directed through the interproximal spaces, or is projected mesiodistally or distomesially instead of at right angles (perpendicularly), the tooth structures in the contact areas will be overlapped; then it will be difficult or even impossible to locate small cavities or decay under restorations, thus defeating the purpose of the bitewing radiograph (Fig. 16–3).

As a rule, the film packet is placed horizontally in the posterior areas and vertically in the anterior ones. Two exceptions are (1) when the posterior portion of the dental arch is very curved or irregular and it is difficult or impossible to find a common angle of projection through the embrasures, and (2) when the patient has severe bone loss, horizontal film placement will not show the extent of periodontal destruction; then the problem of overlapping or failure to show the extent of the bone loss can often be solved by using more films placed vertically.

Care should be taken to ensure that the film is positioned in such a manner that it is evenly divided between the maxillary and mandibular teeth. The curvature of the palate or tongue interference has a tendency to disorient the film packet in its horizontal plane. Once the film is satisfactorily positioned, the patient must close down on the tab or biteblock in an edge-to-edge relationship. Generally the bitetab or biteblock is visible after the film is placed. This serves as a guide for directing the central rays toward the center of the film.

To make the molar bitewing exposure, follow these steps:

1. Attach a bitetab or slip the film into a loop if special film is not available. The standard #2 film is generally most satisfactory. If necessary, slightly soften the film corners to conform to the curvature of the arch.
2. Grasp the tab and position the lower half of the film so that it is centered over the mandibular second molar. Cover the distal half of the second premolar with the front edge of the film.
3. Hold the tab firmly against the occlusal surface of the mandibular teeth. Ask the patient to close the mouth so that the teeth occlude normally. Biting down correctly on the tab is important to obtain the proper relationship of the teeth on the radiograph. Sometimes, practice without the film will help patients understand how to bite. Failure to hold the tab firmly permits the film to drift lingually and distally and increases the possibility that the tongue will move the film. This often results in a slanted occlusal plane. Caution the patient to bite firmly.
4. Center the PID over the point of entry—a spot on the occlusal plane between the maxillary and mandibular first molars. Establish the vertical angulation, usually at +8 degrees, and direct the horizontal angulation toward the recording plane of the film.
5. Make the exposure.

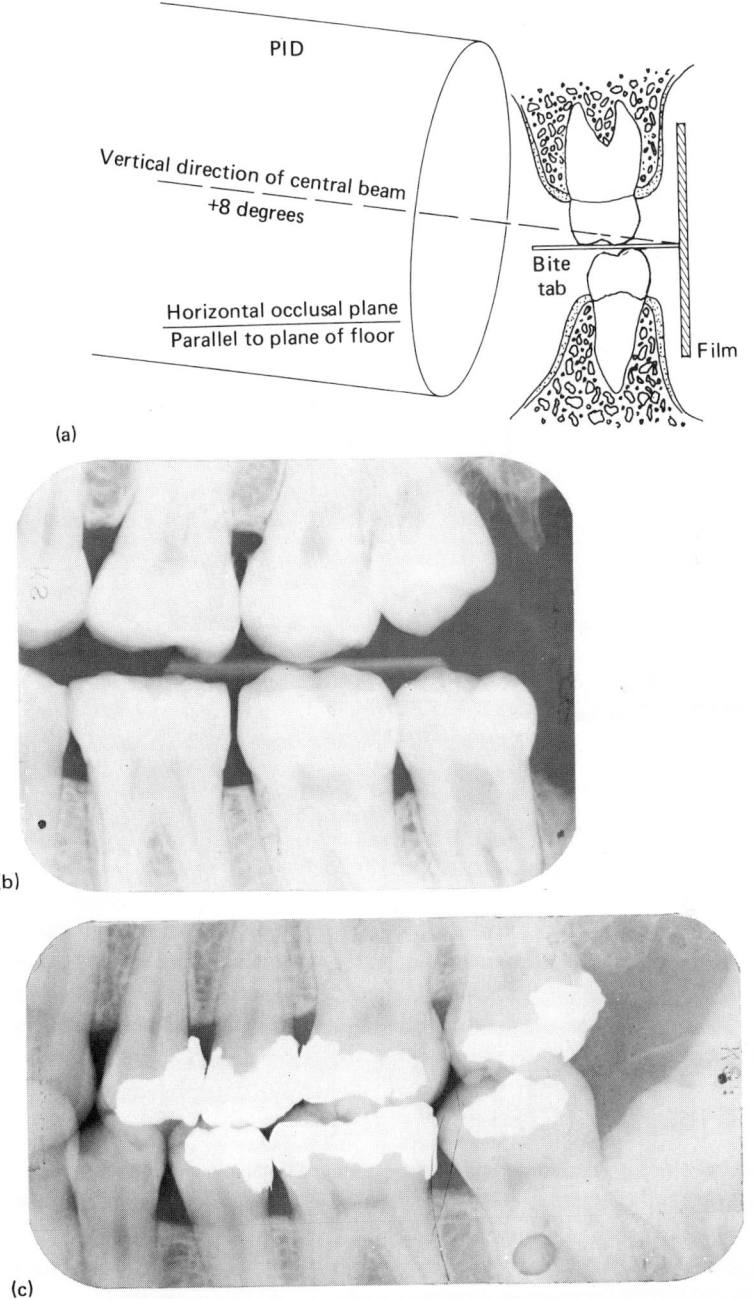

Figure 16–2. Posterior interproximal area. **(a)** Film slips into loop with widest dimension parallel to occlusal plane. Film packet is stabilized by bitetab that rests on the occlusal surfaces of the mandibular teeth. Patient closes on tab to immobilize the film. PID is projected vertically at +8 degrees toward center of film, and the central ray is directed horizontally through the interproximal spaces. Any size film packet from #0 through #3 may be used. **(b)** Radiograph of molar interproximal area made with standard #2 film. **(c)** Radiograph of premolar-molar interproximal area made with the long #3 film.

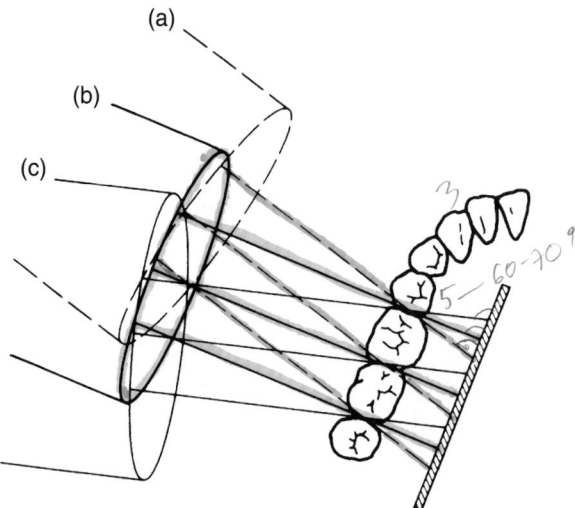

Figure 16–3. Horizontal angulation. **(a)** Mesiodistal projection shown here is deviated from a right angle by about 15 degrees, resulting in large overlapping of the contacts in the distal areas of the radiograph. **(b)** Correct horizontal projection of x-ray beam resulting in no overlapping. **(c)** Distomesial projection shown here is deviated from a right angle about 15 degrees, resulting in large overlapping in the mesial areas of the radiograph.

Since it is critical for the interproximal spaces to be visible without overlapping, it is necessary to understand the anatomy of the molar teeth. The orientation of the maxillary first and second molars to the midsagittal plane is 60 to 70 degrees. The orientation of the maxillary second and third molars to the midsagittal plane is 80 to 90 degrees. The orientation of all mandibular molars to the midsagittal plane is also 80 to 90 degrees. Therefore the horizontal angulation should be 80 to 90 degrees in relationship to the midsagittal plane in order to open all but one of the molar contacts.

The **premolar** bitewing exposure is practically identical to the one described for the molars, with these exceptions:

1. Adjust the occlusal plane if necessary. Center the film over the second mandibular premolar. Cover the distal half of the mandibular canine with the front (anterior) edge of film.
2. Center the PID over the point of entry—a spot on the occlusal plane between the maxillary and mandibular second premolars.
3. Make the exposure.

The **premolar-molar** bitewing exposure is also identical to the exposures described, with these exceptions:

1. Unless the arch is extremely short, use the long #3 film and center it over the embrasure between the mandibular second premolar and first molar.

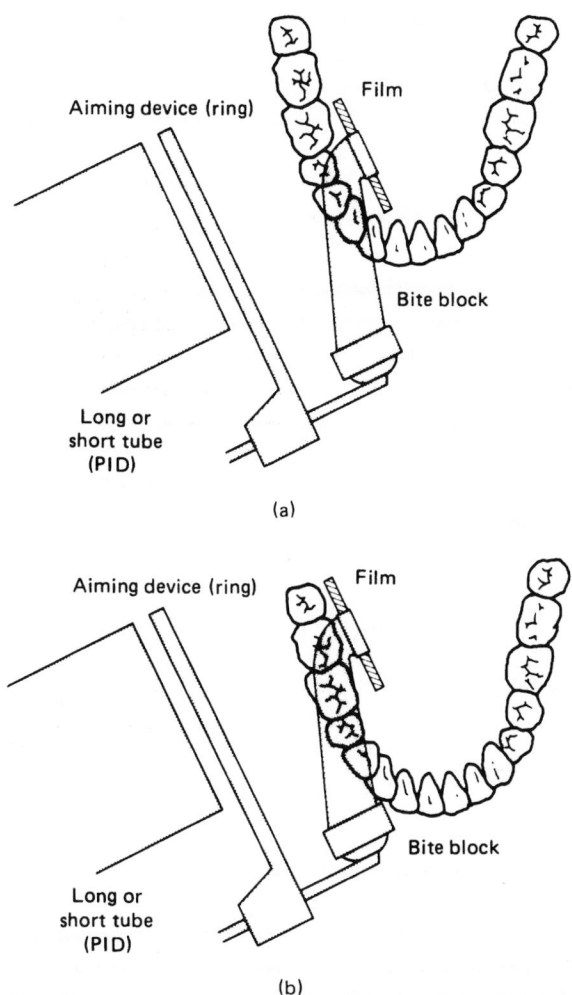

Figure 16–4. Diagrams showing film and PID position with the Rinn bitewing instrument: **(a)** premolar position made in conventional manner, **(b)** recommended molar position. Because the interproximal surfaces of the molar teeth are in a mediodistal relationship to the sagittal plane, conventional positioning of the film parallel to the sagittal plane or to the buccal surfaces will result in overlapping of the contact areas and closure of the embrasure spaces. It is recommended that to avoid this distortion, the film be positioned perpendicularly to the embrasures, resulting in a diagonal placement of the film, with the anterior border at a slightly greater distance from the lingual surface of the teeth than the posterior border. *(Courtesy of Rinn Corporation, Elgin, IL.)*

Cover the distal half of the mandibular canine with the front (anterior) edge of film.
2. Attempt to direct the central rays perpendicularly at the mean tangents of the interproximal spaces of both the premolars and molars. This is not always possible, particularly if the arch curves, and overlapping in the proximal areas may result. That is why it is generally better to expose the premolar and molar areas separately.
3. Make the exposure.

Because the interproximal surfaces of the molars are in a mesiodistal relationship to the patient's sagittal plane, conventional film placement parallel to the buccal surfaces often results in overlapping of the contact areas and closure of the embrasure spaces. In such cases, position the film perpendicularly to the embrasures to avoid this distortion. Place the film slightly diagonally with the front edge of the film farther from the lingual of the teeth than the back part (Fig. 16–4).

A sloping or slanting occlusal plane is a frequent reason for having to retake bitewing radiographs. Probable causes include (1) the failure of the patient to maintain a steady pressure on the bitetab; (2) the patient swallowing while the exposure is being made; (3) anatomical obstructions such as a torus or malpositioned tooth; (4) the top edge of the film contacting the lingual gingiva or curvature of the palate; and (5) poor placement of the bitetab or film holder.

Possible corrections include (1) cautioning the patient not to swallow or allow the teeth to separate; (2) checking for anatomical obstructions before positioning the film packet; (3) if absolutely necessary, slightly bending a corner of the film; and (4) exercising care in selecting and positioning the correct size film.

ANTERIOR BITEWING EXPOSURES

When making anterior bitewing exposures, seat the patient in the same position and establish the horizontal angulation in the same manner as for the posterior exposures. Increase the vertical angulation to +10 degrees. For ease of placement and least distortion, use the narrow #1 film. Use a longer bitetab (about 1 in. [25 mm] long) than is used for the posterior exposures and attach it to the tube side in such a manner that the film can be placed in the mouth with its longest dimension vertically. This allows the film to be placed farther lingually in the mouth and prevents bending of the film in the middle as the tab is pulled forward when the patient is asked to bite with the teeth in edge-to-edge position on the tab.

To make an **incisor** bitewing exposure (Fig. 16–5), follow these steps:

1. Slightly soften all four corners of the film for greater patient comfort. Grasp the bitetab and position the lower half of the film so that it is either centered at the midline, or if two films are to be used, between the central and lateral incisors. Direct the lower edge of the film into the space between the teeth and tongue.
2. Hold the bitetab so that it rests on the incisal edge of the mandibular in-

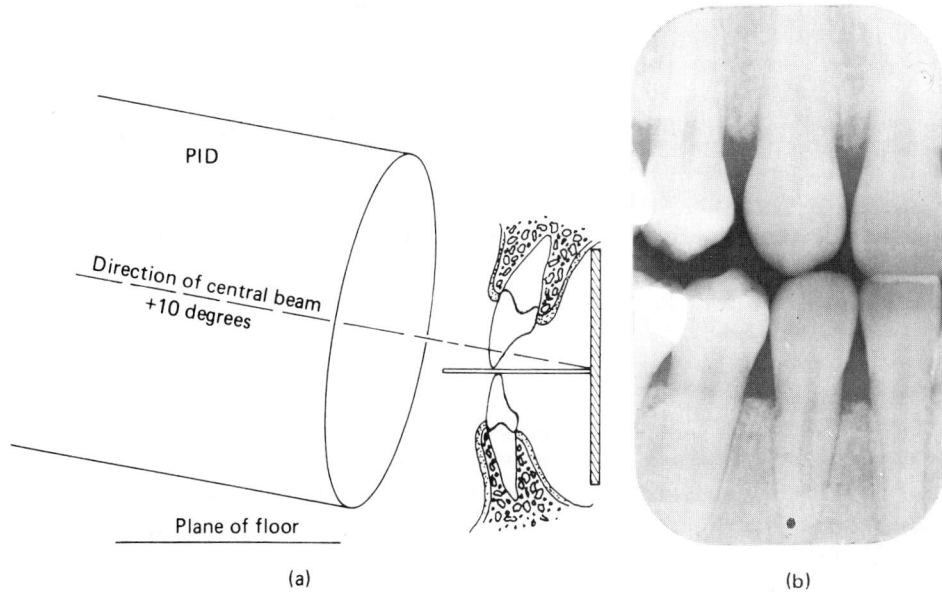

Figure 16–5. Anterior interproximal area. **(a)** Center film packet vertically at midline and stabilize by having patient gently close on tab at incisal edges of teeth. Teeth meet tab in end-to-end position. Suggested vertical angulation is +10 degrees toward the center of the film and horizontally the x-ray beam is directed through the interproximal spaces. **(b)** Bitewing film of the right canine area.

cisor and ask the patient to close gently but firmly on it in an edge-to-edge position. Push the upper part of the film toward the lingual if it appears to prematurely come into contact with the palate. Exert only a gentle pull forward on the tab—just enough to take up any slack and prevent the film from turning.

3. Center the PID over the point of entry—a spot at the incisal line between the maxillary and mandibular incisors. Direct the vertical angulation at about +10 degrees. Establish the horizontal angulation by directing the central rays perpendicularly through the mean tangent of the embrasures between either the central incisors or between the central and lateral incisors toward the plane of the film.

4. Make the exposure.

To make the **canine (cuspid)** bitewing exposure, follow the same procedures as for the incisor area but center the film over the canine, with the front edge of the film including the distal of the mandibular lateral incisor. The point of entry is opposite the maxillary canine at the incisal edge.

CHAPTER SUMMARY

Bitewing films are exposed more often than any other type of dental film. The dentist considers them necessary to detect incipient caries in the tooth contact areas and early resorptive changes in the alveolar bony crest; thus bitewing radiographs not only supplement and complete the full-mouth survey but are also exposed at most periodic checkup examinations.

Any length PID may be used. Some form of film retention—bitetab, film loop, or biteblock—must be used. The patient prevents the film from moving by biting firmly on the tab or block in an edge-to-edge or centric relationship. Although many consider the bitewing exposure to be the easiest to make, it is the one most likely to fail.

Great care must be taken in placement of the film so that the radiograph will show the same amount of maxillary and mandibular structures. Although the vertical angulation is less critical in caries detection, an error in the horizontal angulation will cause an overlapping in the tooth contact areas and render the film useless for diagnostic purposes.

KEY WORDS

Bitetab
Bitewing radiograph
Contact area
Embrasure

Film loop
Interproximal radiograph
Overlapping

REVIEW QUESTIONS

1. How many standard-sized films are recommended to make the full bitewing survey of the posterior teeth? (a) 2, (b) 4, (c) 6, (d) 8.

2. Which of these conditions would not be visible on a bitewing radiograph? (a) incipient caries, (b) recurrent caries, (c) apical abscess, (d) alveolar crest resorption.

3. Which of these factors is most likely to reduce the usefulness of a bitewing radiograph? (a) error in horizontal angulation, (b) error in vertical angulation, (c) ver-

tical instead of horizontal film placement, (d) horizontal instead of vertical film placement.

4. Which size film is used and how is it positioned in the anterior area of a small and narrow adult arch? (a) long-bitewing film placed vertically, (b) narrow film placed horizontally, (c) narrow film placed vertically, (d) standard film placed horizontally.

5. Under what circumstances is the use of #3 film indicated? (a) when the patient is edentulous, (b) when a child does not have permanent teeth, (c) when it is desirable to show impacted third molars, (d) when it is desirable to use a single film for the premolars and molars.

6. What is the approximate vertical angulation for most bitewing procedures? (a) −10 degrees, (b) 0 degrees, (c) +10 degrees, (d) +20 degrees.

BIBLIOGRAPHY

Eastman Kodak: *X-rays in Dentistry.* Rochester, NY: 1985

Rinn Corporation: *Intraoral Radiography with Rinn XCP/BAI Instruments.* Elgin, IL: 1983

CHAPTER 17

The Occlusal Examination

By the end of this chapter the student should be able to

1. Identify the reasons for making an occlusal survey.

2. Compare the topographical with the cross-sectional exposure method.

3. Position the film packet and establish horizontal and vertical angulation for maxillary and mandibular areas.

REASONS FOR MAKING THE OCCLUSAL EXAMINATION

The occlusal examination may be made alone or to supplement periapical or bitewing radiographs. The large #4 occlusal film is very useful for recording information that cannot be adequately recorded on the smaller periapical films—for example, whole lesions. The occlusal film can be used to make a rapid survey of the mouth to locate impacted or supernumerary teeth, fractures, foreign bodies, cysts, and malignancies. It can also reveal the presence of stones (sialoliths) blocking the passage of **Wharton's duct** (exit to the submandibular gland) in the floor of the mouth, indicate the size and shape of tori on the mandible, show the progress of healing in the maxillae following a cleft palate operation, locate retained roots, unerupted teeth, or foreign objects in edentulous arches, and do a variety of other things.

Although an occlusal film may sometimes not provide as complete and satisfactory information as a periapical film, the occlusal film can be used when it is desirable to view the area of interest in its entirety or when placement of periapical films is too difficult. For example, a patient with swollen cheeks may be unable to open the mouth wide enough. Children may misunderstand instructions for holding the film in place or may have tissues so sensitive that they cannot tolerate periapical film. Most children can cooperate in biting on a film, and smaller films than the occlusal should be used for them.

TECHNICAL CONSIDERATIONS

In addition to the large occlusal film generally used to make the occlusal survey, smaller intraoral films may also be used, depending on the area to be examined. The standard #2 periapical film is frequently used with children, either to make a rapid survey of labiolingual or buccolingual unerupted tooth positions or in place of periapical positioning. It is also used on adults when the mouth is too small for the large occlusal film. A variety of film positions can be used to make the occlusal examination. The film may be placed horizontally or vertically. It may also be centered over one small sector, over the anterior portion of the arch, or over the entire right or left dental arch. Placement and size of film depend on how large the mouth opening is and the type of information that the radiograph is intended to reveal.

Most occlusal film packets contain two films. When they do, both films can be developed alike to give duplicate films. If duplicate films are not needed, one film can be developed fully for 5 minutes at 68°F, whereas the other film is developed for only 2 1/2 minutes. The fully developed film will show all details of the hard structures, whereas the underdeveloped film will show the soft structures.

The occlusal exposure can be made with any length position indicating device (PID). The occlusal technique is based on the correlation of certain head positions with specific vertical angulations. Most occlusal exposures are made with the patient's mid-sagittal plane perpendicular to the plane of the floor. When maxillary exposures are made, the occlusal plane of the teeth is parallel to the plane of the floor; however, when the mandibular exposures are made, the patient is reclined in the chair, and the occlusal plane may be perpendicular to the plane of the floor. Regardless of how the patient is positioned, the tube side of the film must always face toward the occlusal surfaces of the teeth in the arch being examined. The film is held in place during the exposure by slight pressure of the teeth of the opposite jaw. When the arches are edentulous, the patient holds the film with the thumbs.

Occlusal radiographs may be either topographical or cross-sectional. When the topographical technique is used the rules of bisecting are followed, and the radiation is directed through the apices of the teeth perpendicularly toward the bisector. Because a larger area is involved and it is not always possible to use the most favorable vertical angle, the images of the teeth generally appear longer than they do on periapical radiographs (Fig. 17–1).

The patient's head position and film position may be identical for making a topographical or cross-sectional exposure. The difference is in the direction of the central ray. In the cross-sectional technique, the central ray is directed toward the area of in-

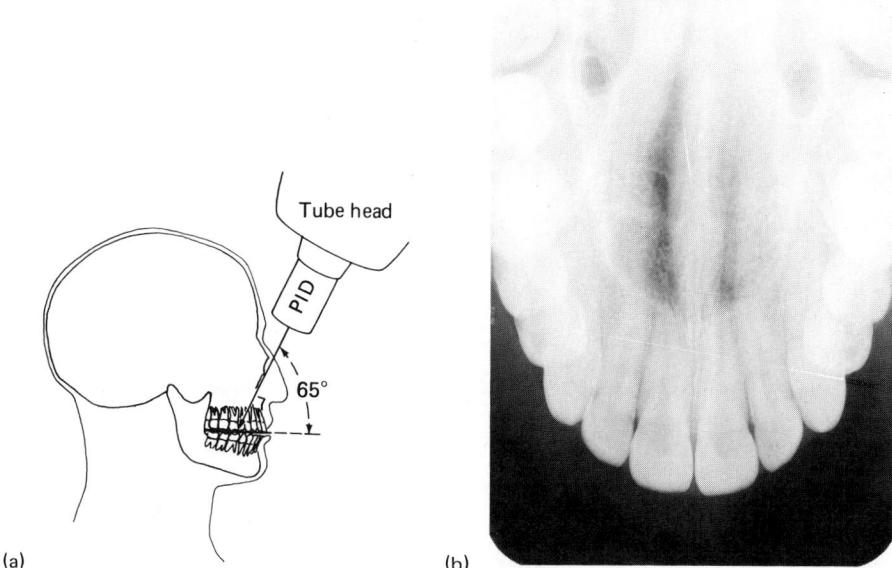

Figure 17–1. (a) Diagram showing relationship of tube head and PID to occlusal film and patient for a topographical view of the maxillary incisor area. Exposure side of film faces maxillary arch with longest film dimension anteroposteriorly. The horizontal central beam is parallel with patient's midsagittal plane, and the vertical angulation is approximately +65 degrees through a point near the bridge of the nose. The radiation beam is directed toward the center of the film. Slight modifications in film placement and angulation can be made when the center of interest is in the canine or molar area or when a cross-sectional view is desired. (b) Typical radiograph of topographical maxillary incisor area.

terest and parallel with the long axes of the teeth and adjacent areas. This results in a circular or elliptical appearance of the teeth on the radiograph (Fig. 17–2).

Film placement, angulation, and exposure procedures vary with the location and type of condition. Only a few simple, common techniques are described in this chapter. Because the film placement and angulation procedures are similar, it is often difficult to determine whether a topographical or a cross-sectional survey would produce the maximum diagnostic yield. Such a decision varies from patient to patient and is influenced by the size and shape of the arches, the alignment of the teeth, the presence or absence of anatomical irregularities, and the type of lesion or area of interest that the dentist desires to view.

A topographical survey generally yields more detail in the alveolar crest and apical areas, whereas a cross-sectional survey yields more information about the location of tori and impacted or malpositioned teeth.

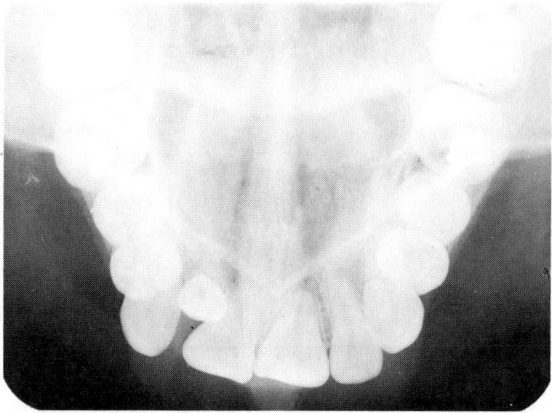

Figure 17-2. Typical radiograph of a maxillary cross-sectional view. Such a view can be made of a specific area or the entire dental arch. The film is placed in the same manner as for the topographical view, but the central ray is directed toward the area of interest parallel to the long axis of the teeth included in the area of interest or directly adjacent to it. The teeth appear as round or elliptical areas on the film.

THE MAXILLARY OCCLUSAL EXAMINATION

The Maxillary Topographical Survey (Fig. 17-1)

The following sequence of steps is suggested to make this exposure:

1. Seat the patient and adjust the headrest so that the midsagittal plane is perpendicular and the occlusal plane is parallel to the plane of the floor.
2. Insert the film packet axis vertically between the occlusal surfaces of the teeth with the tube side toward the palate, gently pushing it back as far as it will go.
3. Instruct the patient to close gently but firmly with the teeth against the film to immobilize it.
4. Establish the horizontal angulation so that the central ray is parallel with the patient's midsagittal plane and is directed through the arch toward the center of the film.
5. Establish the vertical angulation by directing the central rays at +65 degrees toward the center of the film through the point of entry above the bridge of the nose.

The Maxillary Cross-Sectional Survey (Fig. 17-2)

Follow the same procedure as was suggested for the maxillary topographical survey, with these exceptions:

1. Insert the film packet axis horizontally between the occlusal surfaces of the teeth with the tube side toward the palate.

2. Follow same procedure for horizontal angulation but establish the vertical angulation by directing the central rays perpendicularly at +75 degrees toward the center of the film through the point of entry slightly above the bulge of the nose.

The maxillary incisor technique can be modified for exposures of the canine, molar, or sinus areas by making slight changes in film placement and the central ray angulations. To make the canine survey, shift the film laterally to either the right or left side. Direct the central ray horizontally at about 45 degrees to the midsagittal plane and vertically at about +60 degrees. The point of entry is in the canine fossa, at a point near the infraorbital foramen. The film is shifted laterally in the same manner to make the molar survey. Use the same vertical angulation but change the horizontal angulation so it is at 90 degrees to the midsagittal plane. The point of entry is immediately below the outer canthus of the eye. To obtain a sinus survey, establish the horizontal angulation at 0 degrees to the midsagittal plane, and set the vertical angulation at +80 degrees. Direct the central ray toward the center of the film through a point of entry in the canine fossa. In this procedure, the maxillary sinus is directly above the film. This exposure is occasionally made to locate root tips in the sinus.

If the maxillary arch is edentulous, position the film packet axis horizontally. The patient presses the film against the ridge with the thumbs and braces the other fingers against the side of the face to prevent the film from moving. If the patient has a lower denture, it may be left in the mouth to bite against the film.

THE MANDIBULAR OCCLUSAL EXAMINATION

The Mandibular Topographical Survey (Fig. 17–3)

The following sequence of steps is suggested to make this exposure:

1. Seat the patient and adjust the headrest so that the midsagittal plane is perpendicular and the plane of occlusion is at a 45-degree angle to the plane of the floor. This can be done by either tilting the chair back or reclining the backrest.
2. Insert the film packet axis vertically between the occlusal surfaces of the teeth with the tube side toward the floor of the mouth, gently pushing it back as far as it will go.
3. Instruct the patient to close gently but firmly with the teeth against the film to immobilize it.
4. Establish the horizontal angulation so that the central ray is parallel with the patient's midsagittal plane and is directed through the arch toward the center of the film.
5. The problem in establishing ideal vertical angulation is in determining whether the patient has been reclined so that the plane of occlusion is at a 45-degree angle to the plane of the floor. A simple way to establish the vertical angulation is to first parallel the direction of the PID with that of the film and look at the angulation scale on the side of the tube head. Then

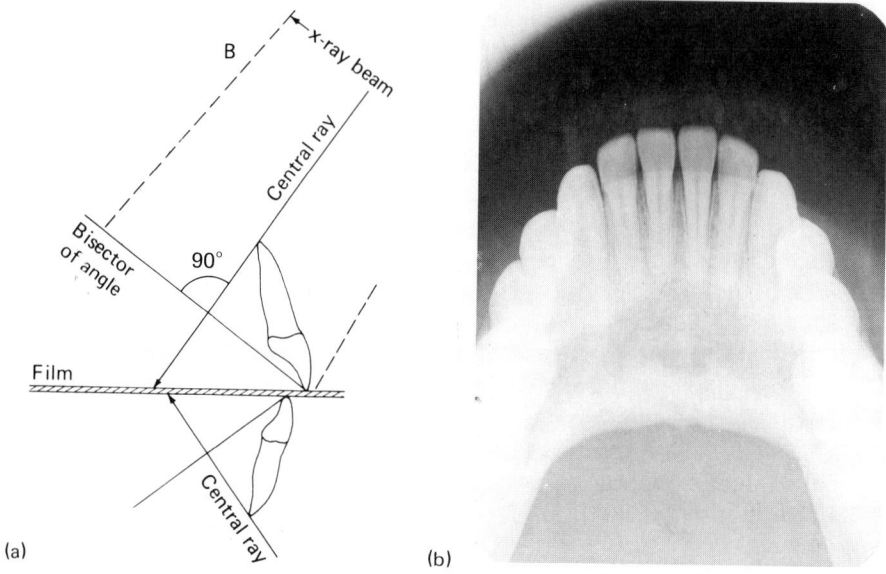

(a)   (b)

Figure 17–3. (a) Diagram illustrating angulation theory of topographic projections. A topographic radiograph appears similar to ordinary periapical film except that it is larger. Angulation rules for topographical projections are identical to those for the bisecting technique. The central ray is directed through the apex of the teeth at right angles to the bisector. Vertical angulations are increased when examining areas in the distal part of the palate. **(b)** A typical radiograph of a mandibular anterior exposure. *(Reproduced with permission from Wuehrmann, AH, Manson-Hing, LR: Dental Radiology, 5th ed. St Louis, MO: CV Mosby, 1981.)*

subtract 60 degrees from whatever reading is shown. For example, if the reading shown is +40 degrees and 60 degrees are subtracted, the new reading is –20 degrees (PID is tilted upward). At that angle, direct the central rays toward the middle of the film through a point of entry at the tip of the chin.

The Mandibular Cross-Sectional Survey (Fig. 17–4)

Follow the same procedure as for the mandibular incisor survey, with the exceptions noted below. A cross-sectional view is produced.

1. Place the patient in a reclined position and insert the film packet axis horizontally in the mouth.
2. Establish the horizontal angulation at 0 degrees to the midsagittal plane and set the vertical angulation at 0 degrees and parallel to the plane of the floor.
3. Direct the PID toward the center of the film through the point of entry, approximately 1 in. (25 mm) below the point of the chin.

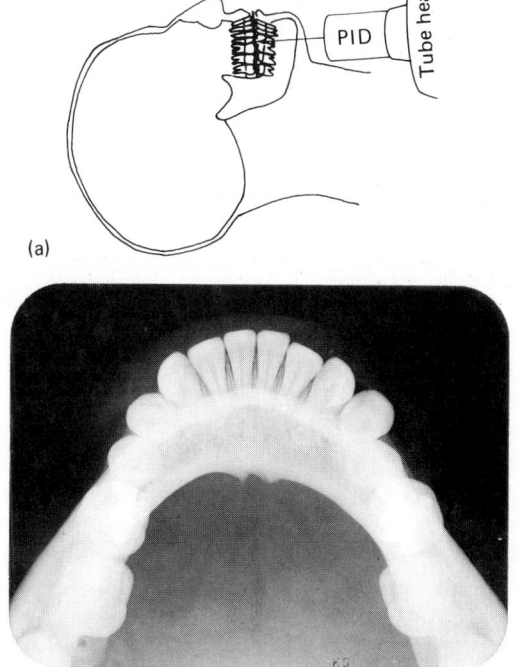

(a)

(b)

Figure 17–4. (a) Diagram showing relationship of tube head and PID to occlusal film and patient for a cross-sectional view of the entire mandibular arch. Exposure side of the film faces the mandibular arch with the widest dimension (longest) at right angles to the midsagittal plane. The central ray is directed perpendicularly to the occlusal plane through the inferior aspect of the mandible toward the center of the film. Slight modifications of this position must be made when the center of interest is in the canine or molar area or when a topographical view of the incisor area is desired. **(b)** Typical radiograph of cross-sectional view of the entire mandibular arch.

The technique for the mandibular incisor survey, with slight changes in film placement and in horizontal and vertical angulations, will give a canine, molar, or floor of the mouth survey.

If the patient is edentulous, position the film packet axis horizontally. The patient places the forefingers against the anterior border of the film to keep it from sliding forward and upward. If the patient has an upper denture, it may be left in the mouth to bite against the film.

Exposure procedures vary slightly according to the lesion or structure to be examined. For special results or in special situations, other head positions, film positions, or angulations may be used. Always use the fastest speed film. The patient's size, age, and the density of the bone structures must be considered when determining the exposure factors. Small intraoral cassettes with intensifying screens to reduce the exposure time may be used in special situations where dense cranial structures must be penetrated.

EXTRAORAL EXPOSURES MADE WITH OCCLUSAL FILMS

Occlusal film is sometimes used extraorally to show areas that are larger than intraoral film can show or when swelling or injury makes intraoral film placement difficult or inadvisable. The use of occlusal film for extraoral viewing of impacted or partially impacted third molars is fully described in Chapter 20 in the section Extraoral Exposures Made with Intraoral Film.

CHAPTER SUMMARY

The occlusal survey is made by inserting a film packet vertically or horizontally between the occlusal surfaces of the patient's teeth. Although it can be made alone, it is usually made to supplement the periapical survey. If the mouth opening is large enough, the #4 occlusal packet is preferred.

Advantages of the occlusal survey are the following: (1) a larger area than is possible on a periapical film can be visualized in its entirety, (2) a three-dimensional effect can be obtained by viewing an occlusal and periapical radiograph simultaneously, and (3) the film packet is easy to position on a disturbed or uncooperative patient.

Two angulation techniques are employed: (1) the topographical—based on a modification of the bisecting principle—used to view fractures and large lesions, and (2) the cross-sectional—based on directing the central rays toward the film at a right angle—used to establish buccolingual dimensions and to locate impactions or erupting teeth that are out of normal alignment.

KEY WORDS

Cross-sectional technique
Occlusal radiographs
Topographical technique

REVIEW QUESTIONS

1. Which of these film sizes is known as the occlusal film? (a) #1, (b) #2, (c) #3, (d) #4.

2. How many films are generally inside the occlusal packet? (a) 1, (b) 2, (c) 3, (d) 4.

3. What term best describes the appearance of the image of the occlusal surfaces of the teeth when the cross-sectional technique is used for making the occlusal survey? (a) overlapped, (b) elongated, (c) elliptical, (d) foreshortened.

4. During which of these occlusal exposures is it advisable to use an intraoral cassette? (a) maxillary sinus survey, (b) maxillary incisor survey, (c) mandibular incisor survey, (d) mandibular molar survey.

5. In which of these situations is an occlusal survey not indicated? (a) to determine the shape of the dental arch, (b) to locate the position of an impacted canine, (c) to reveal a fracture, (d) to reveal the extent of periodontal lesions.

6. When comparing the images of the teeth as shown on an occlusal topographical survey with the same images on a periapical survey, what will the images shown on the occlusal film appear to be? (a) foreshortened, (b) elongated, (c) tilted mesially, (d) tilted distally.

BIBLIOGRAPHY

Eastman Kodak: *X-rays in Dentistry*. Rochester, NY: 1985

Goaz PW, White SC: *Oral Radiology Principles and Interpretation*, 3rd ed. St Louis, MO: CV Mosby, 1994

CHAPTER 18

Radiography for Children

OBJECTIVES

By the end of this chapter the student should be able to

1. Show the importance of making radiographic examinations on children.
2. Identify the factors that determine when radiographs on children should be made and what type of film is best suited in each instance.
3. Differentiate the procedures involved in exposing radiographs on children and adults.

IMPORTANCE OF RADIOGRAPHY FOR CHILDREN

Children have the same basic needs for dental treatment as do adults. It may sometimes be more difficult to treat young children than adults, but the proper care of children's teeth is one of the dentist's basic responsibilities. From a materialistic point of view, too, child patients are important to a growing practice. Treated as children, they may return as adults.

Unfortunately, many parents have not received adequate dental education. Often they consider their children's teeth—particularly the deciduous teeth—to be of little value. More and more parents, however, are bringing in their children for dental examinations and preventive care, instead of only for emergencies. Dental education of the parents is the key to solving problems caused by dental neglect of children. Just as parents have been taught to accept vaccinations to prevent disease, they must be taught to accept dental radiography to detect dental infections, dental caries, and disfigurations produced by premature loss or prolonged retention of the teeth.

Dentists must direct their principal effort toward prevention rather than correction of conditions caused by neglect. In the area of prevention, radiography plays an important role, and perhaps no place in dental practice is good radiography more important than with children. The best time to prevent dental problems is in childhood.

One frequent problem is infected teeth, which can seriously affect a child's health. Hidden infections are often unsuspected. The longer the source of infection remains undisclosed, the greater the effect on the patient. **Deciduous teeth** that are lost too early or retained too long may cause severe damage to the occlusion and other conditions that are difficult to correct later. Hidden lesions can only be detected by frequent periodic examinations including radiographs. Without them, proper diagnosis, intelligent treatment planning, and corrective measures are nearly impossible.

ROLE OF RADIOGRAPHY IN PROTECTING THE DECIDUOUS TEETH

Many explanations are given for dental decay: bacterial action, faulty metabolism, excess acidity, neglect, faulty dental hygiene, and heredity. Whatever the reason, one fact is clear—dental caries are most prevalent in children. Although the teeth form and begin to calcify in the prenatal stage, much of the rapid growth of teeth and facial bones takes place between birth and 6 years. It is during the formative years that the danger of permanent damage from dental neglect is greatest. At this stage, radiography is vital to both prevention and treatment. Through the use of radiographs, the dentist can locate carious lesions in their beginning stages, check how well treatment is progressing, and see signs of further decay. Aside from dental caries, often unnoticed during a visual inspection, a radiograph shows the roots of the deciduous teeth as well as the developing permanent teeth within the alveolar bone. Timely and adequate dental treatment can often avert the premature loss of the deciduous teeth and the subsequent malocclusion, which can turn the child into a dental cripple. Moreover, disturbances in normal development, such as **amelogenesis imperfecta** (failure of the enamel to develop fully), **anodontia** (absence of teeth), the presence of **dentigerous cysts** (sacs containing fluid or producing teeth), **supernumerary (extra) teeth,** and a host of other conditions can be discovered only through radiographs.

WHEN TO EXPOSE RADIOGRAPHS ON CHILDREN

Unless an accident, toothache, or some other unusual circumstance causes a parent to bring a child to the dentist sooner, the first radiographic survey is often made soon after all the deciduous teeth have erupted at 3 years. Several factors determine how often the child's teeth should be x-rayed and the size and number of films used. These include the dental needs of the child, the cooperation and emotional stability of the child, the size of the mouth opening, the size and shape of the teeth and the dental arches, the operator's ability to position the film, and the child's ability to retain the film and keep it still.

In the past it has been the policy in many dental offices to routinely make radiographs at specific periodic intervals. In line with our increased awareness of radiation protection, the practice of making routine exposures is no longer acceptable. The present position of the American Dental Association is that radiographs should only be made when, in the opinion of the dentist, there is a valid reason that they would benefit the patient.

A second complete radiographic survey may be made when the child is about 6 years old, the age when the first deciduous teeth are shed and the first of the permanent teeth erupt. A third survey may be made at 9 years, when the child has a combination of deciduous and permanent teeth. The fourth survey is often made between 12 and 14 years, when the last deciduous teeth are lost. After this, film placement, size, and number are the same as for adults.

Except in emergencies, bitewing surveys are made as needed between complete surveys to detect caries or other incipient lesions.

SUGGESTED TECHNIQUES FOR PEDODONTIC RADIOGRAPHY

Methods for exposing radiographs on children are basically the same as those for adults. Although either the bisecting or paralleling technique can be employed, many children are too small for periapical film positioning or often cannot manage film holders.

Special consideration must be given to the child whose oral tissues are still in the formative stage. The oral mucosa of the young child is extremely sensitive to even the slightest pressure, especially when teeth are erupting or about to be shed. The newer soft film packets are helpful. If film holders are used, they should not be too bulky or heavy. The plastic backing plate on some holders can be cut down to a smaller size. The oral cavity should be examined thoroughly for loose or erupting teeth, any **parulis** (**fistula** or gum boil), **pulp polyps, herpes labialis** (cold sores), **aphthous ulcers** (canker sores), or swollen salivary glands.

Small mouths and difficult behavior can make it hard to radiograph children. Competence helps, but the operator may also need to approach a child differently from an adult. Of course, children differ, just as adults do, in the size, shape, and location of anatomical structures and in temperament and behavior as well. As always, technique and approach must fit the individual.

First impressions are always important and lasting. Unless an emergency makes it impossible, the young child's first visit to the dental office and the x-ray room should be pleasant and informative. Most children are extremely curious. Unless they have been frightened by an unpleasant experience in a hospital or medical or dental office, they are far more curious than apprehensive. Usually it is best to greet and take the child from the reception room to the x-ray room without the parents. Talking to and showing the child some of the equipment to be used and radiographs of other children will help in gaining the child's confidence. Since the child's first experience with radiography is such an important one, the visit should not be hurried and the operator must

refrain from showing signs of impatience. The radiographic survey should be explained to the child in simple terms. For example, the x-ray machine can be explained as a camera that takes pictures of the teeth. The child should be given a film packet to feel and to handle. It may be unwrapped so that the child can see where the film is. If a film holder is to be used, the child should be allowed to examine and handle it, perhaps to put it in the mouth to become convinced that it is not an object to be feared. The entire procedure should be carefully explained and rehearsed. If necessary, the operator should demonstrate how to hold and keep it still. No exposure should be attempted before the child is emotionally prepared for the experience and understands what is to be done.

The easiest and most comfortable exposures—normally radiographs of the anterior teeth—should be exposed first to gain the child's confidence and to get the child accustomed to having a film in the mouth. A young child's span of attention is not very long, and one must repeat instructions with each exposure. Young children are often fidgety and restless, so when the child is finally ready, exposures should be made as rapidly as possible.

Most children react favorably to the authority of a confident, capable operator. Occasionally, a stubborn or frightened child proves difficult to manage. If such a child does not respond to firmness, a parent or older brother or sister may accompany the child into the x-ray room. In fact, if the child is too small to understand instructions or unable to hold the film, a parent or accompanying adult may have to hold the film while it is being exposed. The dentist, the dental hygienist, or the dental assistant should never hold the film in the mouth of a patient.

Only in emergencies should a child ever be forced to have any dental treatment. It is much better to delay until the second or third visit than to instill a lasting fear of dentistry. If the child remains uncooperative after the third visit, a telephone call to the child's physician may be advisable to arrange for sedation. The sedative should be administered shortly before the appointment.

Both intraoral and extraoral films are used in making the radiographic survey on a young child. The choice of film size and type depends on the age of the patient and the area to be examined. As a rule, best results are obtained on a young patient when a combination of techniques and films is used. Periapical film placement is not always possible, and extraoral films provide much essential information about the growth and development of the jaws.

One problem in using periapical films is the distortion caused by the flatness of the palate and the floor of the mouth in children. Because of it, films lie flatter than they do in the mouths of most adults. This position results in an increase in the size of the angle between the teeth and the films, requiring an adjustment to compensate. When bisecting methods are used, the steepness of the vertical angulation is increased.

This problem can be solved by use of paralleling methods. The biteblocks on the XCP instruments can be modified by reducing the size of the backing plate with shears or a knife to accommodate the #0 film. If the child objects to the film holder in the mouth or has difficulty biting hard enough to stabilize it, have the child hold the film with the thumb or index finger, guided by the radiographer. When the child is too small to be seated in the dental chair, the child can sit on the parent's lap in the chair and the parent can hold the film. Under no circumstances should the radiographer hold the film packet.

A lead apron should always be placed over the patient. Special small lead aprons are available. As the bone structure on a child is smaller and less dense than that of an adult, average exposure time can be reduced by about one third.

FILM REQUIREMENTS FOR THE PEDODONTIC RADIOGRAPHIC SURVEY

Various combinations of periapical, bitewing, occlusal, or extraoral films are suggested, depending on the child. As usual, the survey should be thorough but as comfortable as possible. Ideally, the survey includes a minimum of 12 radiographs, 10 periapical and 2 bitewing exposures. However, there is never a required number of films

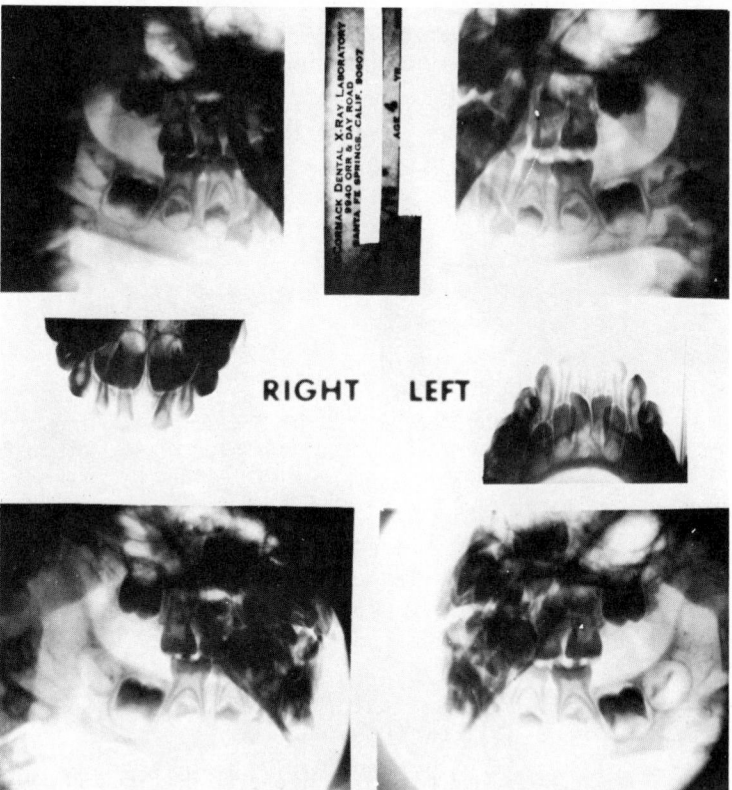

Figure 18–1. Combination of occlusal radiograph of incisal area and extraoral lateral jaw radiographs of the posterior areas of a 4-year-old child. *(Courtesy of McCormack Dental X-ray Laboratory, Santa Fe Springs, CA.)*

for a survey. The number and type of film are determined by the needs of the child so that a proper diagnosis can be made.

The periapical films are exposed in each of the four molar and canine areas and in the two incisor areas. Occlusal and extraoral exposures are included when requested by the dentist. However, small size, tongue resistance, and gagging can be a problem in small children, and occlusal and extraoral films make an acceptable substitute on a 3- or 4-year-old child (Fig. 18–1). At this age, it is often advisable to expose more than four films, one occlusal film in each jaw in the area of the anterior teeth and an extraoral film of each of the lateral jaw areas. Although not as effective as periapical or bitewing films in detecting caries, these show the formation of the permanent tooth buds and the relationship between deciduous and developing permanent dentition. Most children at that age do not object to occlusal and extraoral films, as they cause a minimum of discomfort.

At 6 years, the first permanent teeth have begun to erupt. As the child is now more mature, it may be possible to make the periapical exposures of all tooth areas. If using periapical films is still not feasible, the survey can be made with a minimum of six films—two occlusal, two extraoral, and two bitewings.

Another technique that is gaining in acceptance, as more panoramic x-ray units are available in dental offices and pedodontic clinics, is to make a panoramic exposure

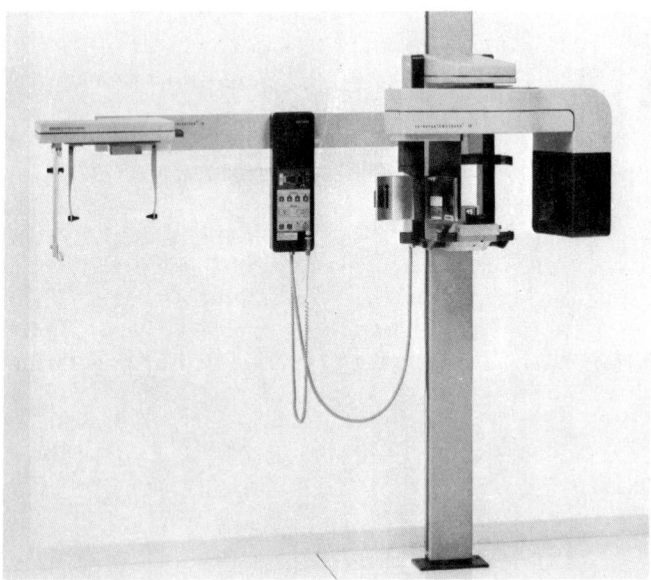

Figure 18–2. Photograph of Orthoceph 10. By having the child stand in position and adjusting the ear plugs for size and height, it is possible to make cephalometric lateral skull and posteroanterior radiographs. The loaded cassette is inserted into the adjustable cassette holder and positioned parallel to the child's face. The head positioner can be rotated as needed. *(Courtesy of Siemens Medical Systems, Inc., Dental Division, Iselin, NJ.)*

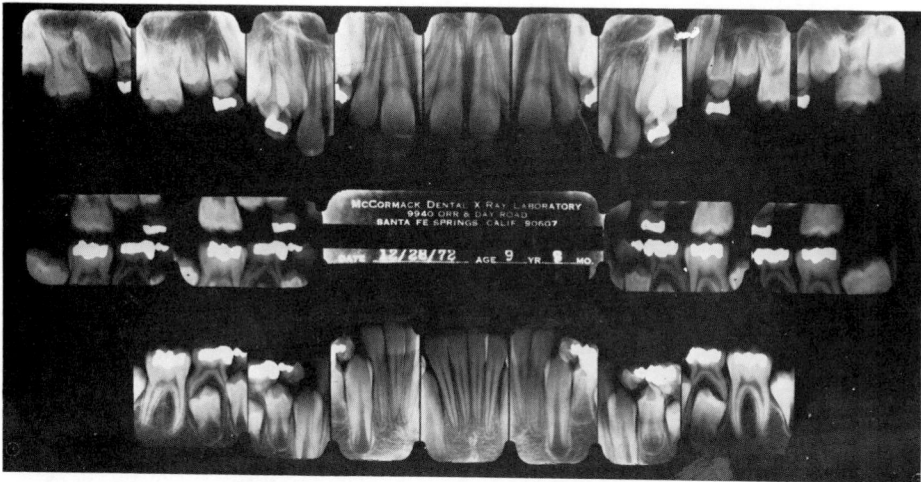

Figure 18–3. Complete radiographic periapical and bitewing series on a 9-year-old child. Depending on the size of the child, fewer films or films of several sizes may be used to make such a survey. *(Courtesy of McCormack Dental X-ray Laboratory, Santa Fe Springs, CA.)*

of the entire dentition to view the overall jaw development and growth of the teeth (Fig. 18–2). Such large radiographs may be supplemental to periapical exposures or may serve as the chief source of diagnostic information and be supplemented by a periapical or bitewing films.

At 9 years, the child has a mixed dentition. This examination may be made with as few as 6 and as many as 18 exposures. The larger #2 periapical films can often be used at this age; however, the smaller film sizes are most frequently used (Fig. 18–3).

Between 12 and 14 years of age, the child may have all permanent teeth except the third molars. It is during this preadolescent period that growth is most rapid and metabolic changes occur that heighten the possibility of dental caries and increase the need for vigilance and preventive care. This survey may be made with 14 periapical and 4 bitewing films. It is the same as that for the adult, and larger films can be used.

BITEWING AND PERIAPICAL EXPOSURES FOR CHILDREN

With few minor exceptions to compensate for the child's smaller mouth, the same technical procedures described in Chapters 15 and 16 are used when exposing radiographs on children. The main difference is in the use of smaller films and shorter exposure times. In addition, in some areas a slightly steeper vertical angulation than is customary in adults is used to compensate for the flatter palate and shallower floor of the mouth during bisecting. Other minor changes in technique are listed below for each of the exposures commonly made in a full-mouth series of radiographs for children.

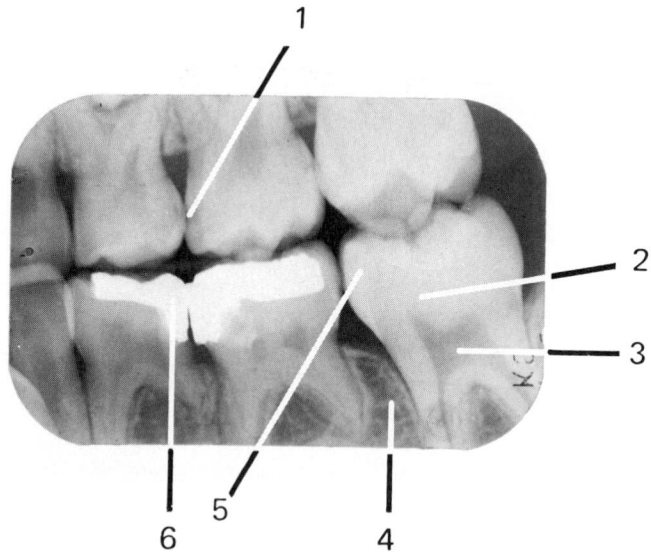

Figure 18–4. Posterior bitewing radiograph of mixed dentition exposed on #0 film shows **1** incipient caries in the interproximal areas between the maxillary first and second deciduous molars, **2** normal-appearing dentin in mandibular first permanent molar, **3** pulp chamber, **4** alveolar bone, **5** normal-appearing enamel covering of crown, and **6** metallic restorations on mandibular deciduous first and second molars.

The Posterior Bitewing Survey (Fig. 18–4)

Only one bitewing film is required on each side unless the second permanent molars have already erupted. Many dentists prefer two films on each side if the child has permanent molars. The front edge of the film should cover the distal half of the mandibular canine. Corners of the film packet may be softened so as not to bruise the delicate oral tissues. If the bisecting technique is used, the vertical angulation is increased from +8 to +10 degrees—to compensate for the reduced curvature of the child's palate. Depending on the age and the size of the child, the exposure time is normally one third less than used for making bitewing or periapical exposures on an adult.

The Mandibular Incisor Survey (Fig. 18–5)

Depending on the technique, the film is placed in the mouth vertically and held in place by the child's finger, or it is placed vertically in the biteblock on which the child closes. The average vertical angulation for bisecting is –20 to –25 degrees. Center the film at the midline and allow about 1/8 in. (3 mm) of the film to protrude above the incisal edge to leave an incisal margin. Refer to Chapter 15 for procedures on the periapical exposures.

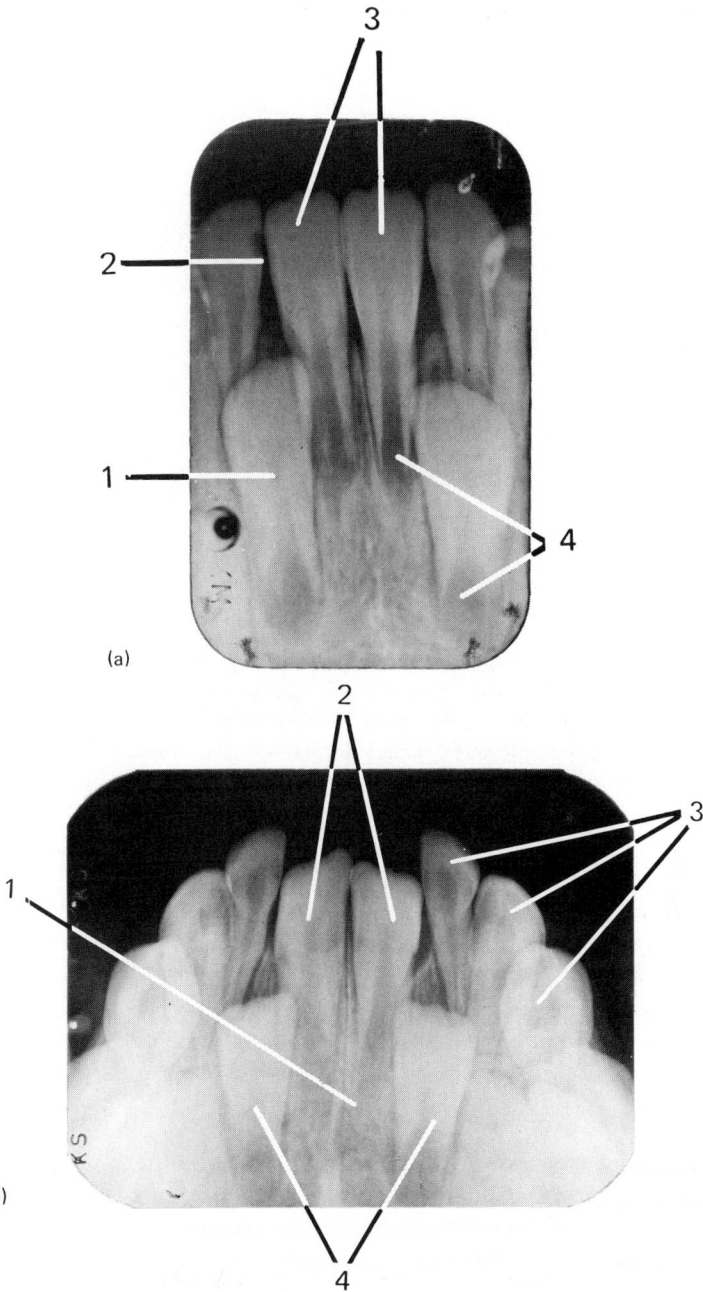

Figure 18–5. Radiographs of the mandibular incisor areas. **(a) 1** unerupted permanent lateral incisor, **2** incipient caries on mesial surface of deciduous lateral incisor, **3** fully erupted permanent central incisors, and **4** large open apex area on all permanent teeth, indicating that root formation is still in progress. Root formation is generally not complete until about 2 or 3 years following tooth eruption. **(b)** An alternate method of exposing the mandibular anterior teeth is to use the occlusal technique with a standard size #2 film. Observe the following: **1** alveolar bone; **2** partially erupted permanent central incisors; **3** deciduous teeth, soon to be exfoliated; and **4** unerupted permanent lateral incisors.

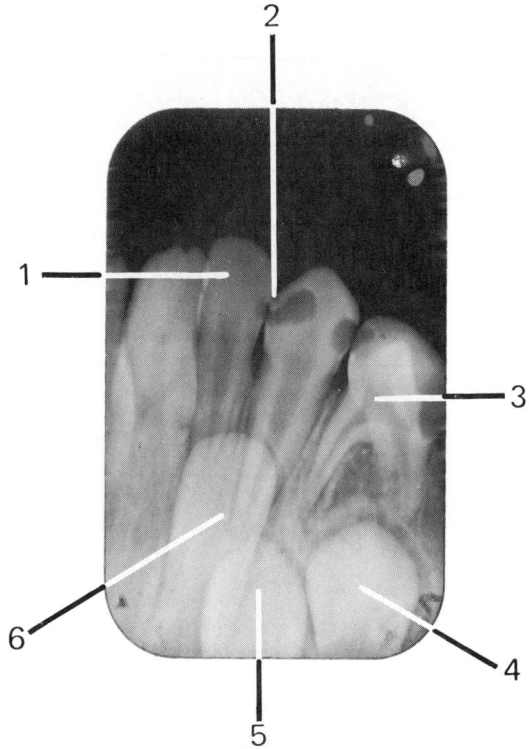

Figure 18–6. Radiograph of mandibular canine (cuspid) area shows **1** deciduous lateral incisor; **2** radiolucent areas on mesial and distal of deciduous canine, which appear to be restored with silicate or acrylic resin; however, this must be confirmed by visual examination because the aesthetic filling materials and dental caries often look similar on radiographs; **3** deciduous first molar; **4** unerupted first premolar; **5** unerupted canine; and **6** unerupted permanent lateral incisor.

The Mandibular Canine Survey (Fig. 18–6)

Except for minor positioning and angulation changes, follow the same procedures as for the mandibular incisors. The front edge of the film should extend forward to cover the distal portion of the mandibular lateral incisor. Increase the average vertical angulation to –25 to –30 degrees if using the bisecting method.

The Mandibular Molar Survey (Fig. 18–7)

The film is positioned horizontally and held by the child's finger or is placed horizontally in the biteblock on which the child closes. The film is centered over the mandibular molars. If possible, the front edge of the film should cover the distal half of the mandibular canine. Increase the average vertical angulation to between –15 and –20 degrees.

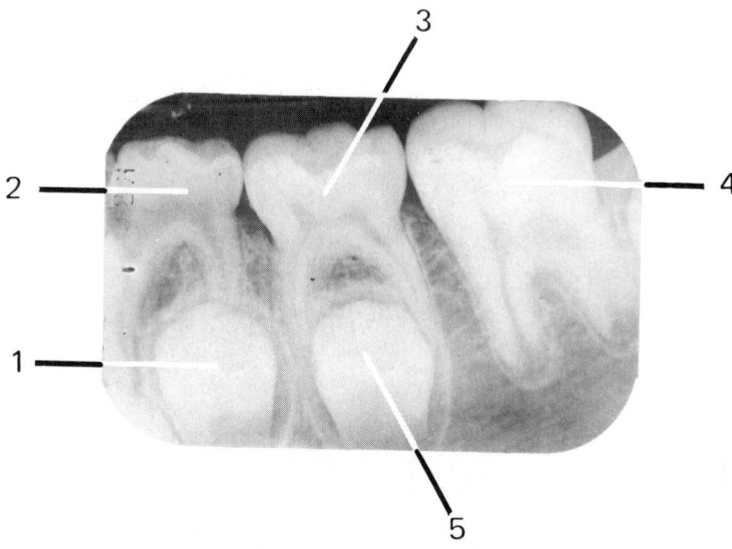

Figure 18–7. Radiograph of mandibular molar area—mixed dentition—shows **1** unerupted first premolar; **2** deciduous first molar—observe partial resorption of distal root; **3** deciduous second molar; **4** permanent first molar; and **5** unerupted second premolar.

The Maxillary Incisor Survey (Fig. 18–8)

Follow procedures for the mandibular incisor survey. The film is positioned vertically and centered at the midline. Increase the average vertical angulation to about +45 to +50 degrees if using the bisecting method.

The Maxillary Canine Survey (Fig. 18–9)

Follow the same procedure as for the maxillary incisor survey but shift the film laterally so that it is centered over the long axis of the maxillary canine. Place the front edge of the film so that it covers the distal half of the maxillary lateral incisor. For the bisecting technique, the average vertical angulation ranges from +55 to +60 degrees.

The Maxillary Molar Survey (Fig. 18–10)

As with the mandibular molar exposure, position the film horizontally over the molar area with the front edge covering the distal half of the maxillary canine. For the bisecting technique, the average vertical angulation ranges from +30 to +55 degrees.

When making any of these exposures for the first time, review how to use the film holders (Chapter 15) and modify these procedures for the child patient. The paralleling technique is the method of choice.

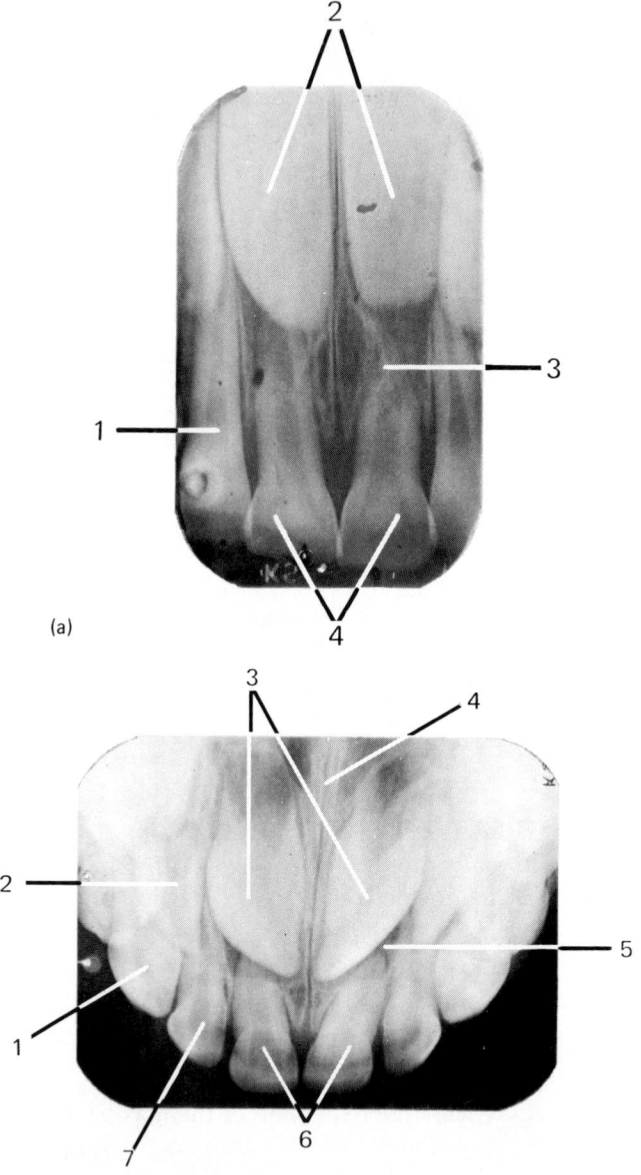

(a)

(b)

Figure 18-8. Radiographs of maxillary incisor areas. **(a)** Exposure with #0 film shows **1** fully erupted deciduous lateral incisor, **2** crowns of unerupted permanent central incisors, **3** roots of deciduous central incisors showing signs of natural resorption, and **4** deciduous central incisors. **(b)** An alternate method of exposing the maxillary anterior teeth is to use the occlusal technique with a standard #2 film. Observe the following: **1** deciduous canine; **2** crown of permanent lateral incisor; **3** unerupted permanent central incisors—note that root formation has not started yet; **4** thin radiolucent line indicating the location of the median palatine suture; **5** partially resorbed root of deciduous central incisor; **6** deciduous central incisors; and **7** deciduous lateral incisor.

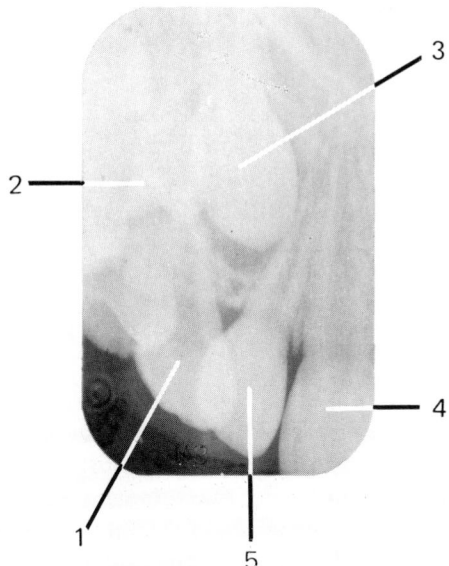

Figure 18–9. Radiograph of maxillary canine area shows **1** deciduous canine; **2** crown of first premolar; **3** unerupted permanent canine—note that part of crown is still in a follicle as indicated by radiolucent area around the tip of the crown; **4** permanent central incisor; and **5** permanent lateral incisor, which appears to be tipped distally and overlapping with deciduous canine.

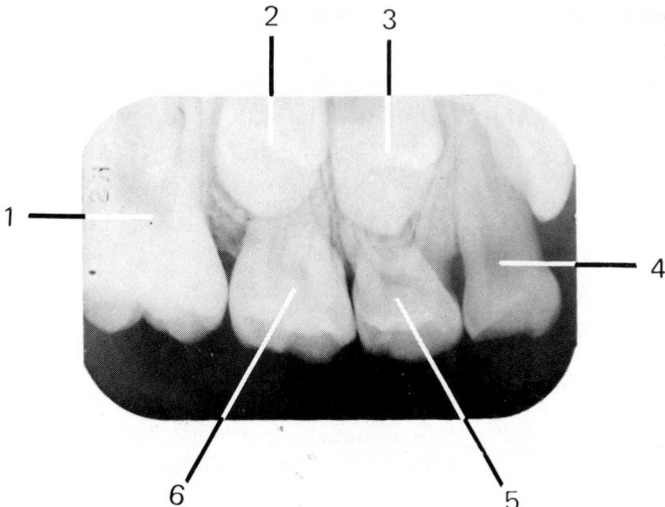

Figure 18–10. Radiograph of maxillary molar area shows **1** permanent first molar; **2** crown of unerupted second premolar; **3** crown of unerupted first premolar; **4** deciduous canine; **5** deciduous first molar—notice that the roots are almost completely resorbed; and **6** deciduous second molar—notice that the shadow of the still unresorbed lingual root is superimposed on the crown of the still unerupted second premolar.

THE OCCLUSAL SURVEY FOR CHILDREN

The occlusal technique is the same for children as for adults, except that the exposure time is decreased. Although the film may be positioned several ways, the maxillary and mandibular topographical surveys described in Chapter 17 are the two variations used most often if the large occlusal film is used. When the child's mouth is too small to accommodate the occlusal film, a smaller film—usually the #2 posterior—is positioned in whatever direction will give the maximum coverage of the desired area.

THE LATERAL JAW SURVEY FOR CHILDREN

The technique for making the lateral jaw exposure is fully described in Chapter 20. The exposure can be made with any size extraoral film or with an occlusal film placed against the cheek when the child is small or the dentist is interested only in a limited area of the teeth. If an occlusal film is used, line up the longest dimension of the film so that it is flush with the lower border of the mandible and line up the front edge of the film with the corner of the mouth. Place the tube side of the film against the cheek and ask the child to hold it with the fingers or palm of the hand. Use the ala–tragus line as a guide to parallel the child's occlusal plane with the plane of the floor, and press against the top of the child's head gently until the head is tipped about 20 degrees toward the side of the film. Then ask the child to close the mouth so that the upper and lower teeth touch each other. Direct the central ray through a point of entry toward the center of the film at a vertical angulation of about –10 degrees from a point slightly behind and below the angle of the opposite mandible.

When extraoral films are used, the size depends on the size of the child's head and the structures the dentist wishes to include. Place the tube side toward the cheek and center the film so that it covers all structures of interest. Several head positions are used with extraoral films; the child may be upright or supine, or the cassette may be laid flat on a table and the child sits in front of it and bends the head until the face contacts the tube side. With some practice each operator develops a favorite technique.

CHAPTER SUMMARY

Good radiographs are essential if the dentist is to provide proper care for the child patient. Without them, incipient caries would be overlooked during a mirror and explorer examination, and studies of facial growth and development or tooth eruption could not be accurately made. Any size film, in whatever number suits the purpose, may be used. The first exposures should be preplanned, rather than occurring in frightening emergency situations, and at a preschool age—preferably when the child is about 3 years old.

The procedures may vary—intraoral or extraoral—with slight modifications due to the smaller size of the face, the dental arches, and the teeth, but they are similar to those performed on adults. A major difference is in the psychological approach. The child has a natural curiosity combined with a fear of the unknown. Securing the child's confidence and cooperation is absolutely essential because the radiograph is completely useless if the child moves suddenly or fails to hold the film in position. Greater care must be exercised in positioning the film packet because some of the deciduous teeth may be loose. Because the bony structures are smaller, the exposure time required is about one third shorter.

KEY WORDS

Amelogenesis imperfecta   Fistula
Anodontia   Herpes labialis
Aphthous ulcer   Parulis
Deciduous teeth   Pulp polyp
Dentigerous cysts   Supernumerary teeth

REVIEW QUESTIONS

1. At what age is the first radiographic survey usually made on a child? (a) at age 3, (b) at age 6, (c) at age 9, (d) at age 12.

2. Which of these conditions would not interfere with film packet positioning in a child? (a) herpes labialis, (b) loose teeth, (c) calculus deposits, (d) malpositioned teeth.

3. Which of these factors does not need to be considered when deciding what size film to use on a child? (a) the size and shape of the dental arches, (b) the degree of stain or calculus present, (c) the size and shape of the mouth opening, (d) the age and emotional stability of the child.

4. What is the best time to give a nervous child sedation prior to radiographic procedures? (a) the evening before the appointment, (b) before breakfast on the day of the appointment, (c) at least two hours before the appointment, (d) about 20 minutes before the appointment.

5. What change in angulation is usually required when using the bisecting technique on a child patient? (a) direct the horizontal angulation mesiodistally, (b) direct the horizontal angulation distomesially, (c) increase the vertical angulation, (d) decrease the vertical angulation.

6. Which of these is not a benefit derived from making radiographic surveys on children? (a) incipient carious lesions can be detected, (b) anodontia can be prevented, (c) supernumerary teeth can be detected, (d) abnormal tooth development can be detected.

7. Which film size is generally easiest to position on a 6-year-old child? (a) #1, (b) #2, (c) #3, (d) #4.

BIBLIOGRAPHY

Eastman Kodak: *X-rays in Dentistry.* Rochester, NY: 1985

Nowak AJ, Creedon RL, Musselman RJ, et al: Summary of the conference on radiation exposure in pediatric dentistry. *J Am Dent Assoc* **103**:426–428, 1981

Rinn Corporation: *Intraoral Radiography with Rinn XCP/BAI Instruments.* Elgin, IL: 1983

Radiography for the Edentulous Patient

OBJECTIVES

By the end of this chapter the student should be able to

1. Explain the importance of making a radiographic survey of edentulous areas.
2. Identify the film requirements for an edentulous survey.
3. Differentiate the procedures used for making the survey in a fully or a partially edentulous patient.

THE IMPORTANCE OF RADIOGRAPHY FOR THE EDENTULOUS PATIENT

A complete examination of the edentulous patient includes radiographs along with the visual and digital inspection. **Preventive radiography** is often of great benefit to the fully and partially edentulous because the normal appearance of the **arches (dental ridges)** may conceal problems underneath. Most edentulous persons have lost their teeth through neglect of decay, infection, or untreated periodontal conditions. Although the teeth have been extracted and the ridges have healed in a satisfactory manner, infection may not have been totally eradicated. It can usually be detected and eliminated only if radiographs are made before prosthetic treatments begin. Occasionally, too, oral malignancies existing in elderly patients are first detected on radiographs. Unfortunately, many edentulous patients do not understand why radiographs are needed. Sometimes even the dentist may think that since the patient has been wearing dentures for years, everything must be in order.

Potential sources of difficulty may be present in a substantial number of edentulous ridges that interfere with the comfortable wearing of prosthetic appliances. A recent survey of panoramic radiographs from 448 edentulous patients in need of complete denture treatment showed the following results: Forty-two patients had one or both mental foramina at or near the crest of the residual ridge. Foreign bodies (such as bits of amalgam, buckshot, or broken canal broaches) were found on 17 radiographs. Fifteen of these patients had impacted or unerupted teeth, 5 had roots embedded within the ridges, and 15 showed various radiopacities.

These are only some of the conditions that may exist under an apparently healthy ridge. The list is imposing enough to suggest that making a radiographic survey on an edentulous patient should be considered extremely important. The Dental Radiographic Patient Selection Criteria Panel, sponsored by the Food and Drug Administration, recommends a full-mouth intraoral radiographic or panoramic examination for newly edentulous patients.

FILM REQUIREMENTS FOR THE EDENTULOUS SURVEY

The easiest way of making the **edentulous survey** is with panoramic film (Fig. 19–1). Most edentulous surveys are made in this manner because it is convenient for the patient and requires only one film. All maxillary and mandibular structures can be visualized in proper relationship to each other. Panoramic techniques are explained in greater detail in Chapter 21. If an examination of the panoramic radiograph reveals that unerupted teeth, root tips, or areas of suspected pathology are present, it is advisable to expose supplementary periapical films in those areas to obtain greater definition and detail.

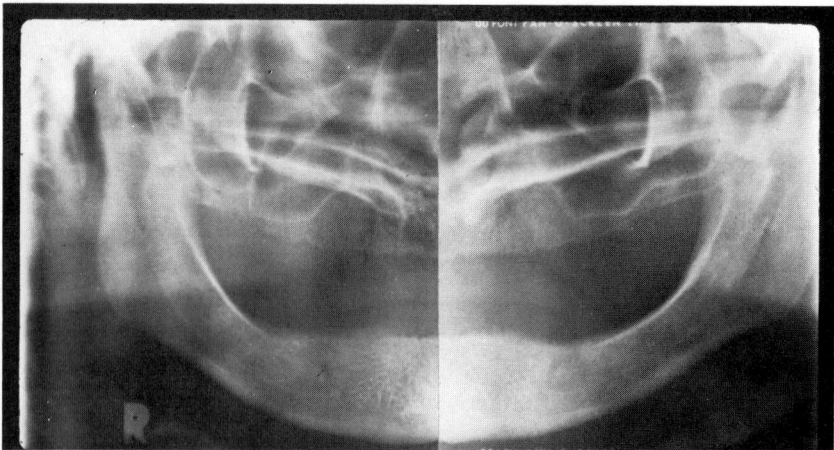

Figure 19–1. Complete edentulous survey made on panoramic-type x-ray machine. Relationship of the maxillary and mandibular structures is shown on a single film. *(Courtesy of UCLA School of Dentistry, Los Angeles, CA.)*

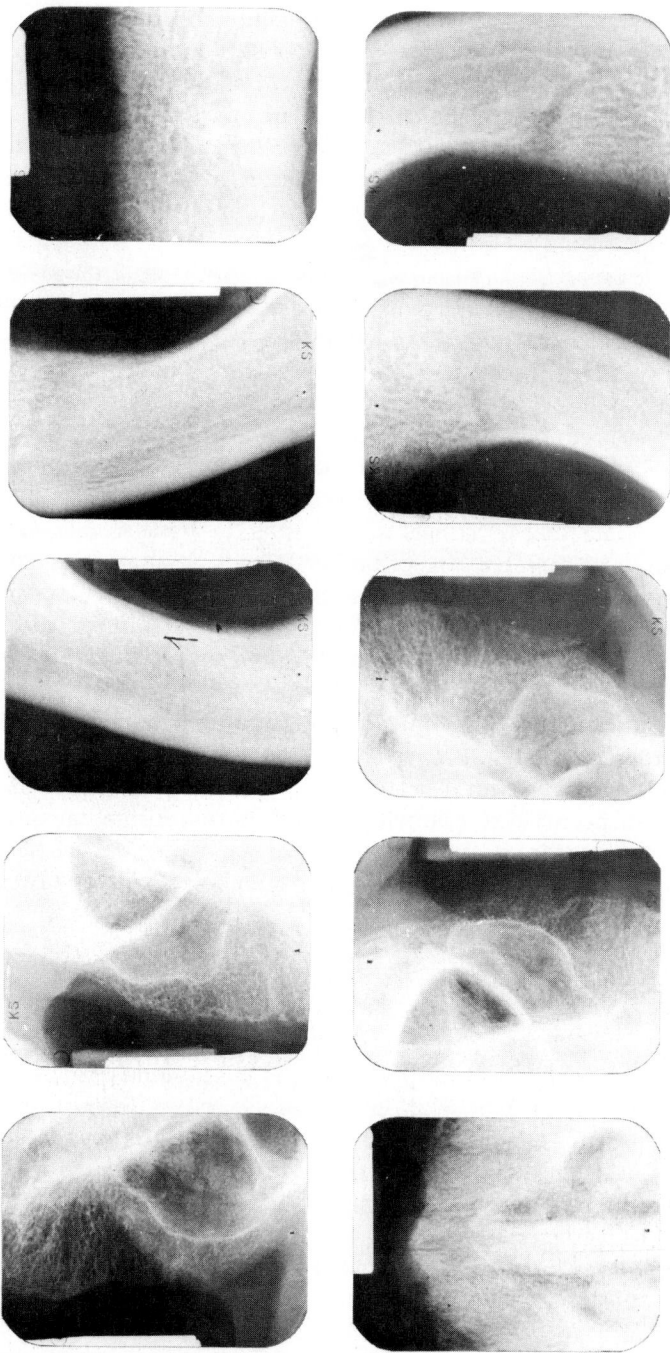

Figure 19–2. Edentulous survey made with 10 standard #2 periapical films. All exposures were made with the paralleling technique, as evidenced by the radiopaque outline cast by the biteblocks. Can you mount these radiographs correctly? *(Courtesy of UCLA School of Dentistry, Los Angeles, CA.)*

Several methods involving various combinations of intraoral, occlusal, or extra-oral films are commonly used for a radiographic survey of the edentulous mouth us-ing the conventional x-ray machine. Some dentists prefer to use 14 periapical films—7 for the maxillary and 7 for the mandibular ridge—placing the films over the same ar-eas of the ridges as they would if the teeth were still present. Others use only 10 films (Fig. 19–2). Still others prefer a total of seven films: two occlusal films (one in each arch) and five periapical films (one in each of the four posterior regions and one in the mandibular incisor region).

In addition to being faster to make and subjecting the patient to less radiation, the latter method has the advantage of pinpointing the location of root fragments, lesions, or other objects because two planes of reference are available instead of one. The oc-clusal film shows a larger section of the jaw structures in relationship to each other and the buccolingual location of teeth or lesions in a horizontal plane, whereas the pe-riapical films show them in a vertical plane.

The occlusal radiograph serves as an excellent guide in establishing the relative position of various structures or lesions to recognizable **landmarks;** however, it may not show some details that periapical radiographs do. Periapical films are used in all four molar areas to supplement the occlusal film, because anatomical restrictions often keep the film from being inserted far enough back to include the third molar area. It is in this region that broken root fragments or unerupted teeth are most likely to be dis-covered. The anterior region of the mandible is also radiographed, because the small size of the mandibular incisors and the denseness of the bone near the front of the mandible often make the identification of small root fragments very difficult on oc-clusal exposures.

Additional films may be used to supplement such a seven-film survey if the pres-ence of some unsuspected object is detected and more information is required. Other effective methods for viewing large edentulous areas involve the use of extraoral films. The conventional x-ray machine may be used to make a lateral jaw exposure on each side.

TECHNIQUES FOR MAKING THE EDENTULOUS SURVEY

Fundamentally, the technique for exposing the 14 edentulous regions of the mandible or maxillae are very similar to the suggested procedures for exposing the periapical re-gions that were described in Chapter 15. These exposures can be made with any size periapical film, but the standard #2 film is generally the film of choice.

Several minor modifications in technique are required for x-raying edentulous ar-eas. Normally, the teeth serve as landmarks to guide film placement. Also, the center of interest is no longer the teeth but the ridge. Because the teeth are no longer present, visualizing the bisecting plane and establishing horizontal and vertical planes are more difficult, particularly when the bisecting technique is used. Fortunately, a fair amount of leeway in horizontal angulation is permissible, because the absence of teeth eliminates the problem of overlapping tooth images. In the bisecting method, since the long axes of the teeth can no longer be used as a guide, one determines vertical angu-

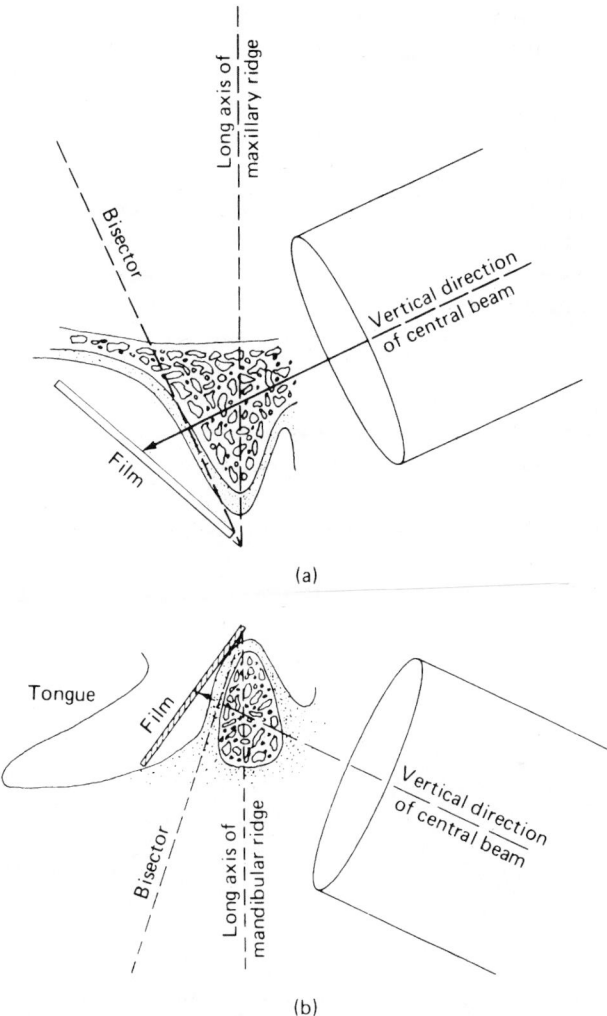

Figure 19–3. Diagrams showing the relationship of the film to the ridge of an edentulous patient. The film packet lies much flatter in the mouth when teeth are missing. Films are placed vertically for anterior and horizontally for posterior exposures. Unless film holders are used, the film is stabilized by the patient's thumb or index finger. When the rules of bisecting are followed, an imaginary line can be drawn vertically through the ridge to substitute for the long axis of the teeth formerly in the ridge. The central ray is directed perpendicularly to the bisector to determine the correct vertical angulation. The correct horizontal angulation is difficult to determine in the edentulous patient; however, it is not a major consideration since the absence of teeth eliminates overlapping. **(a)** Maxillary edentulous ridge. **(b)** Mandibular edentulous ridge.

lation by bisecting the angle formed between the recording plane of the film and an imaginary line through the ridge that substitutes for the long axes of the teeth (Fig. 19–3). Unfortunately, when the patient holds the film with the fingers, it lies much flatter than when teeth are present. This often results in a failure to show all the details of a small area, and in some, dimensional distortion of the visible structure occurs. However, acceptable radiographs can be produced.

The paralleling technique usually gives better results. Radiographic detail is improved and dimensional distortion is minimized when film holders, properly supported by cotton rolls or styrofoam blocks, are used to hold the film parallel to the long axis of the ridge.

When all the teeth are missing, cotton rolls, blocks of Styrofoam, or a combination can be used, with ordinary biteblocks or film holders as the XCP instruments. The thickness of the cotton rolls or Styrofoam will determine the coverage of the edentulous ridge. The film is placed vertically in the anterior biteblocks and horizontally in the posterior biteblocks. Because definite landmarks are seldom present, one must guess the best film position. Obviously, the incisor and molar regions are easiest to locate. Shifting the film distally or mesially is necessary to locate the canine and premolar regions. The biteblock or film holder is then placed in the mouth with the film parallel to the ridge being examined. The patient closes, holding the film in position. The

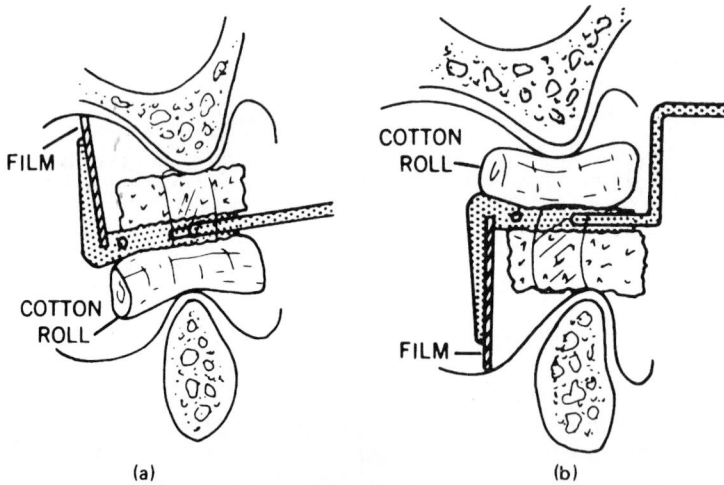

FILM

COTTON ROLL

(a)

COTTON ROLL

FILM

(b)

Figure 19–4. When all teeth are missing, cotton rolls, blocks of Styrofoam, or a combination of both can be used with the XCP instruments. Their thickness will determine the amount of film coverage of the edentulous ridges. The instrument is positioned in the mouth with the film parallel to the ridge area being examined. The patient closes the mouth, stabilizing and holding the film in position, and the standard procedures are followed. (a) Maxillary anterior region—the film holder is rotated so the film is directed upward for the maxillary posterior areas. (b) Mandibular posterior region—the film holder is rotated so that the film is directed down for the mandibular areas. (Courtesy of Rinn Corporation, Elgin, IL.)

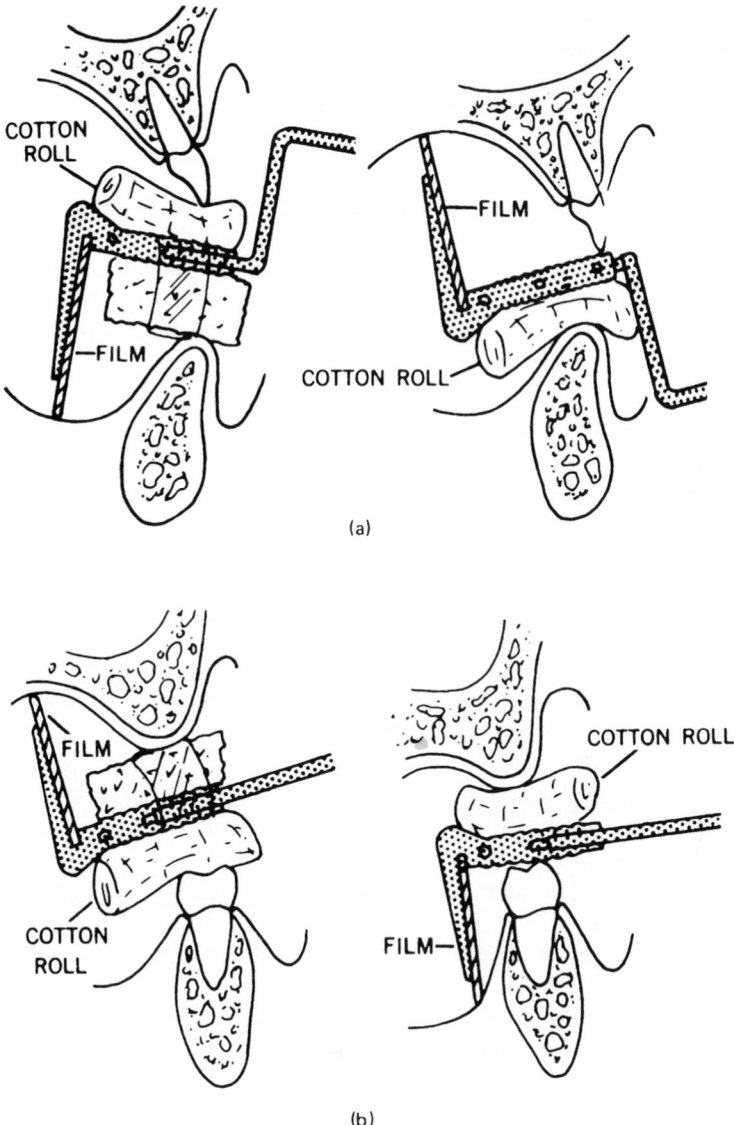

(a)

(b)

Figure 19-5. The versatile XCP instruments can also be used in radiography of the partially edentulous mouth by substituting a cotton roll or block of Styrofoam (or a similar radiolucent material) for the space normally occupied by the crowns of the missing teeth and then following standard procedures. (a) Edentulous mandibular anterior region—opposite placement for the maxillary region. (b) Edentulous maxillary posterior region—rotate the instrument the opposite way for the mandibular posterior areas. *(Courtesy of Rinn Corporation, Elgin, IL.)*

final step is to direct the rays horizontally and vertically toward the center of the film perpendicularly to the mean tangent of the facial side of the ridge and to the plane of the film (Fig. 19–4). As a rule, about 25 percent less exposure is required for an edentulous area than for one with teeth.

One can also modify this technique for use with the partially edentulous patient by substituting cotton rolls or a block of Styrofoam for the space normally occupied by the crowns of the missing teeth and then following the standard procedures (Fig. 19–5).

The dentist may prefer to use larger films to make the edentulous survey. The procedure for making this survey was described in Chapter 17. The methods for exposing the lateral jaw and the panoramic films are described in Chapters 20 and 21.

CHAPTER SUMMARY

It may be difficult to convince an edentulous person that radiographs are necessary, especially if there is no discomfort and the ridges appear healthy. However, the incidence of retained roots, impacted teeth, or other pathological conditions is high, and radiographs are a preventive measure.

The film requirements vary and are somewhat dependent on what equipment and film are available. A rapid survey of both ridges can be made on a panoramic film. By using a single film, all structures are shown in relation to each other. If necessary, supplemental films can be exposed.

Another procedure is to expose a series of 10 to 14 periapical films, preferably by the paralleling method. The absence of teeth or landmarks makes positioning and film identification difficult. Horizontal angulation is less critical because there are no tooth structures to overlap.

It is irrelevant whether the exposures are intraoral or extraoral or a combination of both as long as all ridge areas are revealed. Minor technique modifications are made when the patient is only partially edentulous.

KEY WORDS

Edentulous survey
Landmarks

Preventive radiography
Ridge

REVIEW QUESTIONS

1. Which type of film is best suited to reveal the entire ridge? (a) occlusal, (b) periapical, (c) bitewing, (d) panoramic.

2. How much less exposure time is required when the patient is edentulous? (a) 10 percent less, (b) 25 percent less, (c) 45 percent less, (d) 65 percent less.

3. What type of film is never used when making edentulous exposures? (a) occlusal, (b) periapical, (c) panoramic, (d) bitewing.

4. What is the main cause of dimensional distortion on periapical films placed over edentulous areas? (a) film movement, (b) flat position of film, (c) absence of normal landmarks, (d) shadow cast by Styrofoam block.

5. How is the location of the bisector determined in the edentulous patient? (a) by measuring the width of the ridge, (b) by estimating the long axis of the ridge, (c) by directing the central rays parallel to the ridge, (d) by decreasing the vertical angulation.

BIBLIOGRAPHY

Matteson SR, Joseph LP, Bottomley W, et al: The report of the panel to develop radiographic selection criteria for dental patients. *Gen Dent* **39**:264–70, 1991

Rinn Corporation: *Intraoral Radiography with Rinn XCP/BAI Instruments.* Elgin, IL: 1983

Seals Jr. RR, Williams EO, Jones JD: Panoramic radiographs: necessary for edentulous patients? *J Am Dent Assoc* **123**:74–78, 1992

CHAPTER 20

Extraoral Radiography

OBJECTIVES

By the end of this chapter the student should be able to

1. Identify the types of film used in extraoral radiography.
2. Identify three reasons for making extraoral exposures.
3. Identify the types of surveys that can be performed extraorally.
4. Differentiate between the steps required to make a temporomandibular joint and a lateral skull survey.

INTRODUCTION

Traditionally, most dental radiographs have been exposed intraorally, but such radiographs did not always satisfy the diagnostic needs of the dentist. More information than the periapical or bitewing radiograph revealed was occasionally desired. Thus a series of accessory techniques were developed by which the film was positioned extraorally (outside the mouth at the front or side of the patient's head). As extraoral films were generally ordered by the dentist only in special circumstances, they were considered to be accessory or supplemental films.

The advent, about three decades ago, of the **panoramic** x-ray machines may conceivably reverse the current emphasis on intraoral exposures. Because panoramic exposures are easy to make and require less time to expose than is necessary for a complete intraoral survey, many dentists make the initial examination with a panoramic radiograph. When deemed necessary to obtain better detail in an area of interest, intraoral films are taken to supplement it. Panoramic radiographs are discussed more fully in Chapter 21.

Many dental offices have only the conventional x-ray units because of the high cost of the panoramic x-ray machines. Most of the extraoral techniques described in this chapter can be performed by a trained operator using a conventional x-ray unit.

TYPES OF EXTRAORAL FILM

There is no definite rule governing extraoral film size. Any film that will accomplish the intended purpose may be used. A variety of film, ranging in size from the standard periapical or the occlusal film to the large 5 by 7-in. or 8 by 10-in. (13 by 18-cm or 21 by 26-cm) film, can be used with most conventional x-ray units.

As explained in Chapter 8, only the screen films are intended solely for extraoral use. Because they are extremely light-sensitive and not enclosed in a protective sealed wrapper like the periapical or occlusal films, they must be carefully loaded into a cassette under darkroom safelight illumination. The majority of extraoral exposures are made with **screen film** placed in a **cassette** with **intensifying screens.**

USES OF EXTRAORAL RADIOGRAPHY

Extraoral films are used (1) to show a larger area than an intraoral film can show, (2) when swelling or injury prevents intraoral film placement, (3) when a child will not tolerate films intraorally, and (4) when one wants to show the entire dentition and adjacent structures on a single film. Extraoral radiographs may be used alone to make a facial profile or a cephalometric radiograph, but generally they are used in conjunction with the complete periapical x-ray series.

Periapical film is least used extraorally. Its usefulness is generally limited to very young children. Because of its slightly larger size and the ease of positioning the film packet, occlusal film is more often used. The most common films used for making extraoral radiographs are the 5 by 7-in. and 8 by 10-in. (13 by 18-cm and 21 by 26-cm) screen films. Extraoral radiographs are taken to show large portions of the mandible or the maxilla, a complete posteroanterior view of the skull, a facial profile, a view of the sinuses, or the temporomandibular joint (TMJ). Such radiographs are normally of more value to the oral surgeon, the orthodontist, or the prosthodontist than to the general practitioner. Special-purpose techniques are described in advanced radiography texts and professional journals.

The **posteroanterior** and **lateral jaw surveys** provide an overall view of the facial bones and jaw structures. They are extremely helpful to the oral surgeon in determining the extent of fractures, bone diseases, malignancies, the presence of foreign bodies, and other items of interest. The radiograph of the TMJ is essential in determining the extent of damage caused by tooth loss, injuries, or diseases of this region. The posteroanterior and lateral radiographs of the bones and tooth structures and the profile radiographs of the soft structures show the orthodontist the anatomy of the jaw and the growth and development of the dentition and provide a record of the changes produced by orthodontic treatment.

The prosthodontist frequently makes two facial profile radiographs before the teeth are extracted—one to record the profile of the patient and the other to record the normal relationship of the teeth to each other when the jaws are closed normally. To

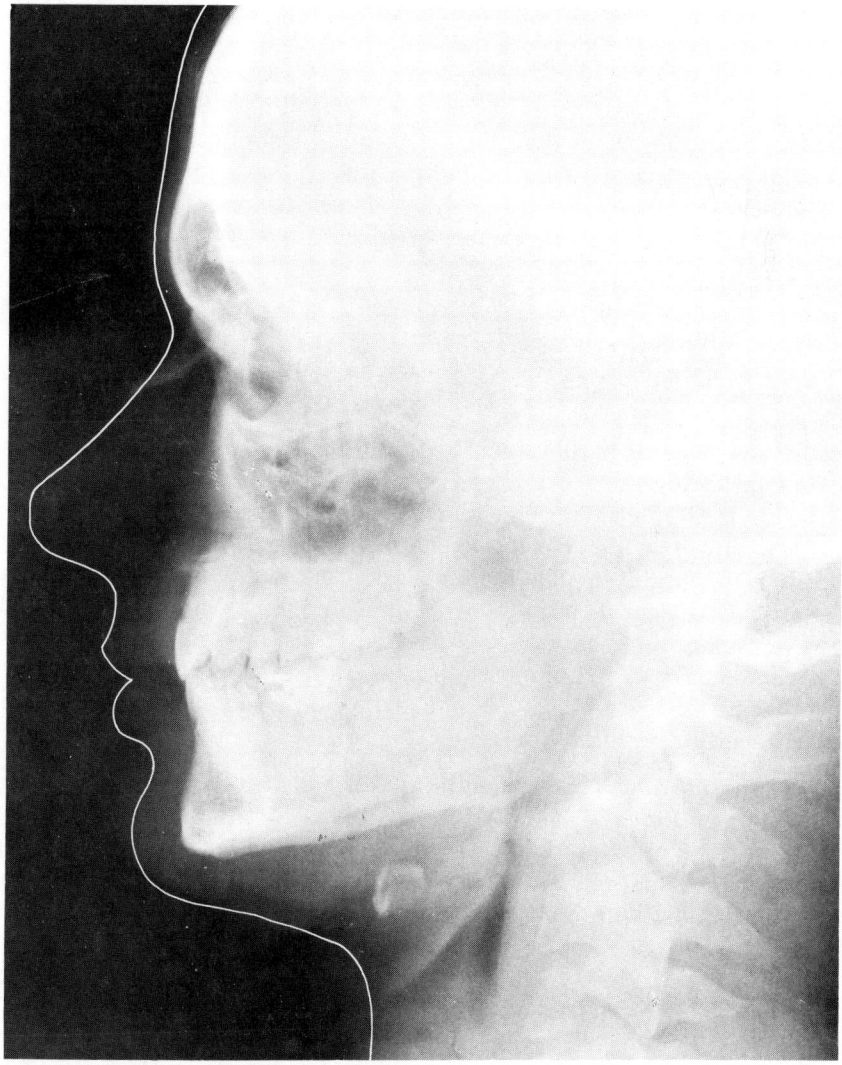

Figure 20–1. Radiograph profile exposed in extraoral cassette. Radiograph was underdeveloped to enhance the outlines of the soft tissues. Template can be made by cutting along the image of the facial outline, which then serves as a guide in maintaining the profile.

do this, two films are placed in a cassette and are exposed together but developed differently. A template to be held against the face as a guide in maintaining the original contour and vertical dimensions of the face can be made by cutting along the outline of the profile on one of the radiographs. The other radiograph is kept as a record. Postoperative radiographs are also frequently used by the prosthodontists to compare the original conditions with the results (Fig. 20–1).

As the larger extraoral films are packaged differently from intraoral films, they require special handling in the darkroom. Types of films and techniques for loading them are fully explained in Chapter 8.

Many film positions and techniques require special equipment and a sound knowledge of the anatomical structures through which the radiation beam is directed. Most of these exposures are made in hospitals, x-ray laboratories, or oral surgery offices by highly experienced operators. Only a few of the simpler exposures are described in this book. For further information about extraoral exposures, consult the Bibliography at the end of this chapter as well as the books in the dental school library.

EXTRAORAL EXPOSURES MADE WITH INTRAORAL FILM

Occasionally, impacted or partially impacted third molars cannot be properly visualized on intraoral radiographs. Complete visualization, evaluation, and final diagnosis can only be made after studying one or more extraoral projections. Such projections can be made in any office that has a conventional x-ray machine. Usually the large occlusal film is used, but the smaller #2 film is also used. Extraoral radiographs of tooth structures are not as clear as intraoral exposures and fail to show many fine details. This, however, is of minor importance when one considers that limited access, gagging, or swelling might make it impossible to expose any films intraorally.

The following steps are suggested in making a survey of an impacted mandibular third molar area using occlusal film extraorally (Fig. 20–2):

1. Adjust the ala–tragus line so that the occlusal plane of the maxillary arch is parallel to the plane of the floor.
2. Position the film extraorally, tube side toward the face, so that it is centered over the mandibular third molar area. Place the widest dimension of the film parallel with the lower border of the mandible and let the front edge of the film extend forward to the corner of the mouth.
3. Tell the patient to hold the film and to thrust the jaw forward to avoid superimposing the vertebrae over the site of the impaction.
4. Tilt the patient's head slightly toward the side of the film and direct the central ray toward the middle of the film at a vertical angulation of about –15 to –20 degrees through the point of entry on the side opposite the film, just below and behind the angle of the mandible. This enables the central ray to pass beneath the mandible without superimposing the structures of one side of the mandible on the other (Fig. 20–2).

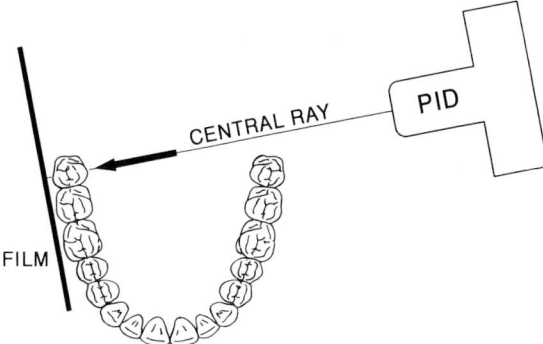

Figure 20–2. Diagram indicating direction of the central ray and placement of the film and PID for the impacted mandibular third molar area. The occlusal film is placed with the widest dimension horizontally (long axis of film parallel to floor). Two changes are necessary to use this technique for the maxillary impacted third molar area. The film is placed vertically so that the upper half is centered over the maxillary third molar, and the central ray is positioned approximately 1 in. (2.5 cm) above the angle of the mandible and just behind the posterior border of the mandible. PID, position-indicating device.

There is a variation of this technique that shows both the maxillary and mandibular impacted third molar areas on the same film. Make two changes to accomplish this: (1) position the film so that its longest dimension is vertical, its front edge extends to the corner of the mouth, and its lower border is even and parallel with the inferior border of the mandible, thus causing the occlusal plane between the maxillary and mandibular third molars to be at the center of the film; and (2) direct the central ray toward the center of the film at a vertical angulation of about –15 to –20 degrees through the point of entry on the side opposite to the film, about 1 in. (2.5 cm) above and 1/2 in. (1.25 cm) behind the angle of the mandible.

As this survey is primarily made to determine the location of the third molars rather than to evaluate the progress of decay, the dimensional distortion and magnification of the image from such an angulation do not detract from the diagnostic value of the radiograph.

EXPOSURES WITH EXTRAORAL FILMS

Many methods can be used to make radiographic surveys of the head and face. Depending on the equipment available, the patient may be upright in a standard dental chair, lying reclined in a contour chair or on a special table, or bending over a table and placing the head on it for stability. In the latter case, plastic bags filled with sand may be used to prop the head at a desired angle and keep it stable during the exposure. It is not within the scope of this book to describe all these techniques.

The Lateral Jaw Survey

The **lateral jaw survey** (Fig. 20–3), also known as the lateral oblique survey, is described first because it is the most frequent extraoral exposure made with the conventional x-ray unit. The lateral jaw survey is especially valuable to use with children (Fig. 20–4), with patients who have fractures or swelling, with patients who are too young or senile to hold intraoral films, and patients with other special problems. The lateral jaw radiograph is often made to evaluate the condition of the bone or locate larger lesions or impacted teeth. Some practitioners consider the lateral jaw survey an essential adjunct to a full-mouth periapical series.

Seat the patient upright in the dental chair with the **midsagittal plane** of the head perpendicular and the **occlusal plane** parallel to the floor. This can be done rapidly by using the **ala–tragus line** as a guide. Some radiographers prefer a slight tilt of the head (about 10 to 20 degrees) toward the side on which the cassette is held. Whether the cassette is positioned with its longest dimension parallel or perpendicular to the lower border of the body of the mandible depends on the size used. Ideally, the front edge of the cassette should protrude slightly beyond the tip of the nose and the chin. Normally the region of the first molars will be near the center of the film. The patient presses the tube side of the cassette firmly against the cheek with the palm of one hand and curves the fingers so that they rest on the top of the head.

Unfortunately, a true projection of the central ray is not possible in the lateral jaw survey. Some magnification and dimensional distortion are unavoidable, because true paralleling is impossible for anatomical reasons. Although the rays can be directed perpendicularly toward the film in a horizontal plane, this cannot be done in the vertical plane because overlapping of the right and left sides would occur. Thus, depending on whether the center of interest is in the region of the body or of the ramus of the mandible, the central ray is directed either slightly underneath the angle of the

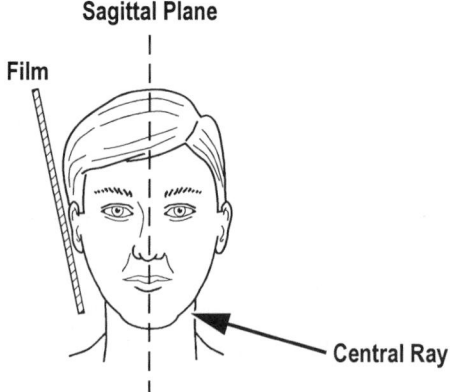

Figure 20–3. Lateral jaw survey (lateral oblique survey). Note the central ray is directed at the cassette slightly underneath the opposite side of the mandible.

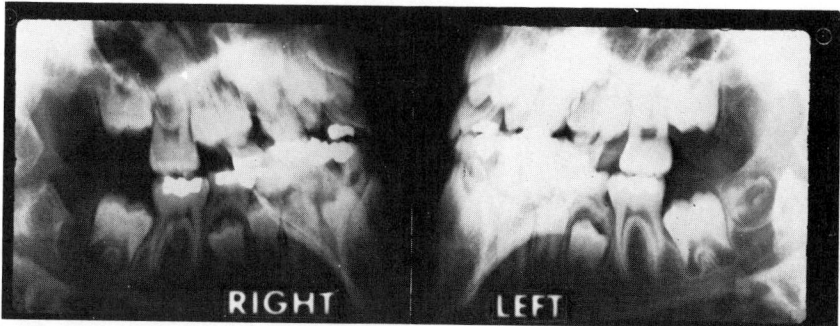

Figure 20–4. Typical lateral jaw radiograph of a child with a mixed dentition. This exposure is generally made with 5 by 7-in. (13 by 18-cm) film on adults.

mandible or 1 in. (2.5 cm) higher and slightly behind the ramus on the side opposite the film. In either case, the trajectory of the central ray is oblique to the vertical plane. A larger area of the maxilla and mandible can be surveyed by projecting the beam from underneath the angle of the mandible than from behind the ramus. However, doing this increases the dimensional distortion because the vertical angulation of the x-radiation is not as steep; therefore more detail of a limited area is observed when the point of entry is behind the ramus.

Figure 20–5 shows four possible centers of interest on the radiograph: the ramus area, the molars, the premolars, and the incisors. To change the center of interest, one varies the angle at which the film is held against the face and the direction of the position indicating device (PID), so that the beam of radiation is directed perpendicularly to the desired area, usually at the level of the occlusal plane. Before making the exposure, ask the patient to thrust the mandible forward so that the vertebrae will not be superimposed on mandibular structures. Estimate the target–film distance and the density of the structures to determine the exposure factors. Follow the manufacturer's recommendations on exposure time according to the type of film used.

The Lateral Skull Survey

The 8 by 10-in. (21 by 26-cm) film used in the **lateral skull survey** (Fig. 20–6) is large enough to give a lateral view of the entire head. It shows the anteroposterior and the superoinferior borders of the skull as well as the relationship of anatomical structures to one another. That is why this survey is so valuable to orthodontists and prosthodontists.

The patient is requested to sit in the conventional upright position. The cassette is held parallel with the midsagittal plane of the head. Center the film with the tube side over the zygomatic arch and make sure that the front edge protrudes about an inch past the tip of the nose.

As with all extraoral exposures, the tube head and position indicating device (PID) are at the side opposite to the film. Direct the central ray at 0 degrees vertical angulation so that it will pass through the **acoustic meatus** of the ear and perpendicu-

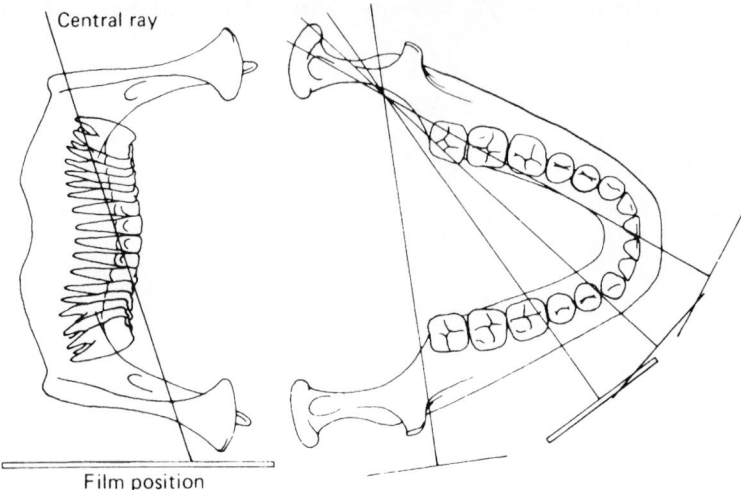

Figure 20–5. X-ray beam direction for the lateral jaw projection. Rays strike the film obliquely in the vertical plane but should be perpendicular in the horizontal plane. A true lateral projection of an entire side of the jaw is not possible because the image of the opposite side would be superimposed on it. The lateral jaw projection must be made with some oblique angulation. The beam of radiation can be directed toward the area of interest from two basic directions: (1) underneath the mandible opposite the one being radiographed or (2) behind the mandible opposite the one being radiographed. *(Reproduced with permission from Wuehrmann AH, Manson-Hing LR:* Dental Radiology, *5th ed. St. Louis, MO: Mosby, 1981.)*

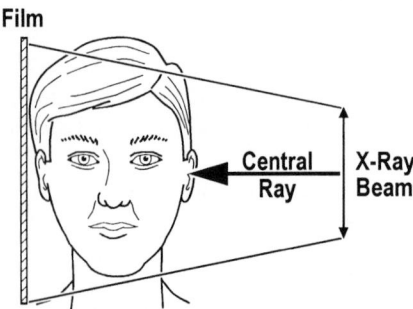

Figure 20–6. Lateral skull survey. The central ray is directed at 0 degrees vertical angulation through the acoustic meatus of the ear and perpendicular to the cassette.

larly toward the center of the film. The target–film distance for this exposure may vary from 36 to 72 in. (0.9 to 1.8 m).

Instruct the patient to keep the jaws in an at-rest position. Set the exposure time as directed by the manufacturer for the type of film used.

The Facial Profile Survey

To make a **facial profile** exposure (Fig. 20–1), seat the patient in the same manner as for the lateral skull survey. Depending on whether only the bone tissues or the details of the soft tissues are to be examined, either one or two films are loaded into an 8 by 10-in. (21 by 26-cm) cassette with an intensifying screen.

The procedure for holding the cassette and the angulation of the central ray are identical to those described for the lateral skull survey. The difference is in the exposure time and the developing. If the objective is to concentrate on the soft tissues, the film is developed for only 1 1/4 minutes at 68°F (20°C). Full development for about 5 minutes at 68°F (20°C) is required to show the bone structures fully.

The Posteroanterior Survey

The **posteroanterior survey** (Fig. 20–7) is not as frequently made as the lateral skull survey. Such a radiograph shows the entire skull in the posteroanterior plane. Because the right and left sides of the bony and facial structures are not superimposed on each other, this survey is often used to supplement the lateral skull survey.

An 8 by 10-in. (21 by 26-cm) cassette with intensifying screen may be held by the patient but preferably is held in a firm position by some form of supporting device. Frequently the cassette is placed flat against the side of the wall, and the patient stands in front of the cassette so that the forehead and nose touch the face of the cassette. The central ray is then directed toward the external **occipital protuberance**—the large bump that can be felt by palpitating the occipital bone near the base of the skull—at a vertical angulation of 0 degrees. The target–film distance is at least 36 in. (0.9 m).

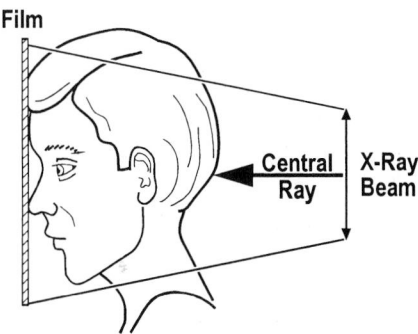

Figure 20–7. Posteroanterior survey. The nose and forehead touch the cassette. The central ray is directed at the occipital protuberance at a vertical angulation of 0 degrees and perpendicular to the cassette.

The Sinus Survey

The **sinus survey** (Fig. 20–8) is also known as the **Waters' projection** and is difficult to make. It is generally made only by commercial x-ray laboratories or in the offices of specialists.

It is similar to the posteroanterior survey except that the center of interest is focused on the middle third of the face. This is accomplished by asking the patient to keep the mouth open as the face of the cassette is touched with the nose and chin. As in the posteroanterior survey, the central ray is directed toward the center of the film through the occipital protuberance at 0-degrees vertical angulation. The target–film distance is usually a minimum of 36 in. (0.9 m).

The Temporomandibular Joint (TMJ) Survey

The most complex of the frequently made surveys is that of the **temporomandibular joint (TMJ)** (Fig. 20–9). The TMJ is very difficult to examine radiographically because the head of the mandibular **condyle** articulates with the **glenoid fossa** in an area where the structure of the temporal bone is extremely dense. There are probably more ways to make this radiograph and more opinions about how to expose it than for any other extraoral radiograph.

Although radiographic examinations of the TMJ area have been made for many years, numerous dentists were unaware of the correlation of TMJ disorders with the patient's dental health. Furthermore, most operators experienced difficulty in positioning the cassette and PID at the correct angle to obtain a film of diagnostic value. Hence few TMJ films were ordered.

The importance of the TMJ survey has been recognized more fully during the last few years and many dentists are now specializing in disorders of the TMJ. Dental manufacturers have produced new devices to assist in determining the correct angle of exposure and simplifying the procedure.

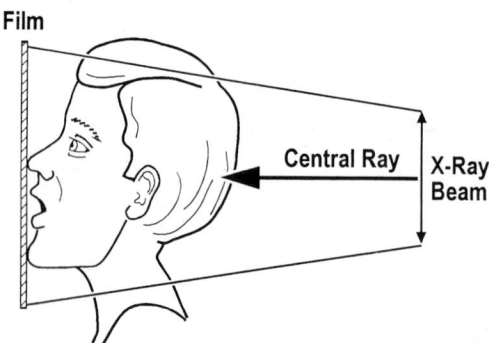

Figure 20–8. Sinus survey (Waters' projection). The nose and chin touch the cassette. The central ray is directed at the occipital protuberance at a vertical angulation of 0 degrees and perpendicular to the cassette.

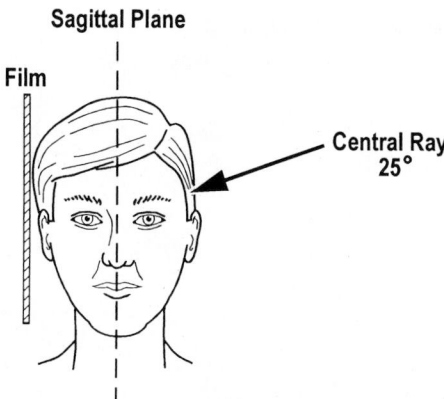

Figure 20–9. Temporomandibular joint survey. The central ray is directed at a vertical angulation of about +25 degrees to the center of the film not covered by lead. The point of entry is located about 2 1/2 in. (6.4 cm) higher and slightly in front of the acoustic meatus of the ear.

Some dentists make only one exposure, whereas others make several—with the mouth closed and the teeth in occlusion, at rest with the teeth slightly separated, and with the mouth fully open (Fig. 20–10). Because this exposure is made from the opposite side, the central ray has to pass first through a series of bones and soft structures. Therefore, the exposure requires extreme care and accuracy in adjusting the cassette to the head position and directing the PID so that the rays will strike the film at the best angle.

A simple technique is to have the patient upright in the dental chair. As the area to be examined is relatively small, a common practice is to use a single large film and make several exposures on it. Parts of the film are covered with lead so that only one part of the film is exposed each time. Thus three or four exposures, with the head of the condyle in a different position each time, can be made consecutively on the same film. Direct the central ray at a vertical angulation of about +25 degrees to the center of the part of the film that is not covered with lead. The point of entry for the central ray is located about 2 1/2 in. (6.4 cm) higher and slightly in front of the acoustic meatus. Caution the patient not to move or change position and follow the manufacturer's suggestions for the exposure time.

The disadvantage of this technique is that it is difficult to stabilize the patient's head and prevent movement. Moreover, without special equipment, it is difficult to repeat the same exposure and get identical results.

The temporomandibular joint survey aids the dentist in diagnosing disturbances of this articulation, such as ankylosis (a stiffening of the joint caused by fibrous or bony union), malignancies, fractures, and tissue changes caused by arthritis. A clear radiograph, or series of radiographs, showing the head of the mandibular condyle in relation to the glenoid fossa of the temporal bone is essential for the dentist to make a diagnostic interpretation.

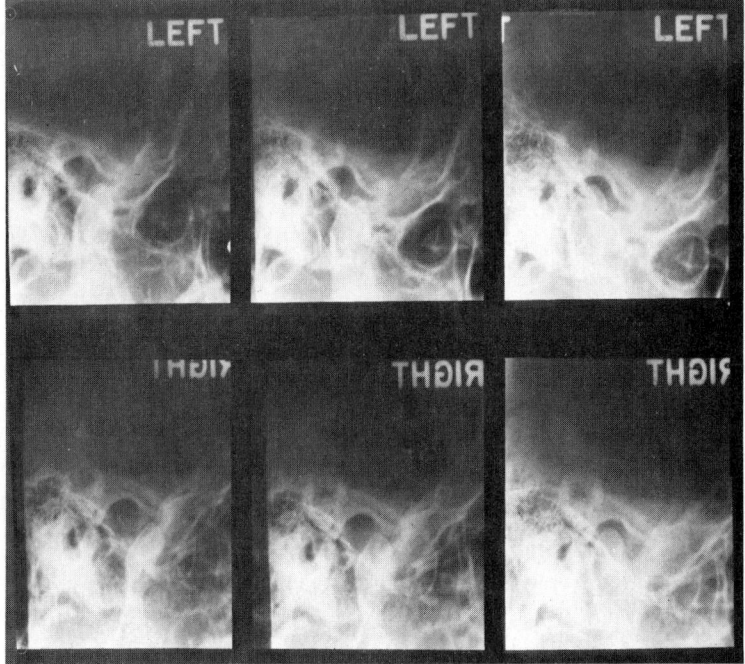

Figure 20–10. Serial radiographs of the temporomandibular joint showing the head of the condyle in the glenoid fossa with the mouth closed, in the at-rest position, and with the mouth open. A stabilizing device of some type is generally required to hold the patient's head in a firm position while the cassette is moved for each exposure on the same side. Such equipment for serial radiography is not available in most offices; however, single exposures can readily be made using techniques similar to those for the lateral jaw exposures. *(Courtesy of McCormack Dental X-ray Laboratory, Santa Fe Springs, CA.)*

CEPHALOMETRIC RADIOGRAPHY

Cephalometric headplates are extraoral radiographs of the head used for making skull and soft-tissue measurements. Although requested occasionally by a general practitioner and more often by a prosthodontist, these are principally required by orthodontists and are an important part of the orthodontic diagnostic survey. Most modern orthodontists now require cephalometric radiographs before treatment, at various stages of treatment, upon completion of treatment, and often as a follow-up procedure. Cephalometric tracings are made from these radiographs. It is now possible to feed the data and measurements derived from these tracings into computers for analysis of the patient's condition or progress. Comparisons are made with similar cases that have already been treated. The orthodontist is thus enabled to establish a preliminary treatment objective and a forecast of the progress.

The word *cephalometric* means "having to do with the measurement of the head." A **cephalometer** is a device used to standardize the placement of the head during exposure. Either conventional x-ray machines modified for cephalometric work or special units may be used. The patient's head must be completely stable, as must the cassette that holds the film. In addition, a cephalometer allows the head to be positioned identically at different times, for a series of identical exposures. To do this, one coordinates the relationship among the direction of the central ray, the patient, and the cassette. Devices called **cephalostats** or **craniostats** are used to stabilize the patient's head parallel to the film and at right angles to the direction of the beam of radiation. Ear rods are pushed into the external openings of the ear. These stabilize the head and also make it possible to secure the same position each time. The cassette with intensifying screens is aligned in a definite relationship to the cephalostats so that the patient's head is between it and the source of radiation. The central ray is directed at 0-degrees angulation toward the patient and the film. On many special units it is possible to turn a knob and move the tube head up or down to correspond to the height of the cassette

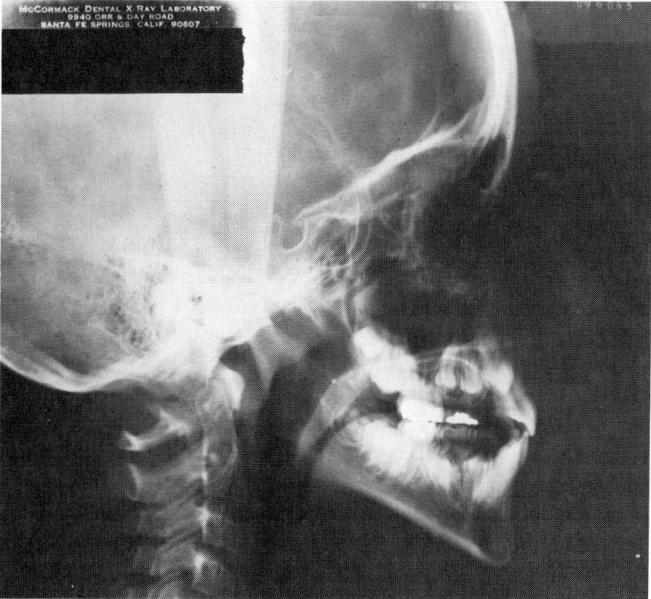

Figure 20–11. Lateral skull cephalometric radiographs are often required by orthodontists for making measurements of the head. Some form of device is essential to position the head to achieve standardization and to establish a fixed relationship among the x-ray tube, the patient's head, and the film cassette. Ear rods are used to stabilize and maintain the head position. The film is positioned in a plane parallel to the midsagittal plane of the patient, and the central ray passes through both ear rods from a target–film distance of 60 in. (1.52 m) or more. Cephalometric tracings may be made from these radiographs. *(Courtesy of McCormack Dental X-ray Laboratory, Santa Fe Springs, CA.)*

when the patient is seated in the chair. Or patients may be required to stand while the cassette and tube head are adjusted to their height as is done when the Orthoceph (a dual-purpose machine that takes both panoramic and cephalometric radiographs) is used (see Fig. 18–2). The target–film distance is normally 60 in. (1.52 m). The exposure time depends on the type of film and intensifying screens used.

Cephalometric radiographs may be either frontal (posteroanterior) or lateral skull projections (Fig. 20–11). Lateral projections (centric soft tissue profiles) are frequently made, sometimes periodically throughout the treatment period. The centric soft tissue profile is used to determine the position and size of the jaws, the steepness of the angle of the mandible, and the relationship of the mandible and maxilla to each other. Tracings of the centric soft tissue profile are made on acetate or special tracing paper with special pencils and pens. The tracing is made after the radiograph and tracing paper are carefully centered over the illuminated viewbox. The procedure is best learned from an experienced teacher or technician.

CHAPTER SUMMARY

Extraoral radiography is the technique of producing radiographs by placing the film at the side of the face or head and positioning the source of radiation on the opposite side. Several advantages to using extraoral radiographs are (1) simplicity and rapidity of procedure, (2) minimum patient discomfort, and (3) large areas can be viewed on a single film.

Three types of x-ray machines are used to produce extraoral radiographs: (1) conventional x-ray machines, (2) panoramic machines, and (3) cephalometric machines.

Extraoral films should be the screen-type, so that the least amount of radiation is used. These films must be loaded into cassettes in the darkroom. Always check the manufacturer's directions for safelight tolerance, exposure time, and processing.

Although extraoral films are exposed for a variety of reasons, the major ones are the following: (1) to show in its entirety a larger area than is possible when intraoral film is used, (2) to make a rapid survey of the teeth and supporting structures, (3) to study areas such as the sinuses or the temporomandibular joints, (4) for studying facial profiles and for measuring the growth and development of the teeth and jaw structures, and (5) for situations where intraoral film placement is inadvisable or impossible.

Initially films were exposed extraorally to supplement the intraoral survey. Several accessory or supplemental techniques that could be used with the conventional x-ray machine evolved. These include techniques for exposing impacted molar areas, the lateral jaw and skull, facial profiles, posteroanterior surveys, the temporomandibular joints, and the sinuses. Cephalometric radiographs are generally exposed at the request of the orthodontist to assist in completing the diagnosis or treatment plan, to make tracings, and to record conditions before, during, and after treatment. Orthodontists, prosthodontists, oral surgeons, periodontists, and pedodontists are major users of extraoral films.

KEY WORDS

Acoustic meatus

Ala–tragus line

Cassette

Cephalometer

Cephalostat

Condyle

Facial profile

Glenoid fossa

Head positioner

Lateral jaw survey

Lateral skull survey

Midsagittal plane

Occipital protuberance

Occlusal plane

Panoramic

Posteroanterior survey

Sagittal plane

Screen film

Sinus survey

Temporomandibular joint (TMJ) survey

REVIEW QUESTIONS

1. Which of these films is most often used in extraoral radiography? (a) periapical film, (b) screen film, (c) occlusal film, (d) nonscreen film.

2. What size film is generally used in cephalometric radiography? (a) 2 1/4 × 3 in. (57 × 76 mm), (b) 5 × 7 in. (13 × 18 cm), (c) 8 × 10 in. (20 × 25 cm), (d) 5 × 12 in. (13 × 30 cm).

3. For which of these purposes is extraoral film least suitable? (a) for detection of interproximal caries, (b) for locating impacted teeth, (c) for viewing the sinuses, (d) for determining the extent of a fracture.

4. Which of these surveys is most frequently ordered by the prosthodontist? (a) sinus, (b) posteroanterior, (c) interproximal, (d) facial profile.

5. Which of these radiographs would best show an impacted mandibular third molar? (a) lateral jaw, (b) bitewing, (c) cephalometric, (d) temporomandibular joint.

6. Which term describes a device used to stabilize the patient's head parallel to the film and at right angles to the direction of the x-ray beam? (a) orbitale, (b) cephalostat, (c) exposure holder, (d) headplate.

BIBLIOGRAPHY

Farman AG, Nortje CJ, Wood RE: *Oral and Maxillofacial Diagnostic Imaging.* St Louis, MO: CV Mosby, 1993

Goaz PW, White SC: *Oral Radiology Principles and Interpretation,* 3rd ed. St. Louis, MO: CV Mosby, 1994

Panoramic Radiography

By the end of this chapter the student should be able to

1. Differentiate between a conventional and a panoramic x-ray machine.
2. Identify the main factor that determines the width of the focal trough.
3. Identify the major factors that affect the geometry of the image.
4. Identify the planes used to position the head correctly.
5. Identify in sequence the basic steps in operating a panoramic x-ray unit.
6. Compare the advantages and disadvantages of panoramic versus intraoral radiographic surveys.
7. Identify five major head-positioning errors that result in faulty panoramic radiographs.

INTRODUCTION

The advent of panoramic radiography has changed and accelerated the use of extraoral films as a major diagnostic aid. The term **panoramic radiography** refers to an important new technique that has been developed and refined within the last three decades. It is also known as **pantomography** (making graphic recordings of contours on radiographic film), **tomography** (making body sections on radiographic film), and **laminography** (from *lamina*, meaning "thin layer," and *graphy*, meaning "to record"), the recording of selected layers of body tissue on radiographic film. The term *panoramic radiography* is most common because the resulting radiograph shows a panoramic view of a large area of the face and lower portion of the head.

Panoramic x-ray machines operate with the patient positioned between the tube head and the cassette that holds the film. The exposure is a continuous one, made as the tube head and cassette rotate slowly about the patient's head during the operational cycle (usually about 15 to 20 seconds). These machines are said to operate on the principle of curved-surface laminography. Lately the term **rotational panoramic radiography** appears to be gaining favor.

By placing an elongated screen film—varying in width from 5 to 6 in. wide and 12 in. long (13 to 15-cm wide and 30-cm long)—in a rigid or flexible cassette that is positioned extraorally, the operator is able to produce an image of the entire dentition, the surrounding alveolar bone, the sinuses, and the temporomandibular joints on a single film. Instead of exposing 16 or more intraoral radiographs, the entire panoramic exposure can be made in less than 3 minutes instead of the 15 minutes usually required for the full-mouth intraoral series. Time is also saved during processing by eliminating the bothersome task of sorting, arranging, and mounting 16 separate films. Not only is the exposure easier and faster to make, but it is also more pleasant for the patient, as pressure against delicate tissues and gagging are eliminated.

 This makes the panoramic radiograph ideal for mass surveys, as are common in the military services and public health clinics, for children, for invalids, and for any situation where a rapid survey is desired. With the aid of a panoramic radiograph, the dentist is able to obtain a complete picture of the area of treatment. Diagnosis is simplified because all the teeth, whether erupted or not, and the sinuses are shown in a consecutive sequence, rather than in a series of separate and overlapping films.

FUNDAMENTALS OF ROTATIONAL PANORAMIC RADIOGRAPHY

During conventional intraoral radiography the x-ray source and the film remain stationary. The opposite happens in **rotational panoramic radiography,** which can be defined as a technique for making radiographic projections by utilizing a narrow beam of x-rays to image a curved layer.

The film in its cassette and the tube head move in opposite directions while the patient stands or is seated in a stationary position (Fig. 21–1). Through a series of rotational points or centers (differing according to the manufacturer), the x-ray beam is directed toward the moving cassette to reveal a select plane of dental anatomy. The **rotational center,** which is defined as the axis on which the tube head and the cassette rotate, is the functional focus of the projection. Unlike the concentric or rectangular beam of x-radiation common in intraoral radiography, the x-rays emerge from a narrow, vertical **slit** opening in the tube head and are constricted to form a narrow band.

The radiation beam then passes vertically through the patient toward the cassette and through another vertical slit in the cassette holder to expose the film that is moving or rotating past (Fig. 21–2). By making use of this narrow opening in the tube head,

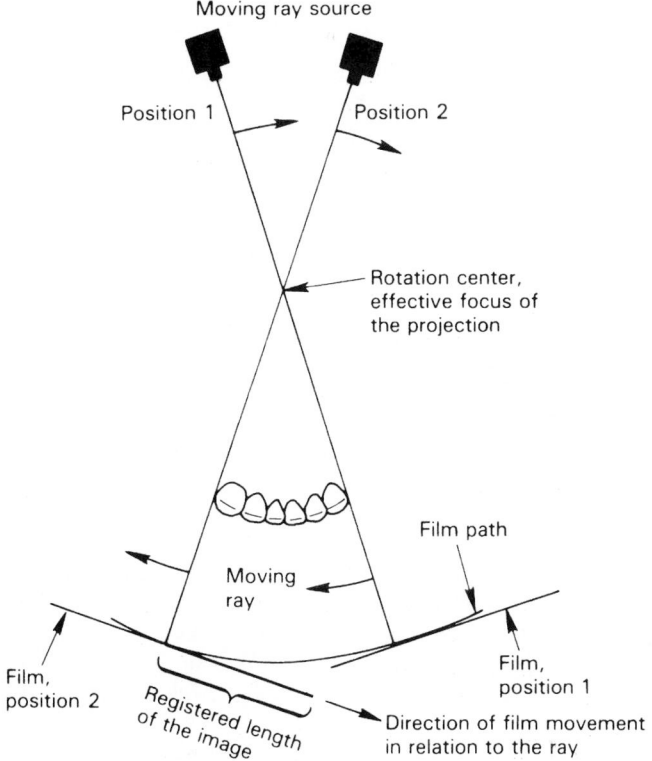

Figure 21–1. Diagram showing the relationship of the moving x-ray beam as it passes through the center of rotation in a horizontal plane toward the path of the moving x-ray film. As the beam scans the object (usually the dental arches), a continuous image is registered on the moving film. *(From a syllabus prepared for a symposium on Panoramic Radiography presented at Anaheim, California, October 3, 1983, by the American Dental Association in cooperation with the University of Texas Health Science Center at San Antonio Dental School. [Particular thanks to the panelists—Drs. Charles R. Morris, W. Doss McDavid, John W. Preece, Robert P. Langlais, Brigit J. Glass, and Olaf E. Langland.])*

the x-ray beam is collimated and much less tissue is irradiated as the x-rays pass through the patient to the slit in the cassette holder. This results in a panoramic radiograph showing a well-defined image of a curved layer of tissue including the teeth and tooth-bearing areas.

Panoramic radiography is still in the process of development. A variety of domestic and imported machines is available. The major differences between the machines are the number and location of rotational centers existing between the x-ray source and film. Following are descriptions of the three basic types, as shown in Figure 21–3.

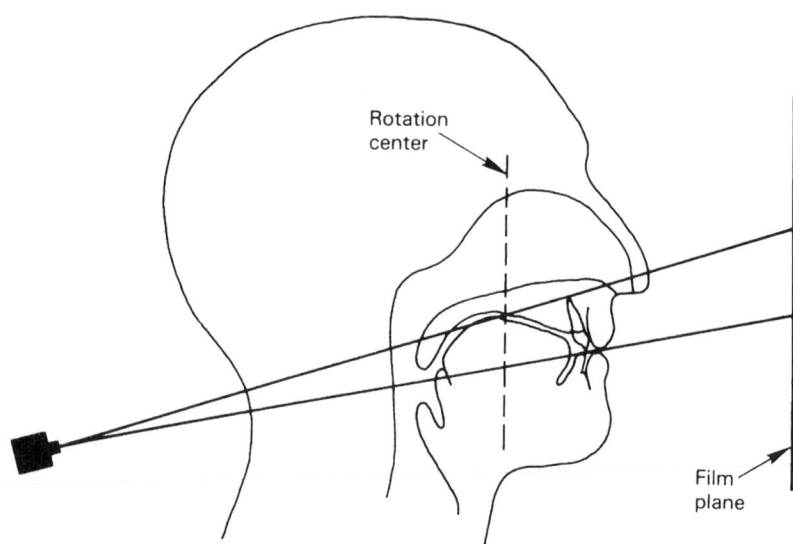

Figure 21–2. Diagram showing the relationship in a vertical plane of the tube head to the center of rotation and the film as the moving x-ray beam passes through the patient's head toward the moving film. *(From a syllabus prepared for a symposium on Panoramic Radiography presented at Anaheim, California, October 3, 1983, by the American Dental Association in cooperation with the University of Texas Health Science Center at San Antonio Dental School.)*

1. **Double-center rotation.** Here the left and right sides of the arc formed by the teeth and jaws coincide with arcs of two circles with centers at X and O (Fig. 21–3a). Two separate exposures are necessary, as the equipment shifts from one center to the other. This results in a "split" film image.
2. **Triple-center rotation.** With this method, three centers of rotation are used, as shown in Figure 21–3b. Although the examination contains three separate segments, the x-ray beam can be shifted from one center to the other with minor interruption, and a continuous image can be made.
3. **Moving-center rotation.** Good diagnostic results can be obtained with the beam rotating around a center that moves continuously in a path that is similar in shape to the anatomy being examined (Fig. 21–3c). This elliptical pattern very closely matches the arc of the teeth and jaws. A continuous image is provided. Both horizontal and vertical magnification of the image are relatively constant, and this system allows adjustment of the size of the elliptical path to match the varying size dental arches.

It is important to be aware that the projections in the horizontal (Fig. 21–1) and the vertical (Fig. 21–2) directions do not have the same focus of projection; in the horizontal plane it is at the center of rotation, whereas in the vertical plane it is located at the target in the tube head. This difference in the location of the foci of projection accounts for the fact that a degree of image distortion is characteristic of rotational panoramic radiographs.

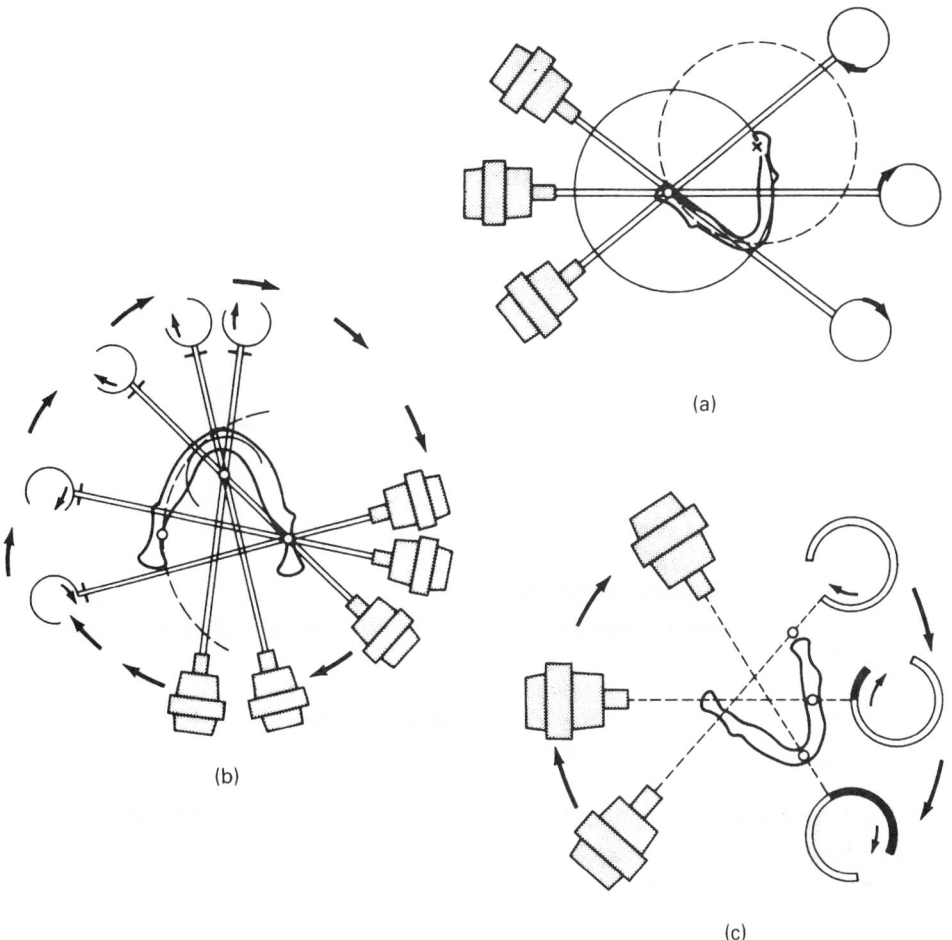

Figure 21–3. (a) Double-center rotation system used by Panorex (made by Keystone X-ray Inc.). **(b)** Triple-center rotation system used by Orthopantomograph (Siemens Corporation, Germany). **(c)** Moving-center rotating system used by Panelipse (Gendex Corporation). *(Panoramic-illustrations reproduced with permission, from Manson-Hing LR: Principles of Panoramic Radiography. Springfield, IL: Charles C Thomas, 1976.)*

CONCEPT OF THE FOCAL TROUGH

The **focal trough** is not an anatomical structure; rather, it is a theoretical concept used in rotational panoramic radiography to determine where the dental arches, the sinuses, or other areas that are to be examined should be positioned in order to achieve the clearest image. The focal trough (Fig. 21–4) is that area of the dental anatomy that is reproduced distinctly on the panoramic radiograph. Theoretically, a plane extends through this trough, and objects in that plane are recorded with diagnostic sharpness.

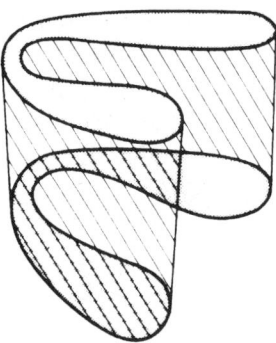

Figure 21–4. Diagrammatic sketch of focal trough. (Panoramic illustration reproduced, with permission, from Manson-Hing LR: *Principles of Panoramic Radiography.* Springfield, IL: Charles C Thomas, 1976.)

Objects located at various distances from the plane become less sharp as they get farther from the plane.

The trough is three-dimensional, and its actual shape varies depending on the equipment used. The size and shape of the focal trough are controlled by the manufacturer. The main factor that determines the width of the focal trough is the distance from the functional center of rotation to the object (the structures to be radiographed). As a general rule the width of the focal trough increases whenever the distance from the rotational center to the object is increased. The width of the focal trough and distance from the rotation center is controlled by the speed of the moving cassette. This means that the manufacturer can program the width and the shape of the focal trough to conform to the shape of an average dental arch by varying the speed of the moving cassette. The drawings in Figure 21–5 show the shapes produced by (a) double-center rotation, (b) triple-center rotation, and (c) moving-center rotation in relation to the patient's jaw.

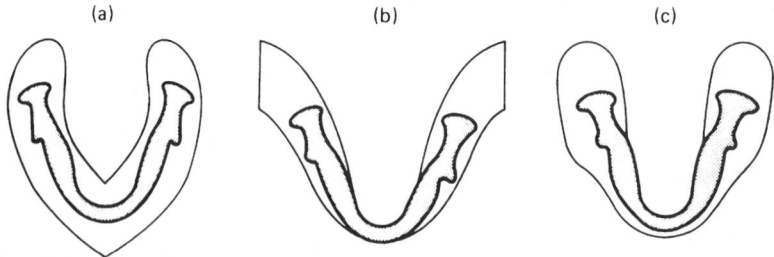

Figure 21–5. Variations in shape of focal trough produced by panoramic x-ray machines having **(a)** double-center rotation, **(b)** triple-center rotation, **(c)** moving-center rotation. *(Panoramic illustrations reproduced with permission from Manson-Hing LR:* Principles of Panoramic Radiography. *Springfield, IL: Charles C Thomas, 1976.)*

The double-center system (Fig. 21–5**a**) trough is wide both anteriorly and posteriorly, with the distal ends of the trough curving medially. The inward curving is unfavorable to obtaining the best sharpness in the temporomandibular joint areas.

The other focal troughs show wide posterior and narrow anterior thickness. The clinical implication is that the anterior teeth must be positioned very accurately.

The distal ends of Figure 21–5**b** flair laterally, whereas in Figure 21–5**c** they extend straight posteriorly. The moving-center system has the widest trough in the posterior areas, facilitating temporomandibular joint studies.

GEOMETRY AND SHARPNESS OF THE PANORAMIC IMAGE

Consideration must also be given to those factors that affect the geometric shape (distortion) and sharpness of the image. Distortion can be defined as unequal vertical and horizontal magnification. In conventional radiography, the x-ray images may be magnified equally in a horizontal and vertical direction by using the paralleling technique. The amount of magnification is proportional to the target–object distance and the object–film distance.

In rotational panoramic radiography, vertical and horizontal magnification are controlled by two different factors. The focal spot in the vertical direction is the actual focal spot in the anode of the x-ray tube, whereas the apparent focal spot in the horizontal direction is the center of rotation (effective rotation center). The magnification in the vertical dimension is proportional to the target–object distance and the object–film distance (the same as conventional radiography). The magnification in the horizontal dimension is controlled by the effective rotation center–object distance and the object–film distance.

If there were no film movement, the amount of magnification would be much greater in the horizontal dimension than in the vertical dimension. But the slow movement of the film compensates for this so that the horizontal and vertical magnification are equal for objects in the focal trough. Therefore, movement of the film not only controls the width of the focal trough, and the shape of the focal trough, movement of the film also compensates to make the horizontal and vertical magnification equal for objects in the focal trough.

It is easier to visualize image geometry if one imagines the focal trough to be that layer of tissues or area of space within the head that is occupied by the teeth and the alveolar bone. The factors of image magnification or diminution are equal if the structures or objects to be viewed are positioned in the center of the focal trough. These same structures or objects, if displaced backward (toward the center of rotation) will appear wider, and if displaced forward (toward the film) will appear narrower (Fig. 21–6).

For the machines that have fixed centers of rotation, the magnification varies within a certain range. The range exists because the object's position relative to the film and x-ray tube is constantly changing. This happens because the curve of the jaw does not identically follow the curve of a circle.

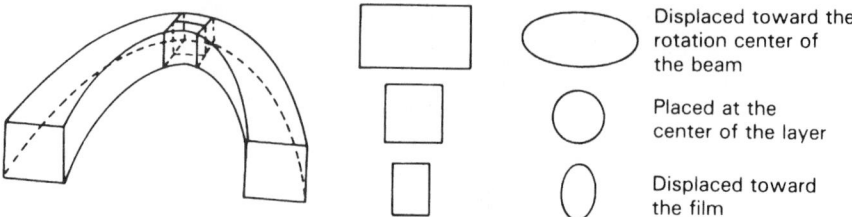

Displaced toward the
rotation center of
the beam

Placed at the
center of the layer

Displaced toward
the film

Figure 21–6. Image geometry. At the center of the layer, the magnification factors in the horizontal and vertical directions are equal. This implies that a small flat object positioned at the center of the layer will be portrayed in proper proportion. Outside the center of the layer, the magnification factors in these two dimensions are unequal. This results in distortion effects. If three planes are cut out from the layer at different object depths, the images of objects in these planes will exhibit different proportions. The plane at the center is correctly depicted. The plane positioned toward the rotational center of the beam will be magnified more in the horizontal than in the vertical dimension and will appear too wide. The plane positioned toward the film will be diminished more in the horizontal than in the vertical dimension and will appear too narrow. *(From a syllabus prepared for a symposium on Panoramic Radiography, present at Anaheim, California, on October 3, 1983, by the American Dental Association in cooperation with the University of Texas Health Science Center at San Antonio Dental School.)*

However, in machines with moving centers of rotation, the object, tube, and film positions are more constant, making the magnification virtually constant. When considering factors that influence the geometry or sharpness of the image, it is helpful to realize that the path of the sliding center of rotation (Fig. 21–7) is predetermined by the manufacturer and cannot be changed by the operator. What can, and unfortunately does, occur is that the operator malpositions the patient's head in relation to the focal trough. When that happens, some of the images may be magnified, diminished, or blurred.

Although undesirable in a panoramic film, a minor degree of magnification of the image is generally acceptable. Blurring or lack of sharpness of the image often reduces the amount of diagnostic information that can be obtained from the radiograph.

The manufacturer gives the film a speed that matches the projected speed of points lying within a selected curved plane. Consequently, these points are sharply depicted on the radiograph. The projection of object points outside the focal trough, either toward the center of rotation or toward the film, has a different projected speed at the film plane from the film itself. Thus, the projection of these points moves in relation to the film and appears blurred. Because the difference between the speed of the film and the speed of the projection of the points in the object (usually the teeth) increases with the distance from the sharply depicted object plane, the lack of clarity increases in both directions from this plane. At some distance, this lack of clarity reaches a level where an object point is no longer visible on the radiograph. This can be avoided by proper head positioning.

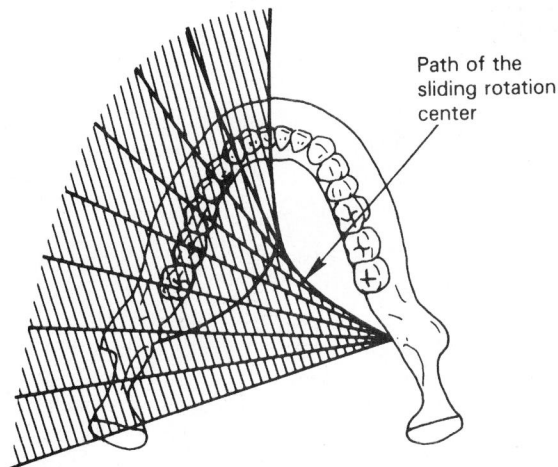

Path of the
sliding rotation
center

Figure 21–7. In systems creating continuous images, several different movement patterns of the beam are utilized to achieve the desired projection of the jaws. The objective is to project each part of the jaws as close to perpendicular as possible. The beam may be given a sliding movement throughout the total excursion, so that the effective projection center (the functional focus) is constantly shifted along a defined path. The central ray of the beam is always at a tangent to this path at some point. The form of the path defines the direction of the beam and hence the projection of each successive part of the jaws. *(From a syllabus prepared for a symposium on Panoramic Radiography at Anaheim, California, on October 3, 1983, by the American Dental Association in cooperation with the University of Texas Health Science Center at San Antonio Dental School.)*

IMPORTANCE OF CORRECT HEAD POSITIONING

The most important factor that can be controlled by the operator is the correct positioning of the patient's head. Failure to do so will result in a radiograph with reduced or no diagnostic value.

The head positioning will vary, depending on whether the major area of interest is in the region of the temporomandibular joints, the sinuses, or the teeth. The manufacturers supply detailed instructions on how each of these areas should be positioned within the focal trough.

Because the area of interest in the majority of panoramic radiographs is centered on the teeth and the surrounding alveolar structures, methods of correctly positioning the dental arches are of prime importance.

Most rotational panoramic x-ray machines have some type of **head positioner** (Fig. 21–8) that assists the operator in determining the optimum position. Each machine is different, and the operator must follow the manufacturer's instructions. Easier-to-adjust head positioners are being introduced. The **Orthopantomograph 10** casts three separate beams of light on the patient's face to indicate the location of important planes. The first beam indicates the position of the **Frankfort plane,** a horizon-

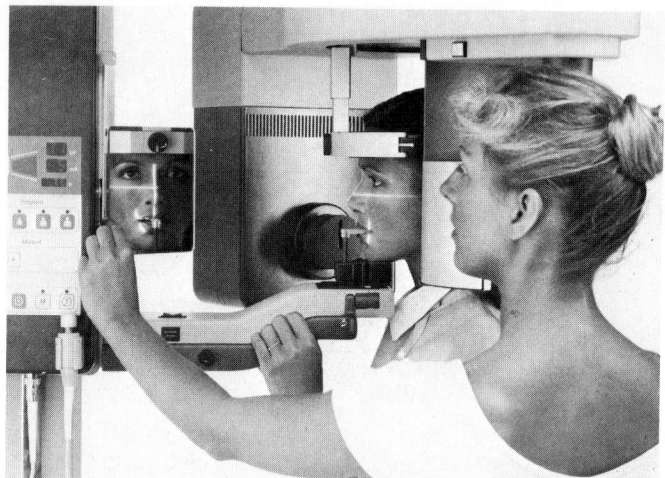

Figure 21–8. Photo of patient with head properly positioned in head positioner of Orthopantomograph 10. The beams of light on the patient's face indicate the location of important planes. *(Courtesy of Siemens Medical Systems, Inc., Dental Division, Iselin, NJ.)*

tal line between the porion and the orbitale. When properly adjusted, this line should be parallel with the floor to give the correct skull inclination. The second beam helps to locate the **sagittal plane,** which must be positioned at midline to locate the vertical center of the focal trough. The third beam indicates to the operator the location of the layer of maximum sharpness in the central incisor region.

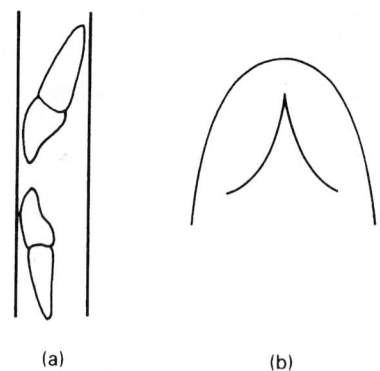

(a)   (b)

Figure 21–9. Correct positioning with equal magnification and sharpness all over the image. **(a)** Anterior teeth in focal trough. **(b)** Relationship of center of rotation to dental arches. *(From a syllabus prepared for a symposium on Panoramic Radiography at Anaheim, California, on October 3, 1983, by the American Dental Association in cooperation with the University of Texas Health Science Center at San Antonio Dental School.)*

Since most panoramic machines have relatively wide focal troughs in the posterior area, the posterior teeth can usually be positioned in the trough. In the anterior region, many of the machines have narrow focal troughs and must be positioned with extreme precision.

If maxillary incisors are to be placed in the trough, the apices must be brought slightly forward. Since mandibular incisors also tend to have their apices placed posteriorly, the operator will have the patient bring the incisors into an edge-to-edge position for better visualization.

The operator may have difficulty checking these head positions when using equipment requiring the patient to face the wall. Extra care must be taken to visualize the midline of the patient's face and the sagittal plane. To maintain image quality and uniform x-ray absorption, the operator should keep the patient's spine as erect as possible. If the patient is seated, rather than standing, the system should have a movable backrest for proper positioning.

When correctly positioned, the anterior teeth are in the focal trough, and there is an equal magnification and sharpness over all parts of the radiographic image (Fig. 21–9). If the patient has been positioned too far forward (toward the film), the anterior teeth are in front of the focal trough and appear blurred and diminished, particularly in width (Fig. 21–10). If the patient has been positioned too far backward (toward the x-ray tube head), the anterior teeth are behind the focal trough and the anterior teeth appear magnified and blurred (Fig. 21–11). If the patient's head has been rotated, the anterior teeth are correctly positioned in the focal trough, but the teeth on the side closer to the film are diminished, whereas those on the side closer to the center of rotation are enlarged (Fig. 21–12).

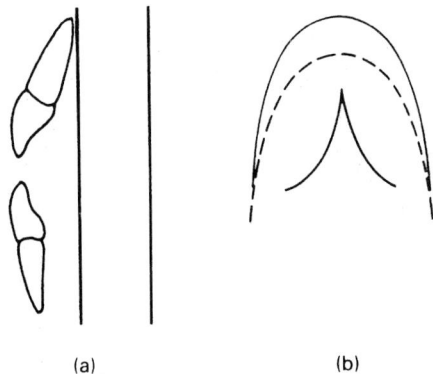

(a)   (b)

Figure 21–10. Incorrect positioning. The patient has been positioned too far forward (toward the film), and the anterior teeth appear blurred and diminished. **(a)** Anterior teeth outside focal trough. **(b)** The dental arches (unbroken line) are positioned forward in relation to focal trough (dotted line). *(From a syllabus prepared for a symposium on Panoramic Radiography at Anaheim, California, on October 3, 1983, by the American Dental Association in cooperation with the University of Texas Health Science Center at San Antonio Dental School.)*

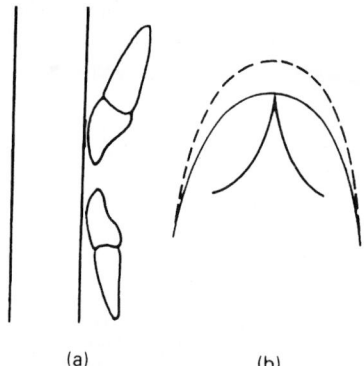

(a)   (b)

Figure 21–11. Incorrect positioning. The patient has been positioned too far backward (toward the x-ray tube head), and the anterior teeth appear magnified and blurred. **(a)** Anterior teeth outside focal trough. **(b)** The dental arches (unbroken line) positioned backward in relation to the focal trough (dotted line). *(From a syllabus prepared for a symposium on Panoramic Radiography at Anaheim, California, on October 3, 1983, by the American Dental Association in cooperation with the University of Texas Health Science Center at San Antonio Dental School.)*

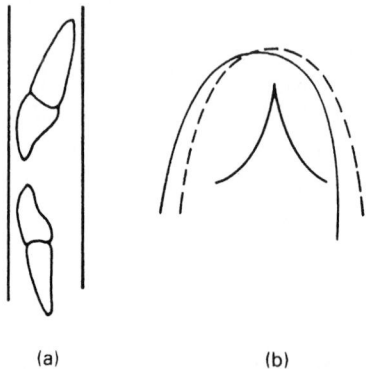

(a)   (b)

Figure 21–12. Incorrect positioning. The patient's head has been rotated. Diminution will be apparent on the side malpositioned toward the film, and magnification will be apparent on the side malpositioned toward the rotation center of the beam. On both sides the distortion will be most marked in the horizontal dimension; the width of the teeth and jaw structures is affected more than their height dimension. **(a)** Anterior teeth correctly positioned in focal trough. **(b)** Dental arches (unbroken line) rotated around the anterior teeth. One side will be malpositioned outside the focal trough (dotted line), and the other side will be malpositioned inside the focal trough. *(From a syllabus prepared for a symposium on Panoramic Radiography at Anaheim, California, on October 3, 1983, by the American Dental Association in cooperation with the University of Texas Health Science Center at San Antonio Dental School.)*

Numerous other position errors, such as tilting the chin up or down, can be made. An exposure should never be made until the operator is satisfied that all planes are correctly aligned.

TYPES OF PANORAMIC X-RAY MACHINES

New types of machines with varying capabilities are being introduced, and changes are being made by the manufacturers so rapidly that it is not feasible to give a detailed description here.

The various manufacturers use trade names such as **Orthopantomograph, Orthoceph,** and **Status X** (Siemens); **Panorex** (Keystone); **Panelipse** (Gendex); **Versaview** (Morita); and others. Many panoramic machines now have cephalometric capabilities.

All the x-ray machines mentioned except the Status X (Siemens) are of the rotational type. As stated previously, rotational panoramic x-ray machines have a mechanism that moves the tube and film in opposite directions simultaneously while the specific tissue layer remains in a fixed relationship to the tube. The film produces a clear image of the layer that is being examined while at the same time blurring and eliminating the images in the adjacent tissues. Hence, when the tissues of the right side are in the path of the x-ray beam, the tissues of the left side are out of focus and do not superimpose on those of the right side and vice versa. This blurring of the other layer is necessary to prevent interference from the structures of the other layers that were not selected for viewing.

A second method of exposure employed in panoramic radiography is to use an intraoral source of x-rays. This method has been tested in Europe and used there but has little following in the United States. It is included here for comparison of exposure techniques. The Status X operates on the principle of using an intraoral source of radiation. The anode is located at the tip of the unit containing the tube and is placed inside the patient's mouth. A complete survey is made with two exposures, one of the mandible and one of the maxillae. An alternative procedure is to make an exposure of the right or left side. The film is placed in a flexible cassette that is positioned on the surface of the face.

OPERATIONAL PROCEDURES WITH PANORAMIC X-RAY MACHINES

Although considerable differences exist in the size and configuration of modern rotational panoramic x-ray units, the operational procedures are similar and relatively simple. Obviously, all manufacturers claim that their unit is the best, and each has features that may have special appeal to one dentist or another. Each manufacturer provides an instruction manual that must be carefully read and followed. Most errors can be avoided, and high-quality panoramic radiographs can be produced, with any modern unit if the operator understands the instructions and follows them correctly.

Although a detailed description of all panoramic x-ray units cannot be given, some major differences are visible at a glance. The unit may be constructed in such a manner that the patient must be seated or remain standing during the exposure, or the chair may be positioned so that the patient faces toward or away from the operator.

For example, the patient remains standing and faces toward the back of the unit on the Siemens Orthopantomograph 10 (Fig. 21–13) and the Morita Versaview; however, it is possible to lower the assembly that controls the height of the tube head, cassette, and head positioner so that a patient seated on a movable stool or wheelchair can be accommodated. By comparison, the patient must be seated and facing the operator during the exposure when the Keystone Panorex 2 (Fig. 21–14) or the Gendex Panelipse II (Fig. 21–15) is used.

Less obvious differences are found in the size and shape of the cassette, the manner in which the positioning system is adjusted, and the method used to stabilize the head (Fig. 21–8) and to determine the zone desired to be in focus. The cassette may be in the shape of a circular drum that rotates, or the chair in which the patient is seated may have an automatic lateral shifting device, such as in the older Panorex models. Midway through the exposure cycle, as the tube passes behind the spinal column, the machine automatically shuts down the radiation, producing a split image (see the clear area in the middle of Fig. 21–16). The Panorex 2 is equipped with a mode selector

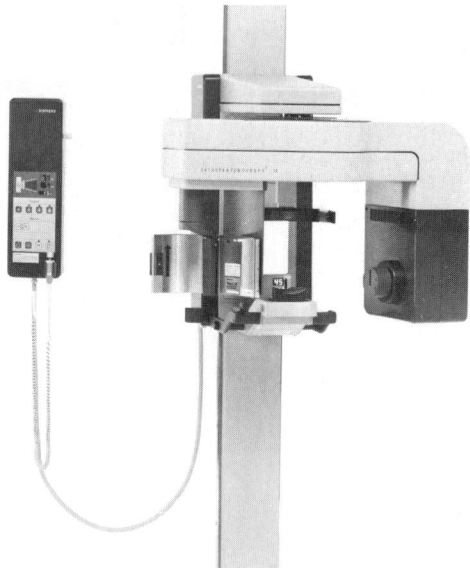

Figure 21–13. Photograph of Orthopantomograph 10. The patient can be examined standing or seated. This unit has a motorized head positioner with digital readout and is height-adjustable. Correct patient head positioning can be controlled in three planes by light beam indicators that show the correct location of the Frankfort horizontal plane, the sagittal plane, and the layer of optimum sharpness in the central incisor region. *(Courtesy of Siemens Medical Systems, Inc, Dental Division, Iselin, NJ.)*

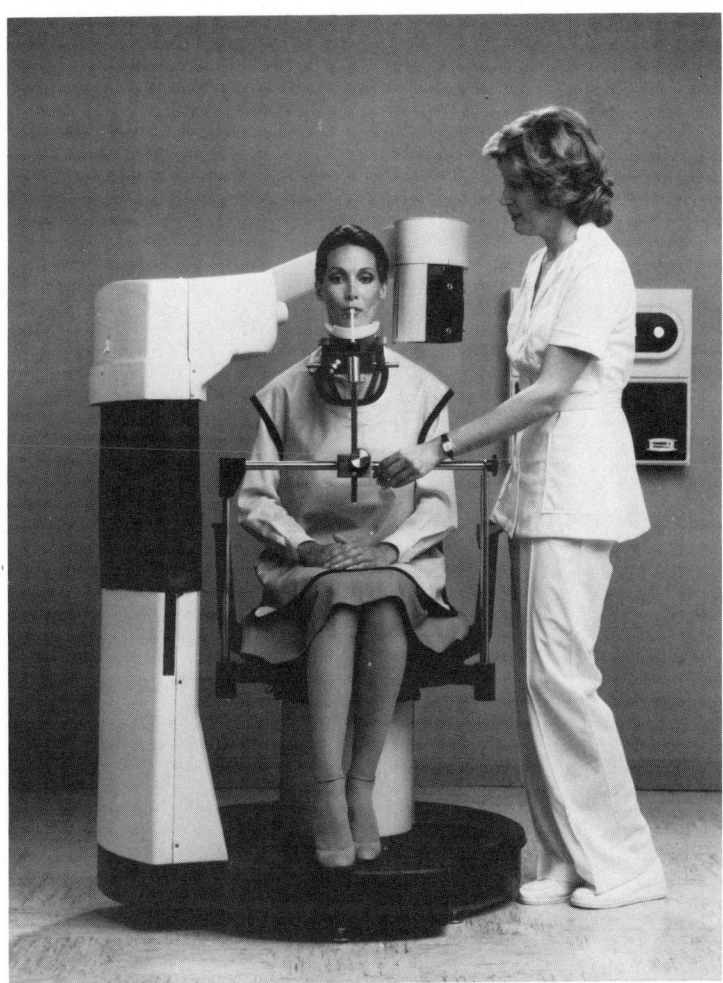

Figure 21–14. Photograph of Panorex 2 with patient seated and facing the operator. Biteblock locates the central teeth in zone focus (focal trough). Shifting of a mode selector determines whether a radiograph with a split or continuous image is produced. *(Courtesy of Keystone X-ray Inc.)*

control, and the operator has the option of producing a radiograph of either a split image or one with a continuous image as shown in Figure 21–17. Most current panoramic x-ray machines produce only continuous image radiographs.

With minor variations, the following operational sequence is required with most panoramic x-ray machines:

1. Load the film into the **cassette** in the darkroom and identify the film. Use only the type of safelight recommended by the film manufacturer.

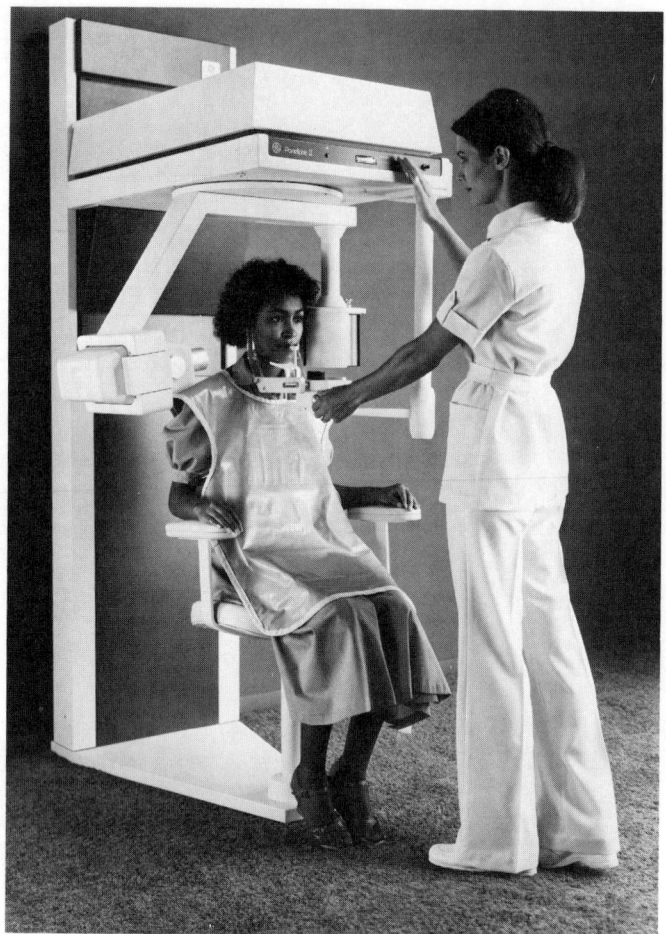

Figure 21–15. The Panelipse II produces an elliptical path of the plane in focus that is adjustable to any size dental arch. All teeth, sinuses, and maxillary and mandibular structures can be displayed in a uniform continuous image. The exposure is made in approximately 20 seconds. *(Courtesy of Gendex Corporation.)*

2. Handle the film carefully. Be sure that it is inserted between the screens of the cassette. Close the cassette completely before leaving the darkroom.
3. Depending on the type of cassette, either place it into the **cassette holder** or securely fasten it to the **drum.** Check that the drum can turn.
4. Turn the machine on to check that it is operational. Raise or lower the overhead assembly, and swing the head positioner out of the way so that the patient can be positioned.
5. Ask the patient to remove glasses, earrings, or other appliances that might become superimposed on the image. This includes necklaces, napkin chains, or any other metal objects on the back of the neck.

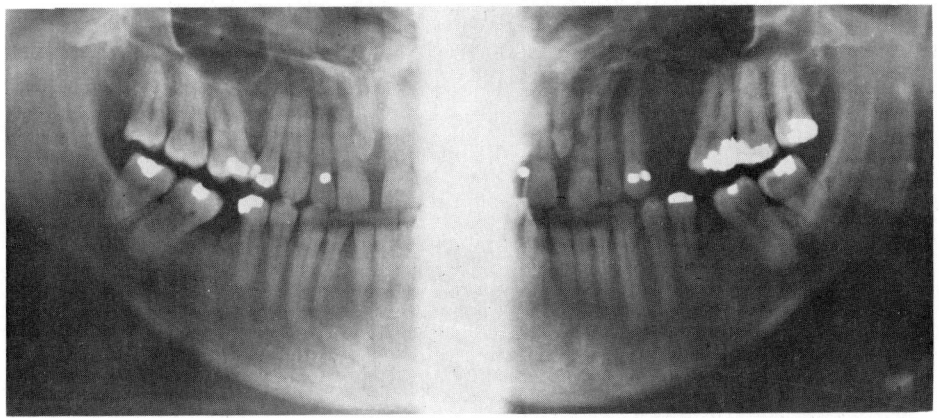

Figure 21–16. Illustration of a panoramic radiograph exposed with a Panorex machine. The blurring in the center of the film and the duplication of tooth structures in the incisor regions are caused by the shift in position of the moving parts of the machine during the middle of the exposure. This, however, does not materially detract from the diagnostic quality of the radiograph.

6. Depending on the machine used, ask the patient to stand or sit up straight. Drape the patient with a lead apron.
7. Swing the head positioner assembly into place. According to the unit used, follow the manufacturer's directions in positioning the patient's head and chin. Make sure that the **midsagittal plane** of the patient's face is perpendicular to the floor.

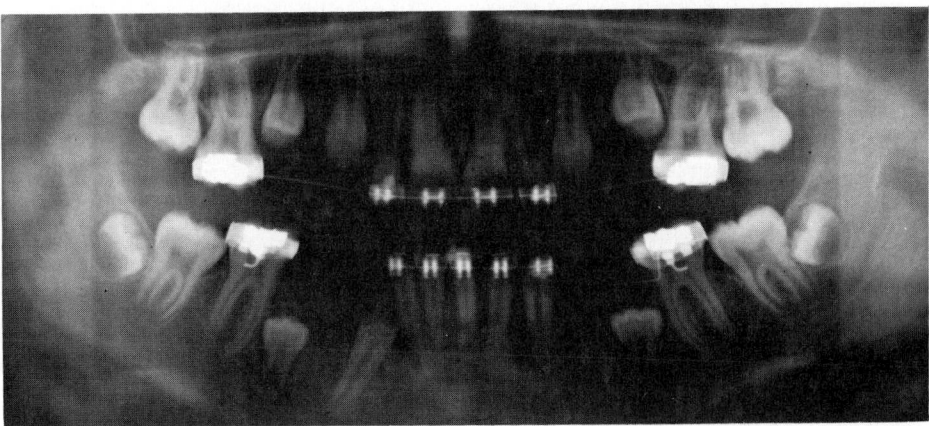

Figure 21–17. Panoramic radiograph produced by Panelipse. Notice the presence of orthodontic bands and wires. Radiograph also shows erupting teeth, impacted teeth, and anodontia. Teeth are shown in an uninterrupted sequence. *(Courtesy of General Electric Company, Medical Systems Division.)*

8. Confirm that the manufacturer's recommendations on mA, kVp, and duration of exposure time are followed. Alert the patient to the fact that certain parts of the machine will revolve around the head. Stress the importance of remaining still during the time required to make the exposure.

9. Make a final check to determine that the anterior teeth are in the proper (edge-to-edge) position, and ask the patient to place the tongue against the roof of the mouth.

10. Stand behind protective covering or an adequate distance away while making the exposure. Watch the patient during this time to make sure that there has been no undesired movement.

11. Swing the head positioning assembly out of the way. Remove the protective apron or collar, and release the patient. Return glasses, earrings, or appliances.

12. Deactivate the x-ray machine, and swing the head positioner back into place. Remove the cassette from the cassette holder or drum.

13. Unload the cassette under proper safelight conditions, and process the film according to the manufacturer's instructions.

The procedures for making the exposures are similar on most panoramic machines. As the complexity of the controls and head holder adjustments varies from unit to unit, read the manufacturer's instructions carefully before attempting to operate an unfamiliar machine. If possible, have someone who is familiar with it give a demonstration. Although the panoramic x-ray machines are larger, costlier, and more complex than the conventional x-ray machines, their operation is much simpler and can be learned in less than one hour.

ADVANTAGES AND DISADVANTAGES OF PANORAMIC RADIOGRAPHY

The panoramic radiograph is extremely valuable to the pedodontist and orthodontist concerned with the eruption of the teeth, their spacing, and the bony development of the supporting jaw structures, to the oral surgeon concerned with possible fractures, impacted teeth, or tumors, and to the periodontist concerned with the conditions of the bony structures and soft tissues surrounding and supporting the teeth. A panoramic radiograph is less confusing to the patient than a series of small separate intraoral radiographs, making it easier for the dentist to explain the diagnosis and the proposed treatment plan in a manner that is clear and understandable to the patient.

Because a much greater area can be examined than is possible by the conventional full-mouth survey, the patient benefits if conditions are revealed that otherwise would not have been detected. However, panoramic radiography has limitations because such factors as magnification, distortion, and poor definition are inherent with panoramic techniques. For example, most dentists agree that incipient caries can be visualized better on periapical or bitewing radiographs. Therefore, it should be emphasized that panoramic radiography is an adjunct or additional diagnostic aid but does not replace conventional radiography.

To summarize, the major advantages and disadvantages of panoramic radiography compared with conventional full-mouth radiography are as follows.

Advantages:

1. The procedure for exposing panoramic films is relatively simple to perform and requires considerably less time.
2. Panoramic exposures are better tolerated by the patient, especially when gagging problems exist.
3. Visualization is greater because all parts of the maxillae and the mandible that lie within the zone of the focal trough of any given panoramic machine can be seen on a single film.
4. The area covered exceeds that of the full-mouth survey and may reveal conditions that otherwise might remain undetected.
5. The radiation dose is relatively low.
6. Less operator time is required in processing, as only one film instead of a series must be handled.
7. Mounting time is eliminated. Panoramic film is easier to file and store. The danger of losing or damaging a film of the series is removed.
8. Panoramic film is useful in patient education and as a visual aid. The absence of a series of overlapping films makes it easier for the patient to follow the dentist's explanations.

Disadvantages:

1. Areas of diagnostic interest out of the focal trough may be visualized poorly or not at all.
2. A varying degree of magnification, geometric distortion, and poor definition is inherent in panoramic radiographs.
3. It is common to overlap teeth, particularly in the premolar (bicuspid) area.
4. It is difficult to obtain good images of the anterior teeth when they have a sharp inclination toward either the labial or lingual.
5. The spinal column often becomes superimposed on structures of interest.
6. The amount of vertical and horizontal distortion is not constant—it varies from one part of the radiograph to another.
7. Incipient caries are difficult to detect and are frequently missed. Supplementary films are required for this purpose.
8. Artifacts are common and may easily be misinterpreted.

TECHNIQUE ERRORS RESULTING IN FAULTY PANORAMIC RADIOGRAPHS

The procedures for identification and correction of errors that result in faulty radiographs when intraoral films and conventional dental x-ray equipment are used were explained in Chapter 14. Many of the errors listed apply also to panoramic radiographs. However, panoramic imagery differs vastly from conventional imagery, and some of the errors are unique to it. For instance, because a narrow x-ray beam is used to image a curved layer and only the plane at the center of the layer is reproduced correctly, all errors in positioning the patient or the movable parts of the panoramic unit result in distortion of the image, superimposition of the vertebrae over the anterior region, the inclusion of artifacts, or the formation of "ghost" images. When the head is positioned correctly, all parts of the image have the same degree of magnification and sharpness. Conversely, unequal magnification (or diminution) and unsharpness (blurring) are clear indications of malpositioning.

The following positioning errors are common in rotational panoramic radiography:

1. Patient too far forward, too close to the film (Fig. 21–10). This results in all of the anterior teeth appearing blurred and diminished, particularly in width.
2. Patient too far back toward the tube head (Fig. 21–11). This results in all the anterior teeth appearing blurred and magnified.
3. Chin tipped too low. When this happens the maxillary anterior teeth or the mandibular anterior teeth are placed outside the focal trough and are blurred. When the maxillary teeth are positioned within the focal trough, the mandibular teeth will be blurred and magnified. Conversely, when the mandibular teeth are positioned within the focal trough, the maxillary teeth are blurred and diminished, most prominently in width.
4. Chin raised too high. When this happens, the bottom of the nasal cavity and the palatinal plate form a line of low density that partially overlaps the apices of the maxillary teeth. The maxillary anterior teeth or the mandibular anterior teeth are positioned outside the focal trough and are blurred. When the mandibular teeth are positioned within the focal trough, the maxillary teeth appear blurred and magnified. When the maxillary anterior teeth are positioned within the focal trough, the mandibular teeth appear blurred and diminished, most prominently in width.
5. Patient's head rotated (Fig. 21–12). The teeth on the side closer to the film are diminished, whereas those on the side closer to the center of rotation are enlarged.

Additional, less-common patient positioning errors include the following: failure to position the chin on the chin rest, failure to use the bite guide or failure to use it correctly, setting the machine too high or too low, failure to remove earrings or prostheses, failure of the patient to keep lips closed or to keep the tongue on the palate, and patient movement.

Other errors are caused by improper exposure and film handling. These include improper manipulation and loading of the film, the presence of paper or lint on the intensifying screens, failure to start the film at the proper line, interference of the thyroid collar with the rotation of the cassette, artifacts caused by fingernail pressure or static electricity, chemical stains, the use of "unsafe" safelights, overexposure, underexposure, and double exposure.

CHAPTER SUMMARY

Panoramic radiography is an important new technique that has been refined in the last two decades. Almost all panoramic x-ray machines used in the United States work on a system by which the patient's head is carefully positioned between the tube head and the film. The tube head and film rotate at a predetermined speed around the patient's head. A narrow beam of x-rays is used to project the image on the film.

Several different continuous movement patterns of the x-ray beam (centers of rotation) are built into the machines by the manufacturers to achieve the desired projection of the jaws. The form of the path determines the direction of the beam and hence the projection of each successive part of the jaws. The target in the tube serves as the focus of the projection in the vertical dimension, whereas the center of rotation serves as the functional focus in the horizontal direction. Distortion effects are characteristic of panoramic radiographs because the focus of projection is different in the horizontal and vertical planes.

The panoramic radiograph (often called the **tomograph**) is produced by a special technique used to show in detail the images of structures located within a predetermined plane of tissues, while at the same time eliminating or blurring those structures located in the planes that were not selected. The plane in focus or depth of field—also known as the **focal trough**—is the sharply defined area that in most tomographs corresponds to the size and shape of the dental arches. Correct patient positioning and head and jaw alignment are the decisive determining factors for the quality of the radiograph produced.

The best image is obtained when the teeth and jaws are positioned in the center of the focal trough. Displacement toward rotation center of the beam (backward) causes the anterior teeth to appear magnified horizontally and blurred. Conversely, if displaced toward the film (forward), the anterior teeth will appear narrower and blurred.

The procedure for exposing panoramic radiographs varies from unit to unit but generally involves the following steps: (1) identifying and loading the film into the cassette; (2) activating the unit and attaching the cassette to the holder or drum; (3) preparing the patient, making required head measurements, and positioning the patient's head so that the teeth will be in the focal trough; (4) selecting the proper mA and kVp and holding the button on the hand switch pressed down firmly until the exposure is completed; and (5) deactivating the machine, releasing the patient, and removing the cassette from the holder or drum.

There are advantages and disadvantages to using panoramic radiographs. Among the advantages are the following: (1) simplicity and rapidity of procedure, (2) minimal patient resistance to film positioning, (3) large areas, even sinuses and temporomandibular joints, can be viewed on a single film, (4) useful for making mass surveys, and (5) easier for the patient to visualize and understand the dentist's plan of treatment. Among the disadvantages are the following: (1) loss of radiographic detail, (2) inherent magnification and image distortion, and (3) the difficulty experienced by many operators in correctly positioning the patient's head so that the dentition is centered on the focal trough when using panoramic machines.

Many of the technique errors that result in producing substandard panoramic radiographs are the result of mistakes in film handling and exposure. However, most errors are caused by malpositioning the head. Excellent radiographs can be produced when the operator follows the technique procedures carefully and adheres to the manufacturer's instructions.

KEY WORDS

Cassette

Cassette holder

Drum

Flexible cassette

Focal trough

Frankfort plane

Head positioner

Laminography

Midsagittal plane

Orthopantomograph

Panelipse

Panoramic radiography

Panorex

Pantomography

Rotational center

Rotational panoramic radiography

Sagittal plane

Slit

Tomography

Versaview

REVIEW QUESTIONS

1. A panoramic film shows an unexposed area in the center that was caused by the shifting of the chair. Which make of panoramic machine was used to make the exposure? (a) Orthopantomograph, (b) Panelipse, (c) Orthoceph, (d) Panorex.

2. In what position should the incisors be during a panoramic exposure? (a) mandibular incisors should protrude, (b) edge-to-edge relationship, (c) maxillary incisors should protrude, (d) mouth should be open with incisors at least 1/2 in. (13 mm) apart.

3. Which term describes the area of the dental anatomy that is reproduced distinctly on the panoramic radiograph? (a) focal trough, (b) rotation center, (c) sagittal plane, (d) laminograph.

4. Which of these factors is a disadvantage of extraoral radiography that is often observed when a panoramic and an intraoral film are compared? (a) more teeth are shown on a panoramic film, (b) the sinuses may be shown on a panoramic film, (c) the images are magnified on a panoramic film, (d) the temporo-mandibular joints may be shown on a panoramic film.

5. In panoramic radiography, the focal trough is (a) the slit in the cassette holder, (b) the collimated radiation beam, (c) the zone of sharpness, (d) the path that the cassette holder follows while rotating.

6. A panoramic radiograph is of little value when diagnosing (a) an impacted molar, (b) recurrent caries, (c) a cyst, (d) a supernumerary tooth.

7. Which of these is an advantage of using panoramic instead of periapical film? (a) mounting time is eliminated, (b) the image is magnified, (c) distortion is eliminated, (d) definition is improved.

8. What is the effect on the shape of the focal trough when the distance from the center of rotation to the dental arches is increased? (a) there is no effect, (b) the width increases, (c) it is eliminated, (d) the width decreases.

9. Which type of film is best for detecting incipient caries? (a) extraoral film, (b) bitewing film, (c) occlusal film, (d) panoramic film.

10. Where is the center of rotation located? (a) between the teeth and the film, (b) between the tube head and the film, (c) between the Frankfort plane and the cassette, (d) between the focal trough and the cassette.

11. What is the effect on the image geometry of the central incisors when the patient's head is positioned too far forward? (a) the incisors are diminished and blurred, (b) there is no effect, (c) the incisors are magnified vertically, (d) the incisors are magnified and blurred.

12. In a panoramic radiograph, the teeth on the right side are magnified and the teeth on the left side are very small. This error was caused by positioning the patient's head (a) too far forward, (b) too far backward, (c) to the left of the midline, (d) to the right of the midline.

BIBLIOGRAPHY

Farman AG, Nortje CJ, Wood RE: *Oral and Maxillofacial Diagnostic Imaging*. St. Louis, MO: CV Mosby, 1993

Goaz PW, White SC: *Oral Radiology Principles and Interpretation*, 3rd ed. St. Louis, MO: CV Mosby, 1994

Langland OE, Langlais RP, McDavid WD, et al: *Panoramic Radiology*, 2nd ed. Philadelphia, PA: Lea & Febiger, 1988

CHAPTER 22

Patient Education

By the end of this chapter the student should be able to

1. Explain the necessity for patient education in radiography.
2. Identify the benefits that the patient derives from preventive radiation procedures.
3. Describe several methods by which the patient can be educated to appreciate the value of dental radiography.
4. Identify the goals of the dental radiographer.

VALUE OF PATIENT EDUCATION

One of the greatest services that the dentist, dental hygienist, or assistant can render the patient is dental health education. This includes not only education in oral health and restorative dentistry but education in the value of dental radiography. It is surprising how many patients, even today, do not comprehend the enormous value of an x-ray examination of their teeth.

This deplorable situation is largely the fault of the dental practitioner, who may have been too busy or complacent to have taken the time to explain the reasons for exposing radiographs to the patient. Unfortunately, all too many patients regard radiography as just another method to increase the fees.

The value of **patient education** is twofold. First, by understanding that dental radiographs disclose cavities and lesions that are invisible and can become a source of danger if not treated in time, the dentally educated patient realizes that x-rays are not to be feared but are actually beneficial. Nowhere is the adage "a stitch in time saves nine" more true than in dentistry. Second, the educated patient is more inclined to understand and accept the dentist's treatment plan and prevention program. Such patient acceptance helps to develop a spirit of confidence and mutual trust in the dentist and the staff and launches the patient on the path of improved oral health.

The American Dental Association, through its Council on Dental Materials, Instruments, and Equipment, recently issued updated recommendations intended to promote the safety and effectiveness of diagnostic radiography. It strongly suggested the use of professional judgment to determine the type, frequency, and extent of each radiographic examination. X-radiation for diagnostic purposes should be used only after clinical examination and careful consideration of both the dental and general health needs of the patient. The deciding factor is the total welfare of the patient.

The nature and extent of diagnosis for required patient care, rather than the concept of routine use of x-rays as a part of periodic examination of all patients, constitute the only rational basis for determining whether additional x-rays are required. It should be recognized that each patient is different and, of necessity, the patient's radiographic requirements will differ.

NECESSITY FOR PATIENT EDUCATION IN RADIOGRAPHY

Most dental patients have heard about the bad effects of overexposure to radiation. Rightfully, they are concerned. It is only natural that they may on occasion question the necessity of having more radiographs exposed. It is the responsibility of the dentist or a member of the staff to provide the patient with a clear, concise, and satisfactory explanation.

Periodically a newspaper or magazine article casts doubt on the safety of radiographic procedures. Although undoubtedly sincere and well intentioned, such articles are not always well researched. All too frequently the patients who read them are frightened into avoiding all radiation, thus doing themselves great harm. The result may be pain that could have been avoided, a loss of tooth function, a loss of time, and unnecessary future expenditures.

The problem with many of the articles is that the reporters assigned to write about radiation hazards are frequently not familiar with the complex array of terms and methods used in radiation monitoring and measurement. The figures used to measure the potential output of the x-ray machine are easily confused with the figures for accumulated dose. This is quite understandable as these terms are difficult for the average person working in radiography. Because these terms are primarily used by the radiation physicists, their meaning is quite confusing to anyone who does not have a strong background in physics. No wonder, then, that some of the radiation amounts described are so astronomical—and frightening to the reader.

The dental radiographer—whether dentist, dental hygienist, dental assistant, or radiation technician—must then take the time to educate, or in some instances to re-educate, the patient. The patient may be shown collimated position indicating devices (PIDs), thyroid collars, and protective lead aprons. The patient must be told that the films now used require only a fraction of the radiation previously necessary to expose them and that modern equipment is better constructed to prevent accidental exposure. Further, the radiographer should stress that only enough radiation to be consistent with the patient's diagnostic needs is used and that all standard safety practices as suggested by the National Council on Radiation Protection and Measurements are adhered to in the office. The patient should be assured that everyone in the office who works with radiography is trained in its use and the safety aspects of radiation. If the state issues a license or a certificate of compliance to show that a radiation safety examination has been passed, that can be offered in evidence. Many radiographers display their certificates near the x-ray machine. Regardless of how this information is presented, the patient must be made aware that the timely use of radiographs entails many benefits and few risks.

BENEFITS OF PREVENTIVE RADIATION

It is difficult for most dental personnel to conceive how dentistry was practiced before x-ray examinations were standard procedure. A world without dental x-rays would be like a world without the automobile or telephone. X-rays are a second pair of eyes to the dentist. The older dental practitioner can recollect many embarrassing incidents in his practice that were caused when large interproximal carious lesions remained undetected at the time of the patient's checkup examination. Such carious teeth were often beyond restoration when the patient returned 6 months later. Similarly, restorative work was often performed on teeth that had hidden apical lesions, only to have the traumatic experience of needing to have the restored teeth surgically removed a few days or weeks later.

Almost all modern dental techniques would be unworkable without a supportive x-ray diagnosis. Patients would suffer unnecessary pain if the dentist could not locate the source of their complaints. Radiographs prevent unnecessary removal of teeth, allow diagnosis of conditions in early stages when they can be treated, and even save lives by disclosing malignancies.

Some of the conditions that radiographs can demonstrate are (1) periodontal changes and pathological conditions associated with the loss of bone structure, (2) the damage that can be caused by submarginal and interproximal calculus deposits, (3) the effect on the occlusion caused by premature loss or the prolonged retention of the deciduous teeth, (4) the presence of unerupted or supernumerary teeth, (5) the consequences of losing the permanent teeth and the importance of having them replaced if lost, and (6) the presence or extent of carious lesions not visible to the eye.

Thus the controlled use of dental radiation benefits dental patients by (1) enabling them to feel confident that the dentist has taken all possible steps to institute preventive procedures, (2) minimizing the danger of toothaches or the need for surgical procedures, and (3) saving them time and money while at the same time keeping them in a state of good oral health.

METHODS OF PATIENT EDUCATION

Several methods can be used to educate the patient on the value of **preventive radiation.** What is successful in one office may not be in another. Everyone concerned in the performance of radiation duties shares the responsibility for teaching patients what they should know about radiation. As such, office personnel are urged to devise methods that are consistent with the policies and philosophies of the office. It is important that these are explained in terms that the patients can understand.

One effective method of patient education is to assemble a series of radiographs showing typical dental conditions, both normal and abnormal. Placed in convenient mounts, the radiographs are classified according to condition and shown to the patient on a screen or an illuminated viewer. The viewer-enlarger shown in Figure 10–31 is extremely well suited for enlarging radiographs. Patients are generally able to identify the areas that are pointed out to them on the radiographs better if the images are magnified and the brightness of the light is controlled. Although many trained auxiliaries can interpret radiographs correctly, they should limit their presentations by showing slides or radiographs of someone other than the patient. This avoids the appearance that the auxiliary is making the diagnosis. In the event that the patient's own radiographs are to be shown, the dentist should make the presentation.

Another effective method is to place printed literature in the reception room or to hand it to the patients before their x-ray appointment. Two such pamphlets, *Dental X-ray Examinations: Your Dentist's Advice* and *Dental X-rays: Your Dentist's Advice,* can be obtained from the American Dental Association. These pamphlets explain in simple terms what x-rays can do and how x-rays work for you. Another pamphlet, *Get the Picture on Dental X-rays,* is available from the Bureau of Radiological Health (HFX-28), Rockville, Maryland 20857. This pamphlet was prepared in cooperation with the American Dental Association and contains valuable information for the patient. It has a detachable card on which each patient can keep a record of the date, the type of examination, the name of the referring doctor, and the address where the patient's x-rays are kept. In addition, the pamphlet includes the following advice to the patient:

Don't decide on your own that you need an x-ray.
Don't insist on an x-ray.
If your doctor orders an x-ray, ask how it will help with the diagnosis.
Tell your doctor about any similar x-ray examination that you have had.
Ask if gonad shielding can be used—for yourself and for your children—during x-ray exams near the reproductive organs.
Tell your doctor if you think you're pregnant before having an x-ray examination of the abdomen.

The giving of such a pamphlet to the patient opens the door for two-way communication between the patient and the dentist or staff member on the advisability and necessity of regular radiographic examinations.

Still another extremely effective method is to produce your own brochure to give to the patient. This may require some time, thought, imagination, a degree of artistic ability, effort, and a total dedication to preventive measures. The preparation of such a brochure can be fun, helpful to the patient, and very satisfying. For example, such a brochure could be titled "Why Dental X-rays?" or something similar. The instructive material could be arranged in three or four columns and printed on both sides of a single piece of paper. The brochure is then creased to conform with the width of the columns. The narration should be simple and in language that is professional, yet not overly technical. Depending on the amount of available space, pictures of a few radiographs illustrating conditions that can be identified easily may be shown.

Such a brochure might be constructed by formulating a series of questions and then presenting a very short answer. For example, (1) What is a radiograph? (2) How is it produced? (3) Why is it necessary? (4) What if the patient has no teeth and wears dentures? (5) Should x-rays be taken during pregnancy? (6) Isn't it a waste to take x-rays of children who will soon lose their teeth anyway? (7) What about danger to me? (8) How safe are x-rays? and (9) If x-rays are really safe, why does the operator always leave the room? Obviously, there are many ways of wording these and similar questions—and many ways of answering them.

There are many persons who seldom or never visit the dental office unless an emergency forces them to do so. Such nonpatients are occasionally reached when they attend meetings or lectures devoted to dental health at schools, health centers, or PTA meetings. During such presentations they may learn that certain conditions can be discovered and corrected in time only if radiographs are taken, and they may thus be encouraged to visit the dentist.

Most dental offices do not have a specific method or program by which the benefits of periodic x-ray examinations are taught. All too often the patient is simply told that the doctor requires them and will not treat the patient unless they are taken, or else the explanation is limited to a few short and often unsatisfactory answers.

Whether the patient receives the information at chair-side, in a specially equipped room, or at a talk given at some meeting is irrelevant. A mixture of information presented at chair-side combined with a pamphlet and some form of x-ray slide presentation is probably the most effective.

GOALS OF THE DENTAL RADIOGRAPHER

Everyone who has been properly trained in radiation procedures and safety techniques should develop a professional pride in his or her work, strive for professional improvement, and always keep the patient's well-being as the primary reason for being in dentistry. One achieves this by setting oneself standards of ethics and goals. Such goals are closely related, and all are equally important. One goal is to achieve perfection with each radiograph. This is easier to say than to do. It is accomplished by careful attention to all details. Each step in the process, whether in film placement, exposure technique, or processing and identification, though small, can be significant. A little error at any step can be compounded by others until it ruins the result. A closely related goal is to work rapidly but without undue haste. Haste often makes waste and results in having to retake radiographs.

Another goal is pride in work and professional advancement. This is accomplished by reviewing techniques, reading professional journals and books, and attending lectures and seminars. Still another goal is to keep radiation levels as low as possible. This includes using protective devices that minimize radiation to the patient and remaining in a distant area during the exposure.

An additional goal is to always keep in mind the needs of the patient. Not all patients require the same number of radiographs. Avoid making two exposures when one can produce the same results. A final goal of every radiographer is to develop integrity, dedication, and competence to such a degree that the patient can be motivated and educated. By constantly keeping these goals in mind, the radiographer benefits both the patient and dentistry by rendering the finest professional service.

CHAPTER SUMMARY

Dental health education is not limited to demonstrations on toothbrushing and flossing techniques or to slogans such as "visit your dentist twice a year." It does and must include education in how x-rays can benefit the patient. The emphasis of this education must be on the preventive aspect of radiography. The exposing of interproximal radiographs during the checkup appointment to disclose incipient caries is a perfect example of preventive radiation.

Patient education is necessary not only to secure the patient's cooperation and motivation to return to the office for regular examinations but also to allay any fear about the safety of the procedures involved. Such fears must be recognized and dealt with in a straightforward and professional manner. Although radiation duties are usually delegated by the dentist to the auxiliaries, the responsibility for patient education is everyone's responsibility. Educational efforts are most likely to succeed when the entire staff works together as a team.

The patient must be told or shown why a complete diagnosis is not possible without x-rays, as hidden lesions may remain undetected until it is too late to repair the damage. Dental neglect results in pain, discomfort, loss of function and aesthetics, and a needless expenditure of time and money.

The methods of patient education include oral presentations at chair-side, the distribution of pamphlets, and showing the patient enlarged pictures or slides of radiographs projected on a screen. Lectures may be given to children or adults at schools or at meetings. Often a combination of these measures is most effective, as some patients relate better to the explanations given by the dentist, whereas others communicate better with one of the members of the staff.

Finally, as each person concerned with delivering radiation services develops expertise and establishes a rapport with the patients, a set of standards and goals must be developed. This is essential if the finest service is to be rendered to the patient. These goals include producing radiographs of good diagnostic quality each time, avoiding hasty or careless actions that result in retakes, keeping radiation levels low at all times, and making exposures only when necessary. Additional goals involve continuing education for professional advancement, a desire to pass on knowledge to the patient, and always keeping the patient's interests supreme.

KEY WORDS

Patient education
Preventive radiation

REVIEW QUESTIONS

1. What is the value of patient education? (a) that the dentist can schedule the patients better, (b) that more patients will call for appointments, (c) that an informed patient is inclined to accept the dentist's treatment plan, (d) that the patient will demand more radiographs at each appointment.

2. Why is patient education in radiography necessary? (a) to increase the demand for radiographic services, (b) because it is legally required, (c) to assure the patient that all radiographers are licensed, (d) because patients must be reassured that dental radiation procedures are safe.

3. Why does the patient benefit from preventive radiation? (a) because incipient decay may be disclosed, (b) because radiation inhibits dental decay, (c) because fewer cavities will have to be restored, (d) because radicular cysts can be eliminated by radiation treatment.

4. Which of these is not a method of patient education in radiography? (a) information given orally at chair-side, (b) follow-up letters from the dentist, (c) visual presentation of enlarged radiographs, (d) pamphlets on radiation.

5. Which of the following is not a goal of the radiographer? (a) professional improvement and advancement, (b) reducing the levels of radiation used during an exposure, (c) increasing the demand for dental x-ray services, (d) taking only such radiographs as are needed for diagnosis of the patient's needs.

BIBLIOGRAPHY

Division of Communications: *Dental X-ray Examinations: Your Dentist's Advice.* American Dental Association, 1993

Division of Communications: *Dental X-rays: Your Dentist's Advice.* American Dental Association, 1989

Division of Communications: *Facts About AIDS and Infection Control.* American Dental Association, 1993

Get the Picture on Dental X-rays. Rockville, MD: Bureau of Radiological Health, US Department of Health and Human Services, 1981

Answers to Review Questions

Chapter 1: 1-Wilhelm Conrad Roentgen, November 8, 1895, 2-position-indicating device, 3-dentist, 4-d, 5-c, 6-b, 7-a, 8-c, 9-b, 10-b.

Chapter 2: 1-b, 2-a, 3-d, 4-d, 5-a, 6-a, 7-d, 8-a, 9-c, 10-c, 11-see Figure 2–1, 12-see Glossary.

Chapter 3: 1-see Figure 3–2, 2-c, 3-(1) a source of free electrons; (2) high voltage to impart speed to them; and (3) a target that is capable of stopping them, 4-c, 5-d, 6-thermionic emission, 7-b, 8-square, 9-b, 10-a, 11-a, 12-b, 13-d, 14-b, 15-c.

Chapter 4: 1-d, 2-d, 3-d, 4-d, 5-c, 6-a, 7-b, 8-a, 9-a, 10-d, 11-b, 12-b and d, 13-central ray, 14-contrast.

Chapter 5: 1-a, 2-c, 3-b, 4-d, 5-d, 6-c, 7-d, 8-a, 9-a, 10-b, 11-d, 12-4.5 grays (450 rads), 13-direct hit or target, indirect or poison water, 14-as low as reasonably achievable.

Chapter 6: 1-d, 2-c, 3-b, 4-b, 5-c, 6-d, 7-c, 8-c, 9-d, 10-a, 11-inherent, added, aluminum equivalent, 12-size, shape, 13-aluminum, 14-longer.

Chapter 7: 1-d, 2-c, 3-a, 4-a, 5-c.

Chapter 8: 1-c, 2-b, 3-d, 4-c, 5-d, 6-b, 7-a, 8-c, 9-c, 10-b, 11-periapical, bitewing, occlusal, 12-b.

Chapter 9: 1-b, 2-b, 3-d, 4-c, 5-a, 6-d, 7-c, 8-b, 9-c, 10-b, 11-d, 12-c, 13-d, 14-cross-contamination, 15-x-ray processing chemicals, intraoral film packets and discarded radiographs.

Chapter 10: 1-T, 2-T, 3-F, 4-F, 5-T, 6-F, 7-T, 8-density, 9-sensitometer, 10-saliva, 11-b, 12-b.

Chapter 11: 1-d, 2-c, 3-a, 4-b, 5-c, 6-d, 7-d, 8-a, 9-b, 10-d.

Chapter 12: 1-interpretation, 2-dentist, 3-d, 4-a, 5-b, 6-a, 7-b, 8-c, 9-d, 10-a.

Chapter 13: 1-d, 2-c, 3-a, 4-d, 5-c, 6-a, 7-c, 8-c, 9-a, 10-c.

Chapter 14: 1-c, 2-d, 3-c, 4-d, 5-a, 6-d, 7-d, 8-c, 9-film, 10-paralleling, 11-gloves.

Chapter 15: 1-b, 2-c, 3-b, 4-d, 5-b, 6-c, 7-c, 8-a, 9-b.

Chapter 16: 1-b, 2-c, 3-a, 4-c, 5-d, 6-c.

Chapter 17: 1-d, 2-b, 3-c, 4-a, 5-d, 6-b.

Chapter 18: 1-a, 2-c, 3-b, 4-d, 5-c, 6-b, 7-a.

Chapter 19: 1-d, 2-b, 3-d, 4-b, 5-b.

Chapter 20: 1-b, 2-c, 3-a, 4-d, 5-a, 6-b.

Chapter 21: 1-d, 2-b, 3-a, 4-c, 5-c, 6-b, 7-a, 8-b, 9-b, 10-b, 11-a, 12-c.

Chapter 22: 1-c, 2-d, 3-a, 4-b, 5-c.

Glossary

This glossary includes not only terms used in the text but also terms frequently encountered in other publications on radiography. Many of the following definitions are copied or modified from those that appear in the second edition of the *Glossary of Dental Radiology* published in 1978 by the American Academy of Dental Radiology. The student is encouraged to consult these as supplementary reading. Definitions may vary slightly from source to source. The use of a medical dictionary is also recommended.

Abscess: A localized pus formation often accompanied by swelling and pain. In dentistry an abscess is usually located near the apex of the roots of the infected tooth and may be chronic or acute. Appears radiolucent when large enough to be visible on radiograph.

Absorbed Dose: The amount of energy deposited in any form of matter, such as wood, bracket table, air, teeth, muscles, and so forth, by any type of radiation (alpha or beta particles, x- or gamma rays, etc.). The units for measuring the absorbed dose are the gray (Gy) and the rad (radiation absorbed dose).

Absorption: The process through which radiation imparts some or all of its energy to any material through which it passes.

Acidifier: A chemical (acetic acid) in the fixer solution that neutralizes the alkali in the developer solution and stops further action of the developer.

Acoustic Meatus: The opening at the center of the ear. It is located directly over the temporal bone and shows up on extraoral radiographs as a small radiolucent circle.

Activator: A chemical (usually sodium carbonate) in the developer solution that causes the emulsion on the radiographic film to swell and initiates the reducing action of the developing agents. This sodium carbonate makes the developer alkaline.

Acute: Having a rapid onset, short, severe course, and pronounced symptoms; opposite of chronic.

Acute Radiation Syndrome: Symptoms of the short-term radiation effects after a massive dose of ionizing radiation.

Added Filtration: Added to the inherent filtration built into the x-ray machine. This added filtration is in the form of thin disks of pure aluminum, which can be inserted between the x-ray tube and the lead collimator when the inherent filtration is not sufficient to meet modern radiation safety requirements.

Adumbration: The giving forth of a vague shadow.

Aiming Device (Ring): One of the components of the Rinn XCP and BAI film holders used to determine correct horizontal and vertical alignment (formerly called **locator ring**).

Ala: The wing of the nose. In dental radiography, the depression at which the nostril connects with the cheek.

ALARA: "As low as reasonably achievable," economic and social factors being taken into account.

Ala–Tragus Line (Tragus–Ala Line): An imaginary plane or line from the ala of the nose (a winglike projection at the side of the nose) to the tragus of the ear (the cartilaginous projection in front of the acoustic meatus of the ear). This plane is important in determining the correct position of the patient's head.

Alkalizer: See **Activator.**

Alpha Particle: A common form of particulate (corpuscular) radiation. Alpha particles contain two protons and two neutrons and are positively charged. Symbol α.

Alternating Current: A flow of electrons in one direction, followed by a flow in the opposite direction.

Aluminum Equivalence: The thickness of aluminum affording the same degree of attenuation, under specified conditions, as the material in question.

Alveolar Bone: That portion of the maxillary or mandibular bone that surrounds and supports the roots of the dentition.

Alveolar Process: That portion of the maxillae or mandible that immediately surrounds and supports the roots of the teeth. Appears radiopaque.

Alveolus: In dentistry, that part of the alveolar bone that forms the bony socket in which the roots of the tooth are held in position by fibers of the periodontal ligament.

Amalgam Tattoo: The bluish-purple color to the gingival tissue caused by fragments of amalgam under the tissue.

Ameloblastoma: An odontogenic tumor of enamel origin that does not undergo differentiation to the point of enamel formation.

Amelogenesis Imperfecta: A hereditary enamel deficiency of the teeth. Believed to be caused by a generalized disturbance of the ameloblasts (enamel-producing cells). Also called enamel hypoplasia. The remaining tooth structures are not affected. On radiographs, such teeth lack the radiopaque image of enamel.

Amperage: The strength of an electric current measured in amperes.

Ampere: The unit of intensity of an electric current produced by 1 volt (V) acting through a resistance of 1 ohm (Ω).

Angle of Mandible: The area at the posterior and inferior corners of the mandible, where the body of the mandible meets and joins the ascending ramus of the mandible.

Angström Unit: A unit of measurement that describes the wavelengths of certain high-frequency radiation. One Angström unit (AU or Å) measures 1/100,000,000 of a centimeter. Most wavelengths used in dentistry vary from about 0.1 AU to a maximum of 1.0 AU.

Angulation: The direction in which the central ray and the PID of the x-ray machine are directed toward the teeth and the film. See **Horizontal Angulation, Negative Angulation, Positive Angulation, Vertical Angulation,** and **Zero Angulation.**

Ankylosis: A stiffening of a joint caused by a fibrous or bony union. In dentistry the term applies to a union of the tooth to the alveolus caused by mineralization and hardening of the fibers of the periodontal ligament, which normally surrounds the root and separates it from the alveolus.

Anode: The positive electrode (terminal) in the x-ray tube. This is a tungsten block, normally set at a 20-degree angle facing the cathode, imbedded in the copper portion of the terminal. The x-rays emanate from the point of impact of the electronic stream (cathode rays) from the cathode.

Anodontia: A congenital absence of teeth. Any tooth in the dental arch may fail to develop. The teeth most frequently absent are the third molars, the.premolars, and the maxillary lateral incisors.

Anomaly: Any deviation from the normal.

Anterior Nasal Spine (ANS): The most anterior point on the floor of the nasal cavity. This is located at the midsagittal plane.

Antiseptic: Refers to agents used on living tissues to destroy or stop the growth of bacteria.

Aphthous Ulcer: Small ulcer in the mouth, characterized by whitish spots around a central core. Commonly known as **canker sore.**

Apical Foramen: The opening to the pulp canal at the apex (terminal end) of the root of the tooth. A three-rooted tooth would have three apical foramina.

Area Monitoring: The routine monitoring of the level of radiation in an area such as a room, building, space around radiation-emitting equipment, or outdoor space.

Asepsis: The absence of septic matter, or freedom from infection.

Atom: The smallest particle of an element that has the properties of that element. Atoms are extremely minute and are composed of a number of subatomic particles. See **Proton, Electron,** and **Neutron.**

Attenuation: In radiography, the process by which a beam of radiation is reduced in energy when passing through matter.

Autotransformer: A special single-coil transformer that corrects fluctuations in the current flowing through the x-ray machine.

Background Radiation: Ionizing radiation that is always present. It consists of cosmic rays from outer space, naturally occurring radiation from the earth, and radiation from radioactive materials.

Backscatter: Radiation that is deflected by scattering processes at angles greater than 90 degrees to the original direction of the beam of radiation.

Barrier: Any material that is used to prevent the transmission of infective microorganisms to the patient.

Benign: Not recurrent; favorable for recovery.

Beta Particle: A form of particulate radiation. High-speed negative electrons. Symbol β.

Binding Energy: The internal energy within the atom that holds its components together.

Bisecting Technique (Bisecting-Angle or Short-Cone Technique): An exposure technique in which the central beam of radiation is directed perpendicularly toward an imaginary line that bisects the angle formed by the recording plane of the film and the long axis of the tooth.

Bisector: The imaginary line that bisects the angle formed by the film and tooth. See **Bisecting Technique.**

Biteblock: A small device, usually made of plastic, Styrofoam, or wood, that can be inserted between the teeth and held in place by biting pressure. It functions to hold the x-ray film in position while it is being exposed.

Bitewing Radiograph: A radiograph that shows the crowns of both the upper and lower teeth on the same film.

Bitewing Tab (Bitetab): A piece of heavy paper or linen and paper that is attached at the center of the film packet and on which the patient bites to stabilize the film during a bitewing exposure.

Bremsstrahlung: German word for "braking radiation." The stopping or slowing of the electrons of the cathode stream as they collide with the nuclei of the target atoms.

Buccal-Object Rule: See **Clark's Rule.**

Calcifications: The deposition of calcium salts from the saliva into the tissues surrounding the teeth.

Calculus: In dentistry, a deposition of mineral salts to form a concretion or ring around the root of a tooth or to cover parts of the crown. Also known as *scale* or *tartar.*

Cancellous Bone: See **Trabecular Bone.**

Canthus: The angle at either end of the slit that separates the eyelids. In radiography, the inner canthus is the part of the slit nearest to the nose; the outer canthus is the part farthest from the nose.

Cardboard Cassette: Two pieces of cardboard that are hinged on one end and have a metal clasp on the other end to tightly lock the holder after an extraoral film is inserted into a paper envelope within the holder. Used to make extraoral exposures. (Formerly called *exposure holder.*)

Caries: A disease of the calcified tissues of the teeth. The inorganic portion is demineralized and the organic tissues are destroyed.

Cassette: A rigid film holder consisting of a case with a hinged lid. Cassettes may be designated as extraoral or intraoral. Most cassettes contain a pair of intensifying screens and are intended for extraoral use. Intraoral cassettes have a very limited use.

Cassette Holder: The part of a panoramic-type x-ray machine that holds the cassette.

Cathode: The negative electrode (terminal) in the x-ray tube. The cathode consists of a tungsten filament wire that is set in a molybdenum focusing cup that directs the cathode stream toward the target on the anode.

Cathode Stream (Beam or Ray): The stream of electrons traveling from the heated filament of the cathode toward the target on the anode inside the x-ray tube. This beam of electrons travels at approximately half the speed of light. The speed depends on the electromotive force (kilovoltage) that is applied.

Cementoma: A tumor derived from the periodontal ligament of a fully developed and erupted tooth, usually a mandibular incisor. Early cementomas are radiolucent and appear identical to radicular cysts. In the later stages of development, calcification occurs and cementomas appear as radiopaque masses surrounded by a radiolucent line. The teeth associated with cementomas are vital and need no treatment.

Cementum: One of the four basic tooth structures. The thin layer of bony tissue that covers the root of a tooth. It differs in structure from bone in that it contains a large number of Sharpey's fibers. Because the cementum layer is so thin that it blends into the dentin of the tooth, it is generally radiographically indistinguishable from dentin. When the mass of cementum is large, as in hypercementosis, it appears radiopaque.

Central Beam (Ray): The central portion of the primary beam of radiation.

Cephalometer: A headholder or precision instrument used to stabilize the patient's head during exposure. This usually has cephalostats or craniostats, devices used to standardize the procedure so that identical results may be obtained each time. This holds the head parallel to the film and at right angles to the radiation beam.

Cephalometric Radiographs (Headplates): Lateral and posteroanterior extraoral head films. Frequently used in orthodontic treatment, they are used less often in prosthodontic treatment.

Cephalometric Tracings: Tracings from a cephalometric headplate made on acetate. These tracings indicate the location of various planes and points of interest to the orthodontist. The data are used to measure existing conditions and compare them with future or desirable conditions.

Cephalostat: A device used to stabilize the patient's head in a plane that is parallel to the film and at right angles to the central rays of the x-ray beam. Ear rods that can be pushed into the openings of the acoustic meatus of the ear help to accomplish this. Also called **craniostats.**

Cervical Burnout: A radiolucency often observed on the mesial and distal root surfaces near the cementoenamel junction. The radiolucent appearance is caused by the concave shape of the root at the cervical line and is frequently mistaken for caries when radiographs are being diagnosed.

Characteristic Radiation: A form of radiation originating from an atom following removal of an electron or excitation of the atom. The wavelength of the emitted radiation is specific for the element concerned and the particular energy levels that are involved.

Chromosomes: Structures found in the cell nuclei, which carry the hereditary materials. These are constant in number for each species.

Clark's Rule (Buccal-Object Rule): A rule for the orientation of structures portrayed in two or more radiographs exposed at a different angle.

Collimation: The restriction of the useful beam to an appropriate size; generally, to a diameter of 2 3/4 in. (7 cm) at the skin surface.

Collimator: A diaphragm, usually lead, designed to restrict the dimensions of the useful beam.

Compton Effect (Compton Scattering): An attenuation process for x- and gamma radiation in which a photon interacts with an orbital electron or an atom to form a displaced electron and a scattered photon (x-ray) of reduced energy.

Concrescence: A condition in which the cementum of adjacent teeth is united.

Condensing Osteitis: A term used to describe the formation of compact sclerotic bone within the jaws. Such areas of hardened bone are frequently seen on dental radiographs and appear more radiopaque than the surrounding bone areas. Such areas are generally irregular in shape or location. See **Osteitis.**

Condyle: A rounded knob or projection on a bone, usually where that bone articulates (joins) with another bone. In dental radiography, the condyle of the mandible articulates with the glenoid fossa (depression) of the temporal bone.

Cone (PID): A cone or cylindrical position-indicating device (PID) to indicate the direction of the central beam of radiation. The length of the cone helps to establish the desired target–surface distance. The term cone originated because formerly all PIDs were cone-shaped. The closed, pointed cone caused interference with the passage of the x-ray beam and produced a large amount of scatter radiation. All modern PIDs are open-ended. Although the term is no longer appropriate, some still refer to the PID as a cone.

Cone Cut: A term used to describe a technique error in which the central beam is not directed toward the center of the film. This produces a blank area in the part of the radiograph that was not reached by the radiation.

Contact Area: The area of a tooth surface that touches another tooth. This generally refers to the mesial surface of one tooth making contact with the distal surface of the tooth behind it in the dental arch. The spot where the teeth actually touch is the contact point and the area between the contact point and the gingiva (gum) is called the **embrasure.**

Contrast: The visual differences between shades ranging from black to white in adjacent areas of the radiographic film. A radiograph that shows few shades is said to have short-scale contrast, while one that shows many variations in shade is said to possess long-scale contrast. The use of increased kilovoltage results in the production of a radiograph with long-scale contrast.

Control Panel: The portion of the x-ray machine that houses the major controls.

Controlled Area: A defined area in which the occupational exposure of personnel to radiation is under the supervision of the radiation protection supervisor. The dental office is designated as a controlled area.

Corpuscular Radiation: Minute subatomic particles such as protons, electrons, and neutrons; also alpha and beta particles. These particles occupy space; have mass and weight; and, with the exception of neutrons, have an electrical charge.

Cortical Bone: The solid, outer portion of the bone. Also known as dense or compact bone. Such bone appears very radiopaque (white) on radiographs.

Coulombs per Kilogram (C/kg): A coulomb is a unit of electrical charge (equal to 6.25×10^{18} electrons). The unit C/kg measures electrical charges (ion pairs) in a kilogram of air.

Crest: In radiation, the peak of an electromagnetic wave. The distance from crest to crest determines the wavelength—hence its penetration ability.

Cross-Sectional Technique: A technique used in occlusal radiography, in which the central ray is directed toward the area of interest and parallel to the long axes of the teeth and adjacent areas.

Current: In radiation, a flow of electricity from a point of higher potential to a point of lower potential. The electric current used in most homes and dental offices is spoken of as "line current."

Cutting Reducer: A chemical used to lighten a radiograph that has been accidentally overexposed or overdeveloped. The chemical removes layer after layer of the metallic silver on the radiograph until the desired density is produced.

Cyst: An epithelium-lined sac containing fluid or other fibrous or solid material. If filled with fluid or fibrous material, cysts appear radiolucent. Common cysts in dental radiography are dentigerous, follicular, radicular (apical or periapical), and residual.

"Dead-Man" Switch: A switch so constructed that a circuit-closing contact can only be maintained by continuous pressure by the operator.

Decay Process: In radiography, the radioactive disintegration of the nucleus of an unstable atom by the emission of particles, photons of energy, or both.

Deciduous Teeth: The primary dentition. Teeth that fall out or are exfoliated naturally. The deciduous dentition consists of 20 teeth—8 incisors, 4 canines, and 8 molars.

Definition: In radiography, the sharpness and clarity of the outline of the structures on the image shown on the film. Poor definition is generally caused by movement of the patient, film, or the tube head during exposure.

Dens in dente: A developmental anomaly in which the enamel invaginates within the body of the tooth.

Densitometer: An instrument for measuring the amount of darkening of x-ray film, based on a photocell measuring the light transmitted through a given area of the film.

Density: In radiography, film blackening (the amount of light transmitted through a film). The simplest way to increase or decrease the density of a radiograph is to increase or decrease the milliamperage and exposure time (milliampere/second).

Dentigerous Cyst: A cyst derived from the enamel organ and always associated with the crown of a tooth.

Dentin: One of the four basic tooth structures. The chief substance or tissue of the tooth that surrounds the tooth pulp. It is covered by enamel on the crown of the tooth and by cementum on the root. Appears radiopaque, but not as dense as enamel.

Dentinogenesis Imperfecta: A hereditary condition characterized by imperfectly formed dentin that has an opalescent or amber color.

Depth Dose: The total amount of radiation absorbed at any given point inside the patient or object.

Detail: The point-by-point delineation of the minute structures visible in the shadow images on the radiograph.

Developer: The chemical solution used in film processing that makes the latent image visible.

Developer Agent: Elon and hydroquinone, substances that reduce the halides in the film emulsion to metallic silver. Elon brings out the details and hydroquinone brings out the contrast in the film.

Diagnosis: The art of differentiating and determining the nature of a problem or disease. Dental radiographs are an important factor in evaluating the condition of the dentition and help in finalizing the diagnosis.

Diaphragm: A plate, usually lead, with a central aperture so placed as to restrict the useful beam. See **Collimator.**

Dilaceration: A tooth with a sharp bend in the root.

Direct Current: Electric current that flows continuously in one direction. Unidirectional current is produced in batteries but cannot be used in x-ray machines unless they are modified.

Disinfection: A term used to describe those efforts made to reduce the disease-producing microorganisms to an acceptable level.

Dispenser: In radiography, a lead-lined chute or container from which unexposed film packets can be removed one at a time.

Dosage: The radiation absorbed in a specified area of the body measured in grays or rads.

Dose: The amount of absorbed radiation in grays or rads at any given point. Measurements inside the body are difficult to make. Doses are often spoken of as absorbed, depth, entrance, erythema, exposure, skin, or surface doses.

Dose Equivalent: A term used for radiation protection purposes to compare the biological effects of the various types of radiation. Dose equivalent is defined as the product of the absorbed dose times a biological effect modifying factor. Since the modifying factor for x-rays is one, the absorbed dose and the dose equivalent are equal. The units for measuring the dose equivalent are the sievert (Sv) and the rem.

Dose Rate: The radiation dose received per unit of time.

Dosimeter: A small device, usually the size of a fountain pen, used to measure radiation. This device contains a small ionizing chamber and an electrometer that can be read by the person wearing the dosimeter.

Drum: A part of some panoramic-type x-ray machines to which a flexible cassette can be attached. The drum and attached film rotate when the machine is in operation.

Duplicating Film: A photographic film that appears similar to x-ray film and is used to duplicate x-ray films in a contact-printer–type x-ray duplicating unit.

Duty Cycle: The length of time that the x-ray tube can be energized. A consecutive series of long exposures can overheat and damage the tube.

DXTTR (Dental X-Ray Teaching and Training Replica): A skull with complete dentition that is covered with simulated plastic skin to resemble the head. Contains a hinge mechanism to open and close the mouth. Used by students to practice making radiographic exposures. Also known as a *mannequin* or **phantom.** Sometimes written *Dexter.*

Dysphagia: Difficulty in swallowing.

Edentulous Survey: A radiographic examination of the mouth of a patient without teeth. The mouth may be totally or partially edentulous.

Electrical Potential: See **Potential.**

Electrode: Either of two terminals of an electric source; in the x-ray tube, either the anode or the cathode.

Electromagnetic Radiation: Forms of energy propelled by wave motion as photon. This is a combination of electric and magnetic energy. This radiation has no charge, mass, or weight and travels at the speed of light. These forms of energy differ tremendously in wavelength, frequency, and properties. For convenience they are arranged in diagrammatic form as the electromagnetic spectrum.

Electromagnetic Spectrum: Types of electromagnetic energies arranged in diagrammatic form on a chart. These include radio and television waves, infrared waves, visible light, ultraviolet waves, x-rays, gamma rays, and cosmic radiations. The longer wavelengths are measured in meters and the shorter ones in centimeters or angstroms.

Electromotive Force: The difference in potential between the cathode and the anode in the x-ray tube (generally expressed in kilovolts).

Electron: A small, negatively charged particle of the atom containing much energy and little mass.

Electron Cloud: A mass of free electrons that hovers around the filament wire of the cathode when it is heated to incandescence. The number of free electrons increases as the milliamperage is increased.

Electron Shells: See **Energy Levels.**

Electrostatic: Electric charges at rest (static electricity).

Element: In chemistry, a simple substance that cannot be decomposed by chemical means.

Elongation: A term used in radiography to refer to a distortion of the image in which the tooth structures appear longer than the anatomical size. This is most often caused by insufficient vertical angulation of the central beam.

Embrasure: The space between the sloping proximal surfaces of the teeth. The space may diverge facially, lingually, occlusally, or apically. The interdental papillae normally fill most of the apical embrasures.

Emulsion: The coating on radiographic film, a gelatinous solution containing silver halides.

Emulsion Speed: The sensitivity of the film to the radiation exposure.

Enamel: One of the four basic tooth structures. The white, compact, and very hard substance that covers the dentin of the crown of the teeth. Appears very radiopaque on the radiographs.

Endodontia: The branch of dentistry concerned with the prevention, diagnosis, and treatment of diseases and injuries of the dental pulp and periapical tissues.

Energy: In physics, the ability to do work and overcome resistance.

Energy Levels (Electron Shells or Orbits): A term used in chemistry and physics to denote spherical levels containing the electrons of the atom.

Enhancement: Intensification of detail, making a radiograph easier to interpret.

Enhancer: A device that brings out details on a radiograph. Contains focusing devices and magnifying lenses.

Entrance Dose (Skin Dose): Radiation dosage at the point where it enters the patient.

Eruptive Cyst: A dentigerous (follicular) cyst that is destroyed upon the eruption of the tooth with which the cyst was associated.

Erythema Dose: Radiation overdose that produces temporary redness of the skin.

Exit Dose: The absorbed dose delivered by a beam of radiation to the surface through which the beam emerges from an object.

Exostosis: A bony growth projecting outward from the surface of a bone or tooth. Occasionally encountered on the palate or the lingual surface of the mandible. Also called a torus.

Exposure: A measure of ionization produced in air by x- or gamma radiation. It is the sum of the electrical charges of all of the ions of one sign produced in air when all electrons liberated by photons in a volume element of air are completely stopped in air, divided by the mass of air in the volume present. The units of exposure are coulombs per kilogram (C/kg) and the roentgen (R).

Exposure Rate: The exposure per unit of time.

Extension Arm: Flexible arm from which the tube head of the x-ray machine is suspended.

Extension Cone (Extension Tube): A long cone- or tube-shaped position-indicating device.

External Oblique Ridge (Line): A diagonal ridge of bone on the lateral aspect of the mandible. The ridge runs downward and forward from the anterior border of the ramus to the level of the cervical portion of the molar and premolar roots. This landmark appears very radiopaque.

Extraoral: Outside the mouth.

Extraoral Radiograph: A radiograph exposed outside the mouth.

Farmer's Solution: A chemical reducer used to lighten a dark overexposed or overdeveloped film.

Filament: The spiral tungsten coil in the focusing cup of the cathode of the x-ray tube.

Film Badge: A monitoring device containing a special type of film, which when properly developed and interpreted, gives a measurement of the exposure received during the time the badge was worn. The film badge has been replaced by the **thermoluminescent dosimeter.**

Film Holder: A mechanical device used to hold and stabilize dental x-ray film in the mouth.

Film Loop: A thin, stiff paper constructed in such a manner that a film packet can be slid into the loop portion to hold the film in position while the patient bites on the tab portion. Used in bitewing radiography. Also known as a *bitewing loop.*

Film Mount: A celluloid, plastic, or cardboard holder with frames or windows so arranged that any desired size and number of radiographs can be fastened to the mount for display and viewing of the films.

Film Packet: The intraoral film that is wrapped and enclosed for dental use by the manufacturer. It contains one or two films, a dark protective paper on either side, a thin sheet of lead foil on the back side of the film, and a semimoistureproof outer wrap.

Film Placement: The act of positioning the film packet in the patient's mouth. In horizontal placement, the widest dimension of the film is positioned horizontally, whereas in vertical film placement, the widest film dimension is positioned vertically.

Film Safe: A lead-lined receptacle for storing exposed dental film packets.

Film Sensitivity: See **Emulsion Speed.**

Filter: Absorbing material, usually aluminum, placed in the path of the beam of radiation to remove a high percentage of the low-energy (longer wavelength) x-rays.

Filtration: The use of absorbers for selectively absorbing or screening out the low-energy x-rays from the primary beam. See **Added Filtration, Inherent Filtration,** and **Total Filtration.**

Fistula: A narrow canal or tubular channel leading from an abscess or a diseased lesion within the alveolar bone or soft tissues to the outside of the oral membrane. Fluid in the form of pus or some other serous exudate may be contained within the fistula. Often the fistula leads to a parulis, also known as a *gumboil.*

Fixer: In radiography or photography, a solution of chemicals that stops the action of the developer and makes the image permanently visible.

Fixing Agent: Sodium thiosulfate, also known as "hypo" or hyposulfite of sodium. It is one of several chemical ingredients of the fixer solution and functions to remove all unexposed and any remaining undeveloped silver bromide grains from the emulsion.

Flexible Cassette: A cassette made of plastic or other flexible material so that it can be wrapped around the drum of certain types of panoramic x-ray machines.

Fluorescence: The emission of a glowing light by certain mineral salts when they are struck by particular wavelengths. In radiography, the calcium tungstate that is in the emulsion of the intensifying screen of cassettes glows and gives off a bluish light when the crystals are struck by the x-ray photons.

Focal Spot: A small area on the target on the anode toward which the electrons from the focusing cup of the cathode are directed. X-rays originate at the focal spot.

Focal Trough: A term describing that area of the dental anatomy that is reproduced distinctly on a panoramic radiograph. The size and shape of the focal trough vary with each panoramic x-ray machine.

Focusing Cup: A curved device around the cathode wire filament that is designed to focus the free electrons toward the tungsten target of the anode.

Fog: A darkening of the finished radiograph caused by any of several factors such as old or contaminated processing solutions, exposure to chemical fumes, faulty safelight, or scatter radiation.

Follicular Cyst (or Dentigerous Cyst): A cyst associated with the enamel follicle.

Foramen: A naturally formed hole or passage through a bone or tooth. Often the opening for a canal through which blood vessels and nerves pass. Appears radiolucent on radiograph.

Foreign Body: Any object or material not normally found in the area.

Foreshortening: A term used in radiology to refer to a distortion of the image in which the tooth structures appear shorter than their actual anatomical size. This is most often caused by excessive vertical angulation of the central beam.

Fossa: A depression or hollow area on a tooth or bone. If large enough, it will appear as a radiolucent area on a radiograph.

Fracture Line: A break in a bone that appears radiolucent on the radiograph.

Frequency: The number of crests of a wavelength passing a given point per second.

Full-Mouth Survey: The complete radiographic examination of the mouth in which a film is positioned periapically in each major tooth area. This normally entails a minimum of 14 films and may be over 20 films. Generally such a survey also includes bitewing films.

Fusion: A condition where the dentin and one other dental tissue of adjacent teeth are united.

Gamma Rays: A form of electromagnetic radiation with properties identical to x-rays. Usually produced spontaneously in the form of emission from radioactive substances.

Geiger Counter: A radiation monitoring device that counts the ionizing particles passing through it. A needlelike electrode inside a gas-filled chamber sets up a current in an electric field whenever the gas is ionized by radiation.

Gemination: A single tooth bud divides and forms two teeth.

Genes: The fundamental units of inheritance, arranged on the chromosomes and carrying the individual traits of the organisms.

Genetic Cells: The cells contained within the testes and ovaries, containing the genes.

Genetic Effects: Radiations effects upon the genes and hence upon future generations. It is known that massive exposure of the genes to radiation may produce mutations.

Genial Tubercles: An anatomical landmark situated near the midline on the lingual surface of the mandible about halfway between the alveolar crest and the inferior border of the mandible. There are four of them, and on a radiograph they appear like a very small, doughnut-shaped, radiopaque ring. The lingual foramen is located in the center of this ring.

Geometric Unsharpness: Poor image definition as a result of the penumbra.

Glenoid Fossa: A depression on the temporal bone. The condyle of the mandible fits into this fossa to form the temporomandibular joint. This landmark is seen only on extraoral radiographs.

Globulomaxillary Cyst: A cyst arising between the maxillary lateral incisor and the canine (cuspid).

Granuloma: A tumor or neoplasm made up of granulation tissue. Often follows an abscess. Is usually round or oval and surrounded by a fibrous capsule. Appears radiolucent on a radiograph.

Gray (Gy): A unit for measuring absorbed dose. One gray equals 1 joule (unit of energy) per kilogram of tissue. One gray equals 100 rads.

Grenz Rays: The longest wavelength of the x-rays, known as soft radiation because they have little penetrating power.

Half-Life: The period required for the disintegration of half of the atoms in a sample of some specific radioactive substance.

Half-Value Layer (HVL): The thickness of a specified material that, when introduced into the path of a given beam of radiation, reduces the exposure rate by half.

Halide: A compound of a halogen (astatine, bromine, chlorine, fluorine, or iodine) with another element or radical. In radiography a halide, usually bromide of silver, is suspended in the gelatin that coats the film base.

Hamular Process (Hamulus): A very small hooklike process of bone that extends downward and slightly backward from the sphenoid bone. It appears radiopaque and can occasionally be seen posterior to the maxillary tuberosity.

Hardening Agent (Hardener): Potassium alum, one of the chemicals of the fixing solution. It functions to shrink and harden the wet emulsion.

Hard Radiation: Rays of high energy and extremely short wavelengths. Essential for dental radiography.

Head Positioner: A device used on panoramic and cephalometric x-ray machines to stabilize the head into the most favorable position.

Herpes Labialis: An inflammatory skin disease characterized by the formation of small vesicles in clusters on the lips. Often called fever sores or blisters.

High-Voltage Transformer (Step-Up Transformer): A device consisting of two metal cores and coils so positioned within the circuitry of the tube head that it is capable of increasing the potential of the line current to the high kilovoltage that is required to produce x-radiation.

Horizontal Angulation: The direction of the central beam in a horizontal plane. Faulty horizontal angulation is the main cause of overlapping the proximal structures during exposure.

Horizontal Placement: See **Film Placement.**

Hypercementosis: An excessive development of the cementum of the tooth. It is usually, but not necessarily, confined to the apical portion of the root. Only occurs on vital teeth and is most frequently encountered on premolars. Area involved appears radiopaque.

Identification Dot: A small circular embossed mark on the corner of each x-ray film. The raised side of this convexity is always placed toward the side facing the x-ray beam. The identification dot makes it possible to determine whether the exposure was made on the patient's right or left side.

Image: In radiography, the duplicate in outline form of the structures exposed to radiation. A latent (invisible) image forms on the film when it is exposed. This latent image becomes visible after development and final processing.

Image Magnification: An enlargement of the structures shown on the radiograph over their actual size. Such enlargement is greatest when the target of an x-ray machine is closer to the structures being x-rayed and is decreased when distance is greater.

Impacted Tooth (Impaction): A tooth that is embedded in the alveolar bone in such a manner that its eruption is prevented. An impaction may be partial or total.

Impulse: In dental radiography a measure of exposure time. Many x-ray machines are calibrated to make the exposure in impulses instead of fractions of a second. There are 60 impulses per second.

Incandescence: In radiography, the stage in which the tungsten filament in the cathode becomes red-hot with heat and glows, thus liberating free electrons that swarm around the glowing wire to form the electron cloud.

Incisive Foramen: An important maxillary landmark. It is situated at the midline of the palate immediately behind the central incisors. The nasopalatine nerve and vessels emerge from it. The shape varies but is usually seen as a round pea-shaped radiolucent area. When faulty horizontal angulation is used, the image of the foramen may be superimposed over the apex of the root of the central incisor. It may then be mistaken for an abscess or a cyst.

Indicator Rod (Arm): One of the components of the Rinn XCP and BAI film holders. When properly assembled and positioned in the mouth, this metal rod serves as a guide in determining the correct angulation of the position indicating device (PID).

Infection Control: The prevention and reduction of disease-causing (pathogenic) microorganisms.

Inferior Border of the Mandible: The dense layer of cortical bone that forms the lower portion of the body of the mandible. It appears very radiopaque on the radiograph.

Inherent Filtration: The filtration built into the machine by the manufacturer. This includes the glass x-ray tube envelope, the insulating materials of the tube head, and the materials that seal the port.

Intensifying Screen: A card or plastic sheet coated with calcium tungstate or similar fluorescent salt crystals and positioned in the cassette so that it contacts the film. When exposed to radiation, the fluorescent salts glow, giving off a blue or green light that along with the radiation causes the latent image to form faster than is possible when radiation alone is used.

Interpretation: In dental radiography, the ability to read what is revealed by the radiograph. The final interpretation is the responsibility of the dentist. Dental auxiliaries should be capable of making a preliminary interpretation.

Interproximal Radiograph (Bitewing Radiograph): A radiograph that shows the crowns of both the upper and lower teeth on the same film.

Intraoral: Inside the mouth.

Intraoral Cassette: A very small cassette holding an occlusal film. Its purpose is to reduce exposure time through the action of the intensifying screens.

Intraoral Radiograph: A radiograph produced when the film is placed within the mouth and exposed.

Intrex: Trade name of an x-ray machine that has the tube in a recessed position within the tube head.

Inverse Square Law: A rule stating that the intensity of radiation is inversely proportional to the square of the distance from the source of the radiation to the point of measurement.

Ion: An electrically charged particle, either negative or positive.

Ionization: The formation of ion pairs.

Ionization Chamber: An instrument for measuring ionizing radiation.

Ionizing Radiation: Radiation that is capable of producing ions.

Irradiation: The exposure of an object or a person to radiation. This term can be applied to radiations of various wavelengths, such as infrared rays, ultraviolet rays, x-rays, and gamma rays.

Isotope: An alternate form of an element, having the same number of protons but a different number of neutrons inside the nucleus. Many isotopes are radioactive.

Kilovolt (kV): A unit of electromotive force, equal to 1000 volts. High kilovoltage is essential for the production of dental x-rays.

Kilovolt Peak (kVp): The crest value in kilovolts of the potential difference of a pulsating generator.

Kinetic Energy: The energy possessed by a mass because of its motion.

Lamina Dura: A thin, hard layer of cortical bone that lines the dental alveolus. Appears as a thin radiopaque line around the roots of the teeth on dental radiographs.

Laminography: A type of body-section radiography (tomography). *Lamina* means "thin layer" and *graphy* means "to record."

Landmarks: In dental radiography this term refers to a number of structures located on the bones of the head or face and certain points on the soft tissues of the face or the oral cavity.

Latent Image: The invisible image produced when the film is exposed to the x-ray photons. This image remains invisible until the film is processed.

Latent Period: The time between exposure to radiation and the first clinically observable symptoms. The word latent means "hidden."

Lateral Headplate (Lateral Radiography): Large extraoral film placed against either side of the head and parallel to it.

Lateral Jaw Survey: An extraoral exposure of either side of the patient's face that produces an image of both the maxilla and mandible on the same film.

Lateral Skull Survey: A large radiograph of either side of the skull. See **Lateral Headplate.**

LD 50–30 (Median Lethal) Dose: That dose of radiation that will be lethal for 50 percent of a large population during a specified length of time, usually 30 days.

Lead Equivalence: The thickness of a material that affords the same degree of attenuation to radiation as a specified thickness of lead.

Lead Protective Apron: Apron made of lead or lead-equivalent materials. This covers patients' gonadal areas to protect them from radiation.

Leakage Radiation: The x-rays that escape out of the tube head at places other than the port.

Lethal Dose: The amount of radiation that is sufficient to cause the death of an organism.

Light Fog: Clouding or darkening of radiographic film through accidental exposure to light or prolonged exposure to a safelight.

Line Current: The electric current normally passing through the electric lines in most homes and offices. In the United States, this is generally a 110-volt alternating current.

Line Focus Principle: The method by which the size of the focal spot is reduced to the desired size by the manufacturer. By facing the target at an angle toward the cathode filament, the electron beam is focused into a narrow rectangle on the anode. When viewed from below, as from the position of the film packet, the rectangular area looks like a small square.

Line Switch: The toggle switch that is used to turn the x-ray machine on or off.

Lingual Foramen: A very small opening through which a branch of the incisive artery emerges. It is located in the center of the genial tubercles on the lingual side of the mandible. See also **Genial Tubercles.**

Long-Scale Contrast: The variations in contrast, with many shades of gray, shown on radiographs exposed with high kilovoltage.

Low-Voltage Transformer (Step-Down Transformer): A device consisting of two metal cores and coils so positioned within the circuitry of the tube head that it is capable of decreasing the line voltage to between 3 and 12 volts. Such voltage is required in the cathode to warm up the filament wire.

Mach Band Effect: An optical illusion first described by Ernst Mach in 1865. This effect occurs along boundaries of sharp contrast. There appears to be a darker band along the edge of radiolucent areas and, similarly, a lighter band along the edge of radiopaque areas. The mach band effect is an edge enhancement, created in the eye, that does not result from an actual density change in the film emulsion.

Macrodontia: Very large teeth.

Malignant: Tendency to progress in virulence; tendency to spread and go from bad to worse.

Malposed Tooth: A tooth not in normal location.

Mandibular Canal: A long canal extending from the mandibular foramen on the medial aspect of the ramus of the mandible to the mental foramen on the lateral aspect of the body of the mandible. The canal carries the nerves and blood vessels that supply most of the teeth in the mandible. The canal appears radiolucent. A thin radiopaque line above and below it on the radiograph outline the cortical bone that lines the canal.

Mandibular Plane: A term used in cephalometric radiography. The line of the inferior border of the mandible from the gonion to the menton.

Maximum Permissible Dose (MPD): The maximum accumulated dose that persons who are occupationally exposed may have at any given time of their life.

Maximum Permissible Dose Equivalent: For radiation purposes, the maximum dose equivalent that a person or body part is allowed to receive in a stated period of time. It is the dose of ionizing radiation that, in the light of present knowledge, is not expected to cause detectable body damage to average persons at any time during their lifetime. For whole-body radiation, this is currently established at 0.05 Sv/y (5 rems/y) for radiation workers. Sometimes called Radiation Protection Guide (RPG).

Mean Tangent: The average point where several curved surfaces touch if a ruler is held against them. The labial or buccal surfaces of all teeth have their most prominent point toward the lips or the cheeks and curve toward the mesial or distal. A mean tangent could be established by using a small ruler or any straight edge and attempting to align as many of the teeth as possible. Occasionally four or even five of the posterior teeth will touch the ruler at some point. An imaginary line can be substituted for the ruler, and that is the mean tangent. To establish correct horizontal angulation, the central rays are directed at right angles to the mean tangent.

Meatus: An opening in the bone. The acoustic meatus (the outer opening of the canal of the ear) is often observed on extraoral dental radiographs as a small radiolucent circle.

Median Palatine Suture: An irregular line formed by the junction of the palatine processes of the right and left maxillae. On radiographs it appears as a thin radiolucent line running vertically between the roots of the maxillary incisors.

Mental Foramen: An opening through which the mental nerve and related blood vessels emerge on the lateral aspect of the body of the mandible. The location of this foramen varies and is often not shown on radiographs. When visible, it appears as a small round radiolucent area near the roots of the mandibular premolars.

Microdontia: Very small teeth.

Midsagittal Plane (Midsagittal Line): An imaginary vertical line or plane passing through the center of the body that divides it into a right and left half.

Milliammeter: A device on the control panel of many x-ray machines for determining and controlling the number of milliamperes of electric current flowing through.

Milliampere (mA): The milliampere is one thousandth of an ampere. In radiography, the milliamperage determines the number of electrons available at the filament. See **Ampere.**

Milliampere Second (mAs): The relationship between the milliamperage used and the exposure time in seconds. When one is increased, the other must be correspondingly decreased if the density of the exposed radiograph is to remain the same.

Milliroentgen (mR): One-thousandth of a roentgen. See **Roentgen.**

Modifying Factor (Quality Factor): A factor used for radiation protection purposes and in radiation biology to account for the difference in the biological effectiveness of the various types of radiation (x-, gamma, alpha, beta, etc). Some radiations (such as alpha particles) cause more biological damage than others (such as x-rays). The modifying (quality) factor is used to convert absorbed dose to dose equivalent. The modifying factor for x-rays is 1, for alpha particles it is 10.

Molecule: A chemical combination of two or more atoms that forms the smallest particle of a substance that retains the properties of that substance.

Monitoring: In radiation, the use of any of several devices to determine whether an area is within safe radiation limits or whether a person's exposure is within permissible limits. See **Area Monitoring** and **Personnel Monitoring.**

Monitoring Badge: A device worn by a radiation worker to measure the amount of radiation received in a given period of time. This is most often accomplished by wearing a **thermoluminescent dosimeter (TLD).**

Mutation: A change in the hereditary pattern of an organism. The change itself, if the organism survives, becomes hereditary. It is currently believed that any radiation exposure to the reproductive cells is capable of causing some form of mutation.

Mylohyoid Ridge (Line): A ridge running diagonally downward and forward on the medial aspect of the ramus of the mandible to near the apices of the molar roots. This bony ridge serves for muscle attachments and parallels the external oblique line, but on the lingual surface and about 1/4 in. (6 mm) lower. This line is not always seen on radiographs; when visible, the line is radiopaque.

Negative: A photographic or radiographic film wherein light and dark areas of the subject are shown in reverse.

Negative Angulation (Negative Vertical Angulation or Minus Angulation): Angulation achieved by pointing the tip or end of the PID upward from a horizontal plane.

Negative Ion: An ion that has a negative electric charge. See **Ion.**

Neutron: One form of corpuscular radiation (particulate), or subatomic particle. A neutron has no electric charge and has about the same mass as a proton.

Nonodontogenic Cyst: A cyst that arises from epithelium other than that associated with tooth formation.

Nonscreen Film (No-Screen Film): A form of extraoral film that has an extra-thick coating of emulsion and is sensitive to radiation. See **Screen Film.**

Object: In dental radiography, whatever is being radiographed, usually a tooth or teeth.

Occipital Protuberance: A bulge or prominence at the center of the outer surface of the squamous portion of the occipital bone. The location of this protuberance can be determined by palpating the back of the patient's head.

Occlusal Plane: The plane between the maxillary and the mandibular teeth.

Occlusal Radiographs: Radiographs produced by placing the film along the incisal or occlusal plane and having the patient stabilize it by biting down on it. In addition to the teeth, occlusal radiographs may show surrounding maxillary or mandibular bone structures. Depending on the film placement and angle of exposure, cross-sectional or topographic radiographs are produced. See **Cross-Sectional Technique** and **Topographical Technique.**

Odontogenic Cyst: A cyst that arises from epithelial cells associated with the development of a tooth.

Odontoma: A tumor of odontogenic origin in which enamel and dentin are formed. The odontoma may contain soft tissues that appear radiolucent and also contain a hard calcified mass, sometimes resembling a tooth, that appears radiopaque on the radiograph. **Compound odontoma** refers to odontogenic tissues in normal relationship that resemble teeth. **Complex odontoma** denotes odontogenic tissues arranged in a haphazard manner with no resemblance to normal tooth formation. **Compound–complex odontoma** is a mixture of the two types.

Operator (Radiographer): The person operating any x-ray equipment to make exposures.

Oral Radiographic Survey: An examination of the teeth based on one or more radiographs of the dental area of interest.

Oral Radiography: All the procedures needed to produce radiographs of the teeth or head. These include adjustments of the x-ray machine, preparation of the patient, generation of x-radiation, and film processing and interpretation.

Orthopantomograph: A trade name for a panoramic-type x-ray machine produced by Siemens Corporation.

Ossifications: The pathological or abnormal conversion of soft tissues into bone.

Osteitis: A bone inflammation. In radiography, the term refers to changes in bone density resulting from disease, trauma, or infection. In **rarefying osteitis,** the bone appears more radiolucent, whereas in **condensing osteitis,** the bone structures appear more radiopaque.

Osteoma: Benign tumors composed of bone. They vary greatly in size and appear radiopaque.

Osteomyelitis: An acute or chronic inflammation of the bone or bone marrow, which may sometimes be visible on radiographs.

Output: The amount of radiation that an x-ray machine produces, calculated in coulombs per kilogram per second (roentgens per second), measured at the open end of the PID.

Overlapping: A term used in radiography to refer to a distortion of the tooth image in which the structures of one tooth are superimposed over the structures of the adjacent tooth. This is most often caused by faulty horizontal angulation of the central beam.

Oxidation: In dental radiography, the process during which the chemicals of the developing and fixing solutions combine with oxygen and lose their strength.

Oxidizing Agent: Any substance that produces oxidation in another substance.

Panelipse: A trade name for a panoramic-type x-ray machine produced by the Gendex Corporation.

Panoramic Radiography: Radiographic procedures with a special-purpose x-ray machine that uses a fixed position of the x-ray source, object, and film to produce a radiograph of the entire dentition and surrounding structures on a single film.

Panorex: A trade name for a panoramic x-ray machine produced by Keystone X-ray, Inc. The radiographs taken by this machine can be easily recognized by a 1/2-in. (12-mm) white area in the middle of the film.

Pantomography: The art of making graphic recordings of tissue contours on radiographic film.

Paralleling Technique (Long-Cone Technique or Right-Angle Technique): In radiography, an intraoral technique that requires a biteblock or some type of film holder to hold the film packet parallel to the teeth while the central beam of radiation is directed perpendicularly (at right angles) toward the teeth and the film.

Particulate Radiation: See **Corpuscular Radiation.**

Parulis: A raised swollen area indicating an abscess of the gum. Often called a *gumboil.* A fistula often connects the parulis with the core of the abscess at the apex of the root in the alveolus.

Patient Education: This term refers to effort that is the duty and responsibility of every member of the dental health team—informing the public, and specifically the dental patients, about the values of oral health, preventive dentistry, and good dental care. As used in this text, patient education refers to providing the patient with necessary information on the value of dental radiography and the safety measures employed in the dental office to limit its effects.

Pedodontic Film: The smaller sizes of film packets commonly used for radiographs of children's teeth.

Penumbra: In radiography, a partial shadow or fuzzy outline around the image.

Periapical Radiograph: A radiograph that shows the entire tooth or teeth and surrounding tissues. *Peri* means "around" and *apical* is the root end of the tooth.

Periodontal Ligament: A thin but very dense and strong fibrous tissue that binds the cementum of the tooth to the lamina dura that lines the alveolus. It not only attaches the tooth to the alveolar bone but also acts as a cushion. Radiographically, the periodontal ligament appears as a thin radiolucent line between the lamina dura and the root.

Personnel Monitoring: The occasional or routine measuring of the amount of radiation to which a person working around radiation has been exposed during a given period of time. This is most often accomplished by wearing a monitoring badge, such as a **thermoluminescent dosimeter (TLD).**

Phantom: In dental radiography, a device the size and shape of the head and usually containing parts of the skull and all of the teeth. This is covered with plastic and other materials that resemble the lips, cheeks, tongue, and other facial structures. These materials scatter x-radiation in the same ways the tissues of the body do. The jaws are opened and closed by means of mechanical devices to enable the student to position and expose films in lieu of patients. See **DXTTR.**

Phleboliths: Calcified masses that are observed as round or oval bodies in the soft tissues of the cheeks.

Phosphors: Fluorescent crystals, usually calcium tungstate, used in the emulsion that coats the intensifying screens. These give off light when subjected to radiation.

Photoelectric Effect: An attenuation process for x- and gamma radiation in which a photon interacts with an orbital electron of an atom. All of the energy of the photon is absorbed by the displaced electron in the form of kinetic energy.

Photon (X-Ray Photon): A quantum of energy. Both x-rays and gamma rays are photons.

PID: See **Position-Indicating Device.**

Plane: In dental radiography, a level surface or a straight line connecting two anatomic landmarks.

Pocket Dosimeter: A small personal monitoring device that resembles a fountain pen in size and can be clipped to the garment to measure radiation received. See **Dosimeter.**

Point of Entry: The spot on the surface of the face toward which the central beam of radiation is directed when intraoral exposures are made.

Polychromatic: A term derived from the Greek meaning "having many colors." This term is used in dental radiography to describe the x-ray beam that is composed of many different wavelengths.

Port: An opening in the tube head that is covered with a permanent seal of glass, beryllium, or aluminum through which the x-rays leave the tube head. The port is opposite the window in the x-ray tube and is the place where the PID attaches to the tube head.

Position-Indicating Device (PID): Any device attached to the tube head at the aperture to direct the useful beam of radiation. It can be long or short, pointed, cylindrical or rectangular, and open or closed.

Positive Angulation (Positive Vertical Angulation or Plus Angulation): Angulation achieved by pointing the end of the PID downward from a horizontal plane.

Positive Ion: An ion that has a positive electric charge. See **Ion.**

Posteroanterior Radiograph: A radiograph of the head in which the x-ray film is in front of the face and the x-ray machine is behind the patient; the x-ray beam is directed at the occipital bone and passes through the skull from the back to the front.

Potential: In radiography and electricity, the difference in relative voltage or amount of electric pressure between the negative and positive electrodes.

Preservative: In radiography and photography, one of the chemicals (sodium sulfite) used in both the developer and fixer solutions to slow down the rapid rate of oxidation and prevent spoilage of the solution.

Pressure Mark: A black (radiolucent) line that appears on a processed film at a point where the film packet has been bent or subjected to excessive pressure.

Preventive Radiation: X-rays, through their ability to penetrate tissues, enable the dentist to look within the jaws and the teeth to discover conditions that can be remedied when recognized in time, thus preventing greater future problems to the dental patient. Preventive radiation is also practiced by the medical profession for diagnosis and therapy.

Primary Beam (Primary Radiation or Useful Beam): The original undeflected useful beam of radiation that emanates at the focal spot of the x-ray tube and emerges through the aperture of the tube head.

Primary Protective Barrier: A barrier sufficient to attenuate the useful beam to the required degree.

Primary Radiation: See **Primary Beam.**

Process: In dental anatomy, any prominent outgrowth of bone. May be rounded or pointed. Processes of dental importance include alveolar, coronoid, hamular (hamulus), mastoid, and styloid. These appear radiopaque.

Processing: The act of bringing out the latent image and making it permanently visible. Includes the following darkroom procedures: developing, rinsing, fixing, washing, and drying. See **Developer** and **Selective Reduction.**

Processing Tank: A metal or hard-rubber receptacle divided into compartments for developer solution, water rinse, and fixer solution and used to process radiographs.

Profile Radiographs (Lateral Headplates): Radiographs that record the shadow images of the soft tissues forming the facial curves and the features of the profile and those forming the tongue and palate of the oral cavity. They are used to indicate the facial contours and to indicate the relationship of the soft to the bony tissues.

Protection Survey: An evaluation of the radiation hazards incidental to the production, use, or existence of sources of radiation under a specific set of conditions.

Protective Apron: An apron made of radiation-absorbing material (lead equivalent), used to protect the patient from unnecessary radiation exposure. See **Lead Protective Apron.**

Protective Barrier: A barrier of radiation-absorbing material, used to reduce radiation exposure. See **Primary Protective Barrier** and **Secondary Protective Barrier.**

Protective Tube Housing (Diagnostic Tube Housing): An x-ray tube housing so constructed that the leakage radiation measured at a distance of 1 meter from the target does not exceed 1 millisievert (100 millirems) in one hour when the tube is operated at its maximum, continuous-rated current for the maximum rated tube potential.

Proton: A subatomic particle of the atom. The proton is contained in the nucleus and has a positive electrical charge. The proton has mass and weight. The number of protons determine the chemical element.

Pulp Polyp: A vascular outgrowth of the pulp into the oral cavity when the crown of the tooth is largely destroyed by dental caries. Polyps are frequently observed on children between the ages of six and ten. As a rule such polyps are easily seen on visual examination but have no specific outline on the radiograph because they blend into the radiolucency as an occlusal extension of the pulp chamber.

Pulp Stones: Calcifications that appear in the pulp chamber of the teeth, caused by an abnormal deposition of calcium salts. Often described as nodules or denticles. Seen on radiographs as one or more small, radiopaque, irregularly shaped rounded masses within the pulp chamber.

Qualified Expert: In dental radiation-monitoring terminology, a person having the knowledge and training to measure ionizing radiation, to evaluate safety techniques, and to advise regarding radiation protection needs of dental x-ray installations.

Quality Control: A term used to describe a series of tests to assure that the radiographic system is functioning properly and that the radiographs produced are of an acceptable level of quality.

Quality Factor (Q): A factor used for radiation protection purposes that accounts for differences in biological effectiveness among the different kinds of radiation. For x-rays, $Q = 1$.

Quantum: In the quantum theory, an elemental unit of energy. The theory holds that energy is not absorbed or radiated continuously but discontinuously in definite units called *quanta.*

Rad (Roentgen-Absorbed Dose): A special unit of absorbed dose equal to 0.01 joule (unit of energy) per kilogram of tissue (which is equal to the old terminology of 100 ergs per gram of tissue). For x-rays the rad is approximately numerically equivalent to the roentgen. Doses smaller than a rad are expressed in millirads, with 1000 millirads equaling 1 rad. The rad has been replaced by a new unit for measuring absorbed dose, the gray (Gy). One rad equals 0.01 Gy.

Radiation: The emission and propagation of energy through space or through a material medium in the form of electromagnetic waves, corpuscular emissions such as alpha and beta particles, or rays of mixed and unknown types such as cosmic rays. Most radiations used in dentistry are capable of producing ions directly or indirectly by interaction with matter.

Radiation Field: The region in which energy is being propagated.

Radiation Hazard: The risk of exposure to radiation in an area where x-ray equipment is operating or where radioactive material is stored. Any uncontrolled source of radiation presents a potential danger.

Radiation Hygiene: Methods of protecting persons from accidental injury from exposure to radiation. Also includes techniques used to reduce and control the amounts of radiation used in medical and dental installations.

Radiation Monitoring: See **Monitoring, Area Monitoring,** and **Personnel Monitoring.**

Radiation Protection Supervisor: The person directly responsible for radiation protection and safety measures. In dental offices it is usually the dentist.

Radiation Protection Survey: In dentistry, an evaluation of the radiation safety in and around a dental office.

Radiator: A large mass of copper just outside the x-ray tube and connected to the anode terminal. The radiator functions to carry off the excess heat produced in the energy exchange that takes place when the electrons of the cathode stream are converted into about 1 percent x-rays and 99 percent heat. The radiator conducts the heat away from the target and cools the tube.

Radicular Cyst: A cyst around the apex of a tooth. Generally seen as a small radiolucent circular area that extends away from the apical portions of the root. The sac of the cyst has a distinct wall or capsule that surrounds it and can be distinguished as a faint radiopaque thin line.

Radioactivity: The process whereby certain unstable elements undergo spontaneous disintegration (decay). The process is accompanied by emissions of one or more types of radiation and generally results in the formation of a new isotope.

Radiograph: An image produced on photosensitive film by exposing the film to x-rays and then developing the film so that a negative is produced. Also called an **x-ray film,** *radiogram, roentgenogram,* or *roentgenograph.*

Radiographer: Person who operates an x-ray machine. See **Operator.**

Radiographic Fog: A darkening or clouding of the radiographic film image caused by exposure of the film to stray radiation during storage or by failure to protect the film from radiation while other exposures are made.

Radiography (Roentgenography): Generating and applying x-radiation to film sensitized for the purpose of making shadow pictures.

Radiology: That branch of medical science that deals with the use of radiant energy in the diagnosis and treatment of disease.

Radiolucent: The portion of the processed radiograph that is dark because the exposed structures lack density; also refers to a substance that permits the passage of x-rays with little or no resistance.

Radio-osteosclerosis: An increase in density to the bone that appears radiopaque as a result of excessive ionizing radiation.

Radiopaque: The portion of the radiographic film that appears light; also refers to a substance that resists the passage of radiation.

Radioresistant: Refers to a substance or tissue that is not easily injured by ionizing radiation.

Radiosensitive: Refers to a substance or tissue that is relatively susceptible to injury by ionizing radiation.

Ramus: The ascending portion of each end of the mandible.

Rarefaction: The state of being or becoming less dense, usually as a result of some disease process, indicated by radiolucent areas in the bone structures shown on radiographs.

Rarefying Osteitis: A term used to describe a demineralization of the trabecullae within the alveolar bone. The causes are often difficult to determine and vary considerably. The appearance on a radiograph is as an irregularly shaped radiolucent area.

Rectification: In radiography, the unidirectional current inside the x-ray tube from the cathode to the anode.

Rectifier: A device within the vacuum tube for converting the alternating to direct current.

Reducer: A chemical capable of bringing a salt into its metallic state by removing the nonmetallic elements.

Reduction: In dental radiography, a process in which an overexposed or overdeveloped radiograph is placed in a reducing solution. This lightens the radiographic image by removing one layer of metallic silver at a time from the film surface.

Rem (Roentgen Equivalent Man): A unit used to measure the dose equivalent. It is used to compare the biological effects of the various types of radiation. One rem equals 1 rad times a biological effect modifying factor. Since the modifying factor for x- and gamma radiation equals 1, the number of rems is identical to the absorbed dose in rads for these radiations. The rem has been replaced by a new unit for measuring the dose equivalent, the sievert (Sv). One rem equals 0.01 Sv.

Replenisher: A superconcentrated solution of developer or fixer that is added daily, or as indicated, to the developer or fixer in the processing tank to compensate for loss of volume and loss of strength from oxidation. The act of adding replenisher to the processing solutions is known as replenishment.

Residual Cyst: This is a cyst that remains in the jaw after the tooth that caused the cyst to form is no longer attached to it. During surgical removal of the root or during exfoliation, cysts may become detached from the root and remain within the bone for many years, often undiscovered. Such cysts may become encapsulated with an epithelial lining or may undergo considerable growth. Radiographically the cyst appears radiolucent and the lining of the cyst appears as a thin radiopaque line.

Resorption: Removal by absorption. In radiography, resorption generally refers to a loss of bone or tooth structure. Resorption may be due to natural causes, such as the gradual reduction of size of the roots of deciduous teeth, or it may be idiopathic (the result of unknown causes), as may occasionally be observed by internal or external changes in the size of the pulp chamber or the length of the roots of permanent teeth.

Restrainer: In radiography, the potassium bromide in the developer solution. It slows down the action of the Elon and hydroquinone in the developer and inhibits the tendency of the solution to chemically fog the films.

Retained Root: A root remaining after the tooth has been extracted.

Reticulation: Cracking of the film emulsion caused by a large temperature difference between the developer and the rinse water.

Rhinoliths: Calcifications within the maxillary sinuses.

Ridge (Alveolar): A ridge is an extended elevation or crest of bone. In dental radiography, the term ridge generally refers to the alveolar crests of the mandible or the maxillae. The alveolar ridge may be partially or fully edentulous. On dental radiographs the ridges appear radiopaque.

Right-Angle Technique: See **Paralleling Technique.**

Roentgen (R): The special unit of exposure to radiation measured in air. This is the exposure required to produce in air 2.58^{10} coulombs per kilogram of air. A simpler definition of the roentgen is that it is the amount of x-radiation or gamma radiation required to ionize 1 cc of air at standard conditions of pressure and temperature (2.083 billion ion pairs).

Roentgen Ray: See **X-Ray.**

Rotational Center: In tomographic radiology, the axis on which the tube head and the drum rotate.

Rotational Panoramic Radiography: A specific radiographic projection technique that utilizes a narrow beam of x-rays to image a curved layer.

Rule of Isometry: A geometric theorem stating that two triangles with two equal angles and a common side are equal triangles. The application of this theorem to the bisecting technique was suggested by Cieszynski in 1907 (Cieszynski's law).

Safelight: A special type of filtered light that can be left burning in the darkroom while films are processed. The safelight rays do not affect the film emulsion unless the filter is defective, they are too close to the film being exposed, or they are allowed to shine on the unprocessed film for too long a time.

Sagittal Plane: An imaginary vertical line or plane that bisects the body into a right and left portion. If the plane is exactly at the midline, it is referred to as the midsagittal plane. This is a very important orientation line in determining the ideal position of the patient's head during radiographic exposure.

Sanitation: A term used when microorganisms are reduced to a level of concentration considered to be safe.

Scatterguard: A steel cylinder inserted by the manufacturer into the center of the PID where the PID attaches to the aperture of the tube head. Its purpose is to absorb scattered radiation.

Scatter Radiation: Radiation that has been deflected from its path by impact during its passage through matter. This form of secondary radiation is scattered in all directions by the tissues of the patient's head during exposure to x-radiation.

Scintillation Counter: An area-monitoring device containing a photoelectric cell that helps to measure the flashes of visible light emitted when the radiation that bombards certain salt crystals causes them to fluoresce.

Sclerosis: A hardening of the body tissues as a result of inflammation or an excessive growth of fibrous tissue and deposition of mineral salts. In dental radiography, sclerosis generally refers to a stiffening of the temporomandibular articulation or a mineralization of the alveolar bone. See **Condensing Osteitis.**

Screen Film: A type of extraoral film for use in cassettes with intensifying screens. This film has an emulsion that is more sensitive to the green, blue, and violet lights emitted when the radiation strikes the phosphors in the intensifying screens than to the x-radiation.

Secondary Protective Barrier: A barrier sufficient to attenuate stray radiation to the required degree.

Secondary Radiation: The radiation given off by any matter irradiated with x-rays. This form of radiation is created at the instant the primary beam interacts with matter and gives off some of its energy, forming new and less powerful wavelengths. This is often referred to as scatter radiation.

Selective Reduction: A chemical change that takes place within the film emulsion during development. During this change, the nonmetallic elements are separated from the silver halide of the exposed grains, leaving a coating of metallic silver on the film emulsion while the bromide is removed. The process is called selective because the unexposed grains are not reduced.

Self-Induction: An electrical term referring to the ability of a single coil in an autotransformer to vary the current and potential in a nearby circuit.

Self-Rectification: In radiography, the ability of the x-ray machine to produce x-rays only during the portion of the alternating current cycle when the cathode has a negative and the anode has a positive charge.

Sensitivity: See **Emulsion Speed.**

Sensitometer: An instrument used to measure the sensitivity of films to x-rays.

Sepsis: Infection, or the presence of septic matter.

Septum: In dental radiography, a thin wall of bone that acts as a partition to separate the nasal cavity or the maxillary sinuses. Appears radiopaque.

Shells: See **Energy Levels.**

Shield (Shielding): A protective barrier of structural materials.

Short-Scale Contrast: Variations in contrast, with few shades of gray, as when the differences between blacks and whites on the radiograph are great. Fewer shades are produced when low kilovoltage is used.

Sialolith: A salivary calculus or hardened, stonelike mass that forms within the passage of the salivary ducts. If of sufficient size, such masses appear slightly radiopaque on the radiograph.

Sievert (Sv): A new unit for measuring the dose equivalent that has replaced the rem. The sievert is used to compare the biological effects of the various types of radiation. One sievert equals 1 gray times a biological effect modifying factor. Because the modifying factor for x- and gamma radiation equals 1, the number of sieverts is identical to the absorbed dose in grays for these radiations. One sievert equals 100 rems.

Sinus (Maxillary): A cavity within the body of the maxilla that communicates with the middle meatus of the nose. It is also called the *antrum of Highmore.* All sinuses are lined with a mucous membrane and are filled with air or fluid. The apices of some of the maxillary teeth may occasionally protrude into the maxillary sinus. Sinuses may also be located on the ethmoid, frontal, and sphenoid bones. The sinuses reduce the weight of the skull without greatly weakening it.

Sinus Survey: An extraoral radiograph exposed in such a manner that the maxillary sinus can be examined. This projection is similar to the posteroanterior survey.

Skin Dose: See **Entrance Dose.**

Slit: In rotational panoramic radiography, a vertical opening on the tube head through which the narrow x-ray beam exits or the narrow vertical opening on the cassette where the x-ray beam enters to record the image.

Soft Radiation: Rays of low energy and long wavelengths that have little penetrating power. These have no value in producing dental radiographs and are removed from the polychromatic beam by filtration.

Somatic Cells: All body cells except the reproductive cells.

Somatic Effects: In radiography, the effect of radiation on all body cells except the reproductive cells, especially the effect on the blood, the soft muscular tissues, and the bone.

Source: In radiography, the place where the x-ray photons originate. This is the focal spot on the target of the anode inside the x-ray tube.

Source–Film Distance: See **Target–Film Distance.**

Source–Surface Distance (Source–Skin Distance, Target–Skin Distance, or **Target–Surface Distance):** The distance measured along the path of the central ray from the center of the focal spot (front surface of the target) to the surface of the skin or irradiated object.

Step Wedge (Penetrometer): A device consisting of increments of absorber through which a radiographic exposure is made on film to permit determination of the amounts of radiation reaching the film by measurements of film density. From such data, conclusions may be drawn as to the initial intensity and penetrative power of the radiation.

Sterilization: The total destruction of spores and disease-producing microorganisms.

Stray Radiation: The sum of the leakage and scattered radiation; radiation that emanates from parts of the tube other than the focal spot.

Structural Shielding: The protection afforded by building materials, such as the thickness of a stucco wall.

Subject Contrast: The area-to-area difference in density in a radiograph caused by the differing thicknesses of the tissues or the object radiographed.

Submandibular Fossa: A depression near the angle on the lingual of the mandible, irregular in size, usually below the area of the roots of the molars and extending forward as far as the premolar region. The basal bone of the mandible is so thin and offers so little resistance to the passage of the x-rays that it appears radiolucent.

Supernumerary Teeth: These are extra teeth not normally a part of the dentition. Such teeth may be deciduous but are usually permanent. Many supernumerary teeth resemble normal teeth but the majority have conical crowns and are smaller than the tooth they resemble. Some bear no resemblance to normal teeth. These are often unerupted and malpositioned. Radiographically the tooth structures appear the same as any other tooth.

Surface Dose: The dose of radiation at the skin surface measured in grays or rads.

Survey: A term used in dental radiography to indicate an examination of a complete area with radiography. For example, a complete radiographic inspection of all the teeth is called a full-mouth survey, whereas a single film of one specific area could be a lateral jaw survey, a mandibular molar survey, and so forth.

Symphysis: In dental radiography, the prominent bone area where the right and left sides of the mandible fuse at midline.

Syndrome: A group of symptoms that together characterize a disease or lesion.

Target: The small block of tungsten embedded in the face of the anode, bombarded by the electrons streaming toward it from the cathode. The focal spot is located on the target.

Target–Film Distance (Source–Film Distance or Focus–Film Distance): The distance between the focal spot on the target and the recording plane of the film.

Target–Object Distance (Source–Object Distance or Focus–Object Distance): The distance between the target on the anode in the x-ray tube and the object being radiographed.

Target–Surface Distance (Source–Surface Distance): The distance between the target and the surface of the object being radiographed.

Taurodontia: Teeth characterized by very large pulp chambers and very short roots.

Temporomandibular Joint Radiograph (TMJ Radiograph): An extraoral film used to show in profile the articulation of the head of the mandibular condyle with the glenoid fossa of the temporal bone and the surrounding structures.

Thermionic Emission: The release of electrons when a material such as tungsten is heated to incandescence; specifically, the boiling off of electrons from the cathode filament in the x-ray tube when electric current is passed through it.

Thermoluminescent Dosimeter (TLD): A monitoring device containing certain crystalline compounds (usually lithium fluoride) that store energy when struck by x-rays and then, when heated, give off light in proportion to the amount of radiation exposure.

Threshold Dose: The minimum exposure that will produce a detectable degree of any given effect.

Time Delay: The short interval between the moment the activator button on the x-ray machine is depressed and the instant that the high-voltage current begins to flow across the x-ray tube.

Timer: A mechanical, electrical, or electronic device that can be set to predetermine the duration of the interval that the current flows through the x-ray machine to produce x-rays.

Tomography: A special radiographic technique used to show in detail images of structures located within a predetermined plane of tissue while eliminating or blurring those structures in the planes not selected.

Topographical Technique: A method used in occlusal radiography, in which the rules of bisecting are followed and the radiation beam is directed through the apices of the teeth perpendicularly toward the bisector.

Torus: An outgrowth of bone.

Total Filtration: The combination of the inherent and added filtration in an x-ray machine. Many states require a total filtration of 2.5 mm of aluminum equivalent for x-ray machines operating at or above 70 kVp.

Trabecular Bone (Cancellous Bone): The softer spongy bone that makes up the bulk of the inside portion of most bones. The cells of trabecular bone vary in size and density.

Tragus: The small cartilaginous prominence of tissues located near the center and in front of the acoustic meatus (outer ear opening).

Transformer: One of several types of electrical devices capable of increasing or decreasing the voltage of an alternating current by mutual induction between primary and secondary coils or windings on cores of metal. See **High-Voltage Transformer** and **Low-Voltage Transformer.**

Trough: The low spot in the wave form; the opposite of the crest of the wave.

Tube Head (Tube Housing): The protective metal covering that contains the x-ray tube, the high-voltage and low-voltage transformers, and insulating oil. It is attached to the flexible extension arm by a yoke. The PID attaches to the tube head at the port.

Tube Side: A term used to describe the side of the film packet or the cassette that must be positioned facing the source of x-rays coming from the tube.

Tubercle: A rounded eminence on a bone.

Tuberosity : A broad eminence situated on a bone.

Tumor: A swelling; a growth of tissue.

Tungsten (Wolfram): An element with an atomic number of 74. Owing to its high melting point, this metal is extremely suitable to use as the cathode filament and as the anode target in the production of x-rays.

Useful Beam (Useful Radiation): That part of the primary beam that is permitted to emerge from the housing of the tube and is limited by the port, and the collimator, or other collimating device such as a lead-lined PID.

Vertical Angulation: The direction of the central beam in an up or down direction achieved by directing the tip of the PID upward or downward. See **Negative Angulation** and **Positive Angulation.**

Vertical Placement: See **Film Placement.**

Viewer (Viewbox or **Illuminator):** A device for concentrating or reflecting light; generally, a lamp behind an opaque glass used for viewing radiographs.

Volt: A unit of electromotive force or potential that is sufficient to cause a current of 1 ampere (A) to flow through a resistance of 1 ohm (Ω).

Voltage: Electrical pressure or force that drives the electric current through the circuit of the x-ray machine. See **Kilovolt** and **Kilovolt Peak.**

Voltmeter: A device for measuring the electromotive force (the difference in potential or voltage) across the x-ray tube.

Wavelength: In radiography, the length in Angström units or centimeters of the electromagnetic radiations produced in the x-ray machine.

Wetting Agent: A chemical preparation similar to a detergent that reduces the surface tension of film. A small amount may be added to the developer or the final rinse water to facilitate development and drying of the radiograph.

Wharton's Duct: The excretory duct of the submaxillary gland. The opening of this duct is located under the tongue near the lingual frenulum—the small fold that limits the movement of the tongue. On rare occasions the opening of this duct may be blocked by the formation of a stone or mass of calculus called a **sialolith.**

Window: In radiography, the thin wall of glass in an x-ray tube opposite the focal spot. The primary x-ray beam leaves the tube through this thin area of the tube envelope.

Work Load: In radiography, the total time that the x-ray machine is used, expressed in milliampere seconds per week.

Xeroradiography: A technique combining exposure to x-rays by a conventional x-ray machine with a special dry-processing system resulting in a photolike image rather than a transparent radiograph.

Xerostomia: Dryness of the mouth from lack of normal secretion.

X-Ray (Roentgen Ray): The radiant energy of short wavelength discovered by Wilhelm Conrad Roentgen in Germany in 1895 and designated as x-ray by him. This form of radiant energy has the power to penetrate substances that are ordinarily opaque and to record shadow images on photographic film. The term roentgen ray is more technical than the more commonly used term x-ray.

X-Ray Film: See **Radiograph** or **Film Packet.**

X-Ray Film Hanger: Mechanical device for holding x-ray film during the processing procedures.

X-Ray Timer: A clocklike device that can be set for the time intervals required in processing. It is activated by a lever and rings when the interval has elapsed.

Yoke: The curved portion of the x-ray machine that can revolve 360 degrees horizontally where it is connected to the extension arm. The tube head is suspended within the yoke and can be rotated vertically within it.

Zero Angulation (Zero Vertical Angulation): Angulation achieved by directing the tip of the PID so that the entire PID is parallel with the plane of the floor. When directed in this manner, the central beam travels parallel with the plane of the floor. See **Negative Angulation** and **Positive Angulation.**

Zygomatic Arch: The arch formed by the temporal process of the malar (zygomatic) bone and the zygomatic process of the temporal bone. This forms the outer margin of the cheek prominence.

Index

D

F

Also from Appleton & Lange